THE RESPIRATORY CARE WORKBOOK

THE RESPIRATORY CARE WORKBOOK

HOWARD B. SURKIN, M.A., R.R.T.
Director of Respiratory Care Services
Doylestown Hospital
Doylestown, Pennsylvania

ANNA WEIGAND PARKMAN, M.B.A., R.R.T.
Assistant Professor of Respiratory Care
Respiratory Care Program Director
College of Health Sciences
University of Charleston
Charleston, West Virginia

Printed in the United States of America

Last digit indicates print number: 10 9 8 7 6 5 4 3 2 1

NOTE: As new scientific information becomes available through basic and clinical research, recommended treatments and drug therapies undergo changes. The author(s) and publisher have done everything possible to make this book accurate, up-to-date, and in accord with accepted standards at the time of publication. However, the reader is advised always to check product information (package inserts) for changes and new information regarding dose and contraindications before administering any drug. Caution is especially urged when using new or infrequently ordered drugs.

Library of Congress Cataloging-in-Publication Data

Surkin, Howard B.
    The respiratory care workbook   /   Howard B. Surkin, Anna Weigand Parkman.
        p.   cm.
    Includes bibliographical references.
    ISBN 0-8036-8229-8
    1. Respiratory therapy—Problems, exercises, etc. I. Parkman, Anna Weigand. II. Title.
    [DNLM: 1. Respiratory Therapy—problems.   WB   18   S961r]
RC735.I5S87   1989
616.2'046—dc20
DNLM/DLC
for Library of Congress   89-16982
                                                                                        CIP

DEDICATION

To our parents
John and Anna Weigand
Daniel and Mildred Surkin

To our children
Kate Parkman
Sara Surkin
Jenifer Surkin

To our spouses
Ross Parkman
Ann Marie Surkin

PREFACE

The Respiratory Care Workbook is a comprehensive, well-illustrated review of fundamental and advanced concepts in respiratory care. This workbook is ideal for students in one, two, and four year respiratory care programs who need a study guide that will clarify and reinforce their understanding of the material covered in their textbooks and in the classroom. Moreover, students and practitioners alike can use the workbook to prepare for credentialing examinations. Finally, respiratory care department inservice personnel will find this text invaluable as a guide to assessing new employees, and as a resource for material to be presented during inservice education.

The workbook is divided into two principal units, each of which unfolds respiratory care concepts in a logical and progressive sequence. The eleven chapters of Unit I review the basics: mathematics and science, cardiopulmonary anatomy, cardiopulmonary resuscitation, patient assessment, medical gas therapy, oxygen therapy, humidity and aerosol therapy, therapeutic modalities, airway management, infection control and special procedures.

Advanced concepts are covered in the ten chapters of Unit II: respiratory physiology, arterial blood gases, pulmonary function, hemodynamic monitoring, pharmacology, mechanical ventilation, and electrocardiograms. The advanced unit also includes two chapters that survey neonatal and pediatric respiratory therapy as well as pulmonary rehabilitation and home care topics.

Each chapter of Units I and II begins with an outline, study objectives, and a list of references. Then, theoretical and clinical concepts are presented in a question-and-answer format. The style of presentation is varied to include multiple-choice, fill-in-the-blank and short essay question formats. Students also have the opportunity to label and discuss diagrams and illustrations.

Many of the questions contain specific references to the major textbooks in the field, enabling students to investigate the underlying rationale for each answer. This text-to-text correlation will enhance the workbook's usefulness within any respiratory therapy curriculum, no matter which combination of texts a student may be using. Each chapter concludes with answers to the questions and an NBRC credentialing-style sample quiz.

A concluding section, Unit III, is designed to help students and practitioners prepare for credentialing examinations. The opening chapter (Ch 22) outlines recommended study schedules for both the CRTT and RTT examinations. Of course, sample CRTT and RTT comprehensive exams are included, in Chapters 23 and 24, with answers in Chapter 25. An appendix lists commonly used equations and formulas.

ACKNOWLEDGMENTS

The authors of this text are indebted to the following individuals for their time and effort on our behalf: Phillip Geronimo, Thomas Hon and Michael McDonald. Special mention must be given to Allen Marangoni who edited, criticized, recommended and gave inspiration to the authors. Allen's contribution to this workbook is justly recognized and we thank him. We would also like to acknowledge Jean-François Vilain, who made it possible.

CONTENTS

UNIT III   STUDY GUIDE AND EXAMS

UNIT 1

THE BASICS

Chapter 1

MATHEMATICS AND SCIENCE

Outline

LEARNING OBJECTIVES

Upon completion of this unit, the individual will:

1. Define "an unknown variable" and correctly solve basic algebraic equations.
2. Convert metric system equivalents.
3. Convert from the metric system to the English system and from the English system to the metric system.
4. Define:
   a. element
   b. atom
   c. ion
   d. molecule
5. List/describe the major components of an atom.
6. Distinguish between atomic number and atomic weight.
7. Given the appropriate atomic weights, calculate the gram molecular weights and gram equivalent weights.
8. Explain ionic versus covalent bonding.
9. Define the following:
   a. solution
   b. solvent
   c. solute
10. Describe/calculate the relationships of solvent to solute in the following:
    a. ratio solution
    b. % W/V solution
11. Be able to calculate the final concentration or final volume, given the appropriate information.
12. Define the following:
    a. osmosis
    b. acid
    c. base
    d. neutralization reaction
13. Define the following states of matter:
    a. melting point
    b. boiling point
    c. freezing point
    d. sublimation
    e. critical temperature and critical pressure
    f. evaporation
    g. vapor pressure
14. State the principle of gas pressure and describe how gas pressure is measured.
15. List the appropriate percentage of the following gases:
    a. nitrogen
    b. oxygen
    c. carbon dioxide
16. Be able to convert the following gas pressure measurements:
    a. mmHg to psi, cmH_2O, atmospheres, inHg
    b. psi to mmHg, cmH_2O, atmospheres, inHg
    c. cmH_2O to psi, mmHg, atmospheres, inHg
    d. atmospheres to cmH_2O, mmHg, inHg, psi
    e. inHg, to atmospheres, cmH_2O, psi, mmHg
17. Be able to convert the following temperature measurements:
    a. Fahrenheit to Centigrade, Kelvin, Rankin
    b. Centigrade to Fahrenheit, Kelvin, Rankin
    c. Kelvin to Fahrenheit, Centigrade, Rankin
    d. Rankin to Fahrenheit, Centigrade, Kelvin
18. Explain Avagadro's law and described the relationship to the densities of gases.
19. Calculate the density of any gas, given the gram molecular weight.
20. Calculate the specific gravity of any gas, given the density.
21. Calculate partial pressures and barometric pressure using Dalton's law, given the appropriate information.
22. Identify/calculate the practical application of the following gas laws:
    a. Boyle's law
    b. Charles' law
    c. Gay-Lussac's law
    d. combined gas law
    e. ideal gas law
23. Identify/calculate the practical application of the following gas laws dealing with diffusion:
    a. Henry's law
    b. Graham's law
24. Identify/discuss the following gas principles:
    a. Bernoulli's principle
    b. Venturi's principle
    c. Pitot's principle
25. List/describe two factors that influence the degree of fluid/air uptake by a jet.
26. Explain the difference between laminar and turbulent gas flow within the tracheobronchial tree.

REFERENCES

Egan, DF, Sheldon, RL, and Spearman, CB: Egan's Fundamentals of Respiratory Therapy, ed 4. CV Mosby, St Louis, 1982

Kacmarek, RM, Mack, CW, and Dimas, S: The Essentials of Respiratory Therapy, ed 2. Year Book Medical Publishers, Chicago, 1985.

Malone, LJ: Basic Concepts of Chemistry, ed 2. John Wiley & Sons, St Louis, 1985.

McPherson, SP: Respiratory Therapy Equipment, ed 3. CV Mosby, St Louis, 1985

STUDY QUESTIONS

1. Solve for x.
   a. $x + 4 = 9$
   b. $2x - 6 = 10$
   c. $\dfrac{1}{2x} + 5 = 7$
   d. $\dfrac{8}{x} = 16$
   e. $\dfrac{3x}{4} - 12 = 48$
   f. $3(x - 2) + 6 = 27$

2. Convert the following: (Kacmarek, pp 11–12; Malone, pp 32–41)
   a. 3 mm = _____ cm
   b. 10 km = _____ m
   c. 5 cm = _____ km
   d. 4 mg = _____ g
   e. 12 kg = _____ mg
   f. 7 g = _____ kg
   g. 9 ml = _____ l
   h. 15 kl = _____ ml
   i. 2 kl = _____ l

3. Convert the following: (Kacmarek, p 12; Malone, pp 32–41)
   a. 10 cm = _____ in
   b. 42 oz = _____ g
   c. 840 g = _____ lb = _____ kg
   d. 25 in = _____ cm = _____ km
   e. 100 ml = _____ cc

4. Change to scientific notation. (Malone, pp 29–30)
   a. 8964 = _____

   b. $0.253214 =$ _____

   c. $0.001826 =$ _____

   d. $726,000,000 =$ _____

   e. $9.4 \times 10^6 =$ _____

   f. $1.27 \times 10^{-4} =$ _____

5. Define element. (Kacmarek, p 1; Malone, p 11)

_____

_____

6. An atom is composed of the following: (Kacmarek, p 1; Malone, pp 59–60)

   a. _____   c. _____

   b. _____

7. Differentiate between atomic number and atomic weight. (Kacmarek, p 1; Malone, pp 60–63)

_____

_____

_____

8. An atom of a particular element that has a different number of electrons than a normal atom of the same element is known as an _____. (Kacmarek, p 1; Malone, pp 65–67)

9. Differentiate between a molecule and a compound. (Kacmarek, pp 1–2; Malone, pp 64–65)

_____

_____

_____

10. Calculate the gram molecular weights of the following compounds, given the atomic weights $H = 1$, $C = 12$, $N = 14$, $O = 16$, $Na = 23$, $S = 32$, $Cl = 35$, $K = 39$, $Ca = 40$. (Kacmarek, p 2; Malone, p 194)

   a. H_2O_5: _____

   b. HCl: _____

   c. $NaCl$: _____

   d. $HC_2H_3O_2$: _____

   e. $Ca(OH)_2$: _____

11. In the space provided indicate whether the compound was formed by ionic or covalent bonding. (Kacmarek, pp 3–4; Malone, pp 142–146)

   a. $O + O \rightarrow O_2$ _____

   b. $Na + Cl \rightarrow NaCl$ _____

   c. $Ca + F \rightarrow CaF_2$ _____

   d. $H + O \rightarrow H_2O$ _____

   e. $N + H \rightarrow NH_4$ _____

12. Using the atomic weights in question 10, calculate the gram equivalent weights of the following: (Kacmarek, pp 7–9)

    a. H_2S: _____

    b. $CaCl_2$: _____

    c. KOH: _____

13. Define the following terms: (Kacmarek, p 4; Malone, p 304)

    a. solution: _____

    _____

    b. solvent: _____

    c. solute: _____

14. How many milligrams of solute are there in 2 ml of a 1:300 solution? (Kacmarek, pp 4–5)

    _____

    _____

    _____

    _____

15. How many grams of solute are there in 5 ml of a 1:500 solution? (Kacmarek, pp 4–5)

    _____

    _____

    _____

    _____

16. How many grams are there in 5 ml of a 5% W/V solution? (Kacmarek, pp 5–6)

    _____

    _____

    _____

    _____

17. How many milligrams are there in 6 ml of a 0.25% W/V solution? (Kacmarek, pp 5–6)

    _____

    _____

    _____

    _____

18. How many grams are there in 500 g of a 10% solution? (Kacmarek, p 6)

    _____

19. What volume of water should be added to 150 ml of a 35% solution of HCl to dilute it to a 10% solution? (Kacmarek, pp 6–7; Malone, pp 317–318)

    _____

    _____

20. If 8 ml is added to 0.25 ml of a 20% solution, what is the solution's final concentration? (Kacmarek, pp 6–7; Malone, pp 317–318)

21. Define osmosis. (Kacmarek, p 10; Malone, p 325)

22. Distinguish between and give examples of the following: (Kacmarek, p 11; Malone, p 334–340)

    a. acid: _____

    b. base: _____

    c. neutral reaction: _____

23. Match the changes of state in Column A with their definitions in Column B. (Kacmarek, pp 16–17; McPherson, pp 2–8)

    COLUMN A

    _____ melting point

    _____ boiling point

    _____ freezing point

    _____ sublimation

    _____ evaporation

    _____ vapor pressure

    _____ critical temperature

    _____ critical pressure

    COLUMN B

    a. temperature at which a substance changes from a liquid to a solid
    b. pressure required to convert a gas back into a liquid at critical temperature
    c. changing of a substance directly from a solid to a gas
    d. temperature at which a substance changes from a solid to a liquid
    e. pressure caused by molecules hitting surface of a liquid and escaping
    f. temperature at which gas cannot be converted into a liquid at any applied pressure
    g. molecules overcoming attraction of surface forces in a liquid and convert to a gas
    h. temperature at which a substance changes from a liquid to a gas

24. List the approximate percentage of the following gases in our atmosphere: (Kacmarek, p 20)

    a. Oxygen: _____

    b. Nitrogen: _____

    c. Carbon dioxide: _____

25. Identify Figures 1–1, 1–2, and 1–3. (Kacmarek, pp 20, 364; McPherson, pp 8–11)

    a. Fig. 1–1: _____

    b. Fig. 1–2: _____

    c. Fig. 1–3: _____

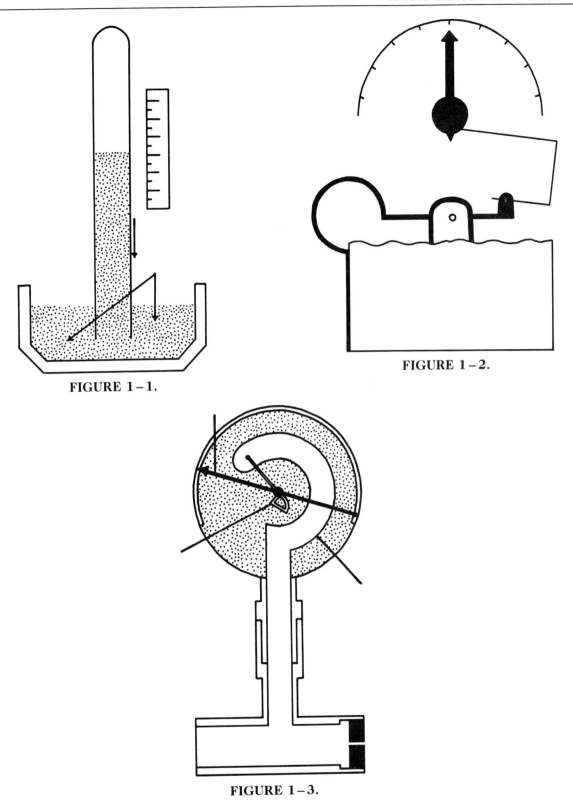

FIGURE 1-1.

FIGURE 1-2.

FIGURE 1-3.

26. Convert the following pressure measurements: (Kacmarek, p 20-21; McPherson, pp 10-11)

   a. 760 mmHg to psi: _____

   b. 1 cmH$_2$O to mmHg: _____

c. 0.5 psi to cmH_2O: _____

d. 6 atm to mmHg: _____

e. 80 inHg to atm: _____

27. _____ is the cessation of kinetic activity. (Kacmarek, p 15; McPherson, p 1)

28. Convert the following temperatures: (Kacmarek, p 9; Malone, pp 45–48)
    a. 78°F to °C
    b. 68°C to °F
    c. 37°C to °K
    d. 895°K to °F
    e. 105°F to °R

29. At 99 feet underwater, the atmospheric pressure would be approximately _____ (Kacmarek, p 21; McPherson, pp 10–11)

30. Define Avogadro's law. (Kacmarek, pp 18–19; McPherson, pp 31–32)

    _____

    _____

    _____

31. What is the density of oxygen? (Kacmarek, pp 19, 31–32)

    _____

32. What is the density of a mixture of 80% oxygen and 20% carbon dioxide? (Kacmarek, p 19)

    _____

33. What is the specific gravity of oxygen? (Kacmarek, p 19; McPherson, p 31)

    _____

    _____

34. How many molecules are there in 2 moles of oxygen? (*Hint*: Use Avogadro's law.) (Kacmarek, p 18; Malone, pp 188–196)

    _____

35. How many moles are there in 453 grams of oxygen? (Kacmarek, 18; Malone, pp 188–196)

    _____

36. Assuming an FIO_2 of 0.21, calculate the following: (Kacmarek, pp 22–23; Malone, pp 254–257; McPherson, pp 19–20)
    a. Partial pressure of oxygen (PO_2) of dry air with a barometric pressure (P_B) of 750 mmHg: _____

    _____

    b. PO_2 of saturated air at P_B of 770 mmHg: _____

    c. The P_B in mmHg with a PO_2 of 140 mmHg in dry air: _____

    _____

37. A gas mixture contains 5% CO_2, 25% O_2, and 70% N_2 at a temperature of 310°K saturated and a barometric pressure of 807 mmHg. What partial pressure would each gas exert if it were present alone? (Kacmarek, pp 22–23; Malone, pp 254–257; McPherson, pp 19–20)

    _____

38. Given a gas cylinder with a pressure of 2400 psig at 20°C, what would be the contents pressure if the cylinder was warmed to 60°C? Whose gas law is this? (Kacmarek, pp 24–25; Malone, pp 247–251; McPherson, pp 17–18)

39. Given 1000 ml of dry gas at 42°C and a barometric pressure of 700 mmHg, what would its volume be at 500 mmHg? Whose gas law is this? (Kacmarek, p 24; Malone, pp 244–247; McPherson, pp 14–15)

40. Given 950 ml of dry gas at 24°C and a barometric pressure of 1 atmosphere, what volume would the gas occupy at body temperature? Whose gas law is this? (Kacmarek; p 24; Malone, pp 247–251; McPherson, pp 15–16)

41. If 750 ml of dry gas at a barometric pressure of 700 mmHg and 37°C, shrinks to 500 ml and 0°C dry, what is the new pressure? (Kacmarek, p 25; Malone, pp 251–252; McPherson, pp 18–19)

42. A volume of saturated gas occupies 400 ml at 37°C and 750 mmHg. What volume will it occupy at STP? (Kacmarek, p 25; Malone, pp 251–252; McPherson, pp 18–19)

43. Given 200 ml of a saturated gas at 800 mmHg and 25°C, what would the pressure be if the gas was saturated at the same volume and 30°C? (Kacmarek, p 25; Malone, pp 251–252; McPherson, pp 18–19)

44. What is the volume of 1.0 mole of a gas at STP? (Boltzmann's constant = 0.0821 L-atm/°K-mole) (Malone, pp 258–260)

45. The rate of diffusion of a gas through another gas is affected by the following: (Kacmarek, pp 25–26; McPherson, pp 21–22)

    a. _____

    b. _____

    c. _____

    d. _____

    e. _____

46. According to Henry's law, the solubility coefficients for oxygen and carbon dioxide at 37°C and 760 mmHg are _____. (Kacmarek, p 26; McPherson, pp 22–23)

47. Whose gas law(s) calculate(s) the diffusibility of a gas? (Kacmarek, p 26; McPherson, pp 22–23)

48. Given the following data, what is the diffusibility of gas B compared with that of gas A? (Kacmarek, p 26; McPherson, pp 22–23)

Gas A	**Gas B**
sol. coefficient 0.30	sol. coefficient 0.70
GMW 25	GMW 64

49. Identify and describe the principle in Figure 1–4. (Kacmarek, pp 33–35, McPherson, pp 24–27)

50. What are the two factors that effect the degree of air/fluid uptake by a jet? (Kacmarek, pp 35–36; McPherson, pp 24–27)

    a. _____

    b. _____

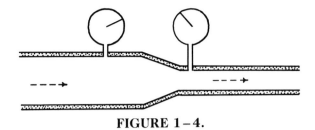

FIGURE 1–4.

51. Identify and describe the principles in Figures 1–5 and 1–6. (McPherson, pp 28–30)

    a. Fig. 1–5: _____

    b. Fig. 1–6: _____

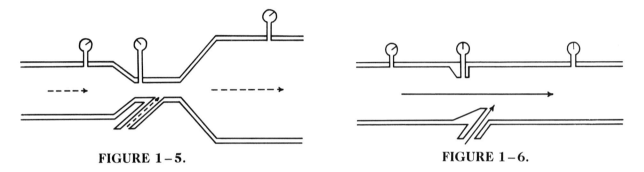

FIGURE 1–5. **FIGURE 1–6.**

52. Describe Figure 1–7 in terms of gas flow through the airways. (Kacmarek, pp 32–33; McPherson, p 33)

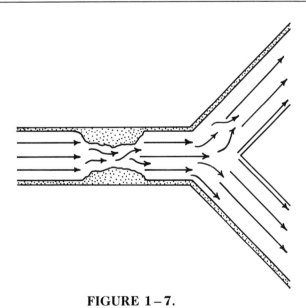

FIGURE 1–7.

ANSWERS TO STUDY QUESTIONS

1. a. 5
   b. 8
   c. 4
   d. $\frac{1}{2}$
   e. 80
   f. 9

2. a. 0.3 cm
   b. 10,000 m
   c. 0.00005 km
   d. 0.004 g
   e. 12,000,000 mg
   f. 0.007 kg
   g. 0.009 l
   h. 15,000,000 ml
   i. 2,000 l

3. a. 3.93 in
   b. 1190.7 g
   c. 1.85 lb, 0.84 kg
   d. 63.5 cm, 0.000635 km
   e. 100cc

4. a. 8.964×10^3
   b. 2.53214×10^{-1}
   c. 1.826×10^{-3}
   d. 9,400,000
   e. 0.000127

5. a substance that cannot be separated into substances different from itself by ordinary chemical processes

6. a. protons
   b. neutrons
   c. electrons

7. atomic number—number of protons and electrons
   atomic weight—average weight of an atom as compared with carbon, which has an atomic weight of 12

8. ion

9. molecule—particle that results from chemical combinations of two or more atoms having neutral charges
   compound—molecule formed from two or more elements

10. a. 82 g
    b. 36 g
    c. 58 g
    d. 60 g
    e. 74 g

11. a. covalent

b. ionic
c. ionic
d. covalent
e. covalent

12. a. 17 g
    b. 55 g
    c. 56 g

13. a. intimate mixture of 2 substances, without reacting (percentage of each substance is the same throughout solution)
    b. medium in which solute is dissolving
    c. substance being dissolved

14. $1:300 = 1$ g to 300 ml
    $$\frac{1000 \text{ mg}}{300 \text{ ml}} = \frac{x}{2 \text{ ml}}$$
    $x = 6.7$ mg

15. $1:500 = 1$ g to 500 ml
    $$\frac{1 \text{ g}}{500 \text{ ml}} = \frac{x}{5 \text{ ml}}$$
    $x = 0.01$g

16. $5\% = 5$ g per 100 ml
    $$\frac{5 \text{ g}}{100 \text{ ml}} = \frac{x}{5 \text{ ml}}$$
    $x = 0.25$ g

17. $0.25\% = 0.25$ g per 100 ml
    $$\frac{2500 \text{ mg}}{100 \text{ ml}} = \frac{x}{6 \text{ ml}}$$
    $x = 150$ mg

18. $500 \text{ g} \times 10\% = 50$ g

19. $V_1 C_1 = V_2 C_2$
    $150 \text{ ml} \times 0.35 = 0.10 \times x$
    $x = 525$ ml
    $525 \text{ ml} - 150 \text{ ml} = 375$ ml

20. $0.25 \times 0.20 = 8.25 \text{ ml} \times x$
    $x = 0.6\%$

21. process by which water moves from an area of high solvent concentration to an area of low solvent concentration through a semipermeable membrane

22. a. compound that has the ability to donate H^+ in solution, for example, HCl
    b. compound that has the ability to accept an OH^- in solution, for example, NaOH
    c. a reaction between an acid and a base that produces a salt and water, for example, $NaOH + HCl \rightarrow NaCl + H_2O$

23. d, h, a, c, g, e, f, b

24. a. 78.08%
    b. 20.95%
    c. 0.03%

25. a. liquid barometer or mercury barometer
    b. aneroid barometer
    c. bourdon gauge

26. a. 14.7 psi
    b. 0.735 mmHg
    c. 35.1 cmH_2O
    d. 4560 mmHg
    e. 2.67 atm

27. absolute zero

28. a. 25.5°C
    b. 154.4°f
    c. 310°K
    d. 1151.6°F
    e. 565°R

29. 4 atmospheres

30. Equal volumes of gases at the same pressure and temperature have the same number of molecules and occupy a space of 22.4 liters. Number of molecules is 6.02×10^{23} and equals 1 gmw of substance or 1 mole of a substance.

31. 32 g/22.4 l = 1.43 g/l

32. (0.80)(32) + (0.20)(44)/22.4 l = 1.53 g/l

33. $\dfrac{1.43 \text{ g/l}}{1.28 \text{ g/l}}$ = 1.12; 1.28 is density of air

34. 2 moles/1 $\times$ 6.02 $\times$ 10^{23} molecules/1 mole
    =12.04$\times$$10^{23}$ molecules

35. 453 g $\times$ 1 mole/32 g oxygen = 14.1 moles

36. a. 157.5 mmHg
    b. 151.8 mmHg
    c. 666.6 mmHg

37. 807 mmHg $-$ 47 mmHg = 760 mmHg
    760 mmHg $\times$ 5% = 30 mmHg
    760 mmHg $\times$ 25% = 190 mmHg
    760 mmHg $\times$ 70% = 532 mmHg

38. $\dfrac{P_1}{T_1} = \dfrac{P_2}{T_2}$

    Temperature must be in Kelvin. Add 273 to the temperature in degrees centigrade.
    $\dfrac{2400 \text{ psig} \times 333°K}{293°K}$ = 2727.6 psig

Gay Lussac's law

39. $P_1V_1 = P_2V_2$
    $\dfrac{700 \text{ mmHg} \times 1000 \text{ ml}}{500 \text{ mmHg}}$ = 1400 ml

Boyle's law

40. $\dfrac{V_1}{T_1} = \dfrac{V_2}{T_2}$
    $\dfrac{950 \text{ ml} \times 310°K}{297°K}$ = 1005 ml

Charles' law

41. $\dfrac{P_1V_1}{T_1} = \dfrac{P_2V_2}{T_2}$
    $\dfrac{273°K \times 700 \text{ mmHg} \times 750 \text{ ml}}{310°K \times 500 \text{ mmHg}}$
    =924.6 mmHg

42. Subtract water vapor pressure if the gas is saturated.
    At 37°C water vapor pressure equals 47 mmHg.
    $\dfrac{703 \text{ mmHg} \times 400 \text{ ml} \times 273°K}{310°K \times 760 \text{ mmHg}}$ = 325.8 ml

43. At 25°C water vapor pressure equals 23.8 mmHg.
    $\dfrac{776.2 \text{ mmHg} \times 200 \text{ ml} \times 303°K}{200 \text{ ml} \times 298°K}$
    =789.2 mm Hg
    At 30°C water vapor pressure equals 31.8 mmHg.
    789.2 mmHg + 31.8 mmHg = 821 mmHg saturated

44. PV = nRT
    R = Boltzmann's constant
    $\dfrac{1 \text{ mole} \times 0.0821 \text{ L-atm°K-mole} \times 273°K}{1 \text{ atm}}$
    = 22.4 l

45. a. concentration gradient
    b. temperature
    c. area available
    d. molecular weight
    e. distance gas has to diffuse

46. 0.023 ml/ml plasma oxygen
    0.510 ml/ml plasma carbon dioxide

47. Henry's and Graham's laws

48. $\dfrac{0.70 \times \text{ square root of } 25}{0.30 \times \text{ square root of } 64}$

$$\frac{3.5}{2.4} = 1.45$$

49. Bernoulli's principle
    As forward velocity of a gas increases, its lateral pressure decreases with a corresponding increase in forward pressure.

50. a. jet orifice size
    b. size of the entrainment port(s)

51. a. Venturi; to restore the delivered (lateral) pressure to its prerestricted value
    b. Pitot; no attempt to restore (lateral) pressure, maintains high velocity and restricted pressures

52. laminar-turbulent flow, mixed because of constant branching of the airways

PRACTICE QUIZ

1. A woman weighing 110 pounds has a weight in kilograms of:
   a. 50 kg
   b. 85 kg
   c. 107 kg
   d. 192 kg
   e. 143 kg

2. In the equation K = AB, how is A related to B?
   a. A is equal to B
   b. A is directly related to B
   c. A is inversely related to B
   d. A does not equal B
   e. A is less than B

3. Calculate the molecular weight of HCO_3, given the following atomic weights: H = 1, C = 12, O = 16.
   a. 28 g
   b. 32 g
   c. 44 g
   d. 50 g
   e. 61 g

4. What would the final concentration of 30 ml of a 10% solution be if we dilute it with 20 ml of water?
   a. 4%
   b. 6%
   c. 8%
   d. 10%
   e. 15%

5. Which of the following gases is found below its critical temperature (liquid form) in everyday use?
   a. C_2H_4
   b. O_2/CO_2
   c. NH_4
   d. He/O_2
   e. none of the above

6. Which of the following is equal to 0.5 psi?
   a. 25.8 mmHg
   b. 1034 cmH_2O

   c. 1 atm
   d. 32.9 inHg
   e. 22.4 ft H_2O

7. Absolute zero means:
   a. absence of molecular motion and heat
   b. point at which water boils on the Kelvin scale
   c. point at which water evaporates on the Kelvin scale
   d. 273°C
   e. triple point for water

8. Approximately how many degrees Kelvin equals 106°F?
   a. 127°K
   b. 140°K
   c. 169°K
   d. 296°K
   e. 314°K

9. Axillary temperature is usually _____ than rectal temperature.
   a. higher
   b. lower
   c. the same
   d. no correlation exists
   e. none of the above

10. Standard temperature and pressure dry means:
   a. 300°K, 760 mmHg, and 0 mmHg H_2O
   b. 0°C, 760 mmHg, and 0 mmHg H_2O
   c. 273°K, 760 mmHg, and 47 mmHg H_2O
   d. 0°F, 760 mmHg, and 47 mmHg H_2O
   e. 0°C, 0 mmHg, and 0 mmHg H_2O

11. At STP 1 gram molecular weight of gas equals:
   a. the molecular weight of a substance times 1 gram
   b. 10 moles
   c. 22.4 g
   d. 6.02×10^{23} molecules
   e. a and d

12. The density of a mixture of 0.70 oxygen and 0.30 carbon dioxide is equal to _____.
   (GMW oxygen = 32 g, GMW of carbon dioxide = 44 g)
   a. 10 g/l
   b. 2.0 g/l
   c. 15.8 g/l
   d. 1.59 g/l
   e. not enough information

13. The Po_2 of dry air at 25,000 feet and a barometric pressure of 300 mmHg is:
   a. 21%
   b. 159 mmHg
   c. 149 mmHg
   d. 63 mmHg
   e. 16%

14. Assuming an F_{IN_2} of 0.78, calculate the barometric pressure in mmHg with a P_{N_2} of 580 mmHg.
    a. 744 mmHg
    b. 760 mmHg
    c. 785 mmHg
    d. 857 mmHg
    e. 903 mmHg

15. If 5 liters of oxygen in a Douglas bag at 740 mmHg is compressed to 2 liters, what is the new pressure inside the bag?
    a. 720 mmHg
    b. 850 mmHg
    c. 980 mmHg
    d. 1520 mmHg
    e. 1850 mmHg

16. Gas flows from one place to another in a closed container because of:
    a. an increase in temperature
    b. diffusion
    c. concentration gradient
    d. osmosis
    e. diffusibility of the gas

17. The principle employed to describe the operation of a jet nebulizer is:
    a. Dalton's law
    b. Charles' law
    c. Stoke's law
    d. Bernoulli's law
    e. Henry's law

18. At a constant temperature, the volume occupied by a quantity of gas varies inversely with the pressure exerted upon it. This is known as:
    a. Charles' law
    b. Henry's law
    c. Gay-Lussac's law
    d. Boyle's law
    e. Venturi's law

19. If the lumen of an airway were reduced by one half by bronchospasm, the pressure required to deliver the same airflow through that airway would be:
    a. 16 times the original
    b. 4 times the original
    c. one half the original
    d. 2 times the original
    e. the same as the original

20. All of the following factors affect the resistance through tubes except:
    a. radius
    b. flow
    c. viscosity
    d. length
    e. diameter

ANSWERS TO THE PRACTICE QUIZ

1. a
2. c
3. e
4. e
5. a
6. a
7. a
8. e
9. b
10. b

11. e
12. d
13. d
14. a
15. e
16. c
17. d
18. d
19. a
20. e

Chapter 2

CARDIOPULMONARY ANATOMY

Outline

Learning Objectives

Upon completion of this unit, the individual will:

1. Describe and identify the anatomic structure of the nose.
2. Identify and describe the three divisions of the pharynx.
3. Describe the structure of the pharynx.
4. Describe the structure of the larynx.
5. List/describe the three unpaired cartilages and the three paired cartilages that compose the larynx.
6. List the various bronchi within the tracheobronchial tree.
7. Describe the respiratory unit, clara cells, Type I cells, Type II cells, and Type III cells.
8. List the generations of airways.

9. Describe the gas exchange unit.
10. Describe the pleura.
11. Locate/describe the following:
    a. ribs
    b. mediastinum
    c. heart
    d. great vessels
    e. lung segments
    f. muscles of respiration
    g. sternum
12. Describe and identify the anatomic structures of the heart.
13. Trace the flow of blood through the heart into the great vessels.
14. Label the muscles of ventilation.

REFERENCES

Burton, G, and Hodgkin, J: Respiratory Care: A Guide to Clinical Practice, ed 2. JB Lippincott, Philadelphia, 1984

DesJardins, TR: Clinical Manifestations of Respiratory Disease. Year Book Medical Publishers, Chicago, 1984

Eubanks, DH, and Bone, RC: Comprehensive Respiratory Care. CV Mosby, St Louis, 1985.

Hagen-Ansert, SL: The Anatomy Workbook. JB Lippincott, Philadelphia, 1986.

Kacmarek, RM, Mach, CW, and Dimas, S: The Essentials of Respiratory Therapy, ed 2. Year Book Medical Publishers, Chicago, 1985.

Shapiro, BA, Harrison, RA, Kacmarek, RM, and Cane, RD: Clinical Application of Respiratory Care, ed 3. Year Book Medical Publishers, Chicago, 1985.

Solomon, EP, and Phillips, GA: Understanding Human Anatomy and Physiology. WB Saunders, Philadelphia, 1987.

STUDY QUESTIONS

1. Locate the following structures on Figure 2–1. (Eubanks, p 46; Kacmarek, p 67)

   _____ manubrium   _____ costal cartilage

   _____ clavicles   _____ rib

   _____ body   _____ xiphoid

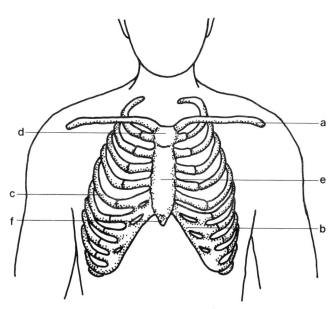

FIGURE 2–1. The sternum.

2. Of which of the following is the thoracic cage composed? Circle the correct letter(s). (Eubanks, p 46; Kacmarek, p 67)

    a. thoracic vertebrae
    b. sternum
    c. ribs
    d. mediastinum
    e. hilus

3. List the four functions of the thorax. (Kacmarek, p 66)

    a. _____

    b. _____

    c. _____

    d. _____

4. Name the three flat elongated bones that compose the structure of the sternum. (Eubanks, p 47; Kacmarek, p 66)

    a. _____

    b. _____

    c. _____

5. Fill in the correct information about the ribs. (Eubanks, p 46; Kacmarek, p 66)

    a. There are _____ pairs of ribs.

    b. There are _____ pairs of true ribs.

    c. There are _____ pairs of false ribs.

    d. There are _____ pairs of floating ribs.

6. The thoracic vertebral column is composed of _____ vertebrae. (Eubanks, p 46)

7. List two functions of the thoracic vertebrae. (Eubanks, p 46)

    a. _____

    b. _____

8. Label Figure 2–2. (Eubanks, p 46; Kacmarek, p 66)

    a. Ribs 1–7 are considered _____ ribs.

    b. Ribs 8–10 are considered _____ ribs.

    c. Ribs 11 and 12 are considered _____ ribs.

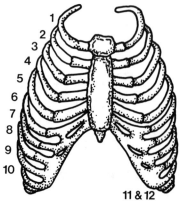

FIGURE 2–2. The thorax.

9. What two layers compose the pleura of the thoracic cage? (Kacmarek, p 61)

    a. _____

    b. _____

10. Which layer of the pleura lines the thoracic wall? (Kacmarek, p 61)

    _____

11. Which layer of the pleura lines the outer surfaces of the lung? (DesJardins, p 37; Kacmarek, p 61)

    _____

12. The potential space between the two layers of the pleura is termed the _____ _____. (DesJardins, p 38; Kacmarek, p 61)

13. What is the function of the small amount of fluid found between the two pleura? (DesJardins, p 38; Kacmarek, p 61)

    _____

14. The heart lies in the mediastinum within the _____. (Eubanks, p 58; Kacmarek, p 104)

15. List the four chambers of the heart. (DesJardins, p 124; Eubanks, p 58; Kacmarek, p 106)

    a. _____

    b. _____

    c. _____

    d. _____

16. Indicate which of the following are True and which are False. (Eubanks, p 58; Kacmarek, p 104)

    _____ The valve located between the right ventricle and the right atrium is the pulmonic valve.

    _____ The most muscular chamber of the heart is the right ventricle.

    _____ The aortic valve allows for coronary blood flow.

    _____ The chamber responsible for receiving oxygenated blood from the lungs is the left atrium.

    _____ The chordae tendineae are responsible for coronary circulation.

17. Label the anatomic structures of the heart as seen in Figure 2–3. (DesJardins, p 124; Eubanks, p 58; Kacmarek, p 107)

    a. _____ i. _____

    b. _____ j. _____

    c. _____ k. _____

    d. _____ l. _____

    e. _____ m. _____

    f. _____ n. _____

    g. _____ o. _____

    h. _____ p. _____

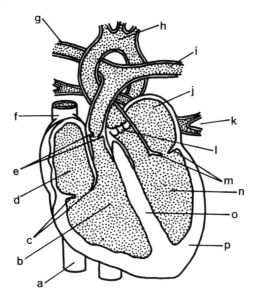

FIGURE 2-3. The heart.

18. The circulation that feeds the heart itself, is termed the _____ circulation. (Eubanks, p 63; Kacmarek, p 106)

19. The three bony plates that project from the lateral wall of each nasal cavity are termed _____ _____ . (Kacmarek, p 39)

20. The _____ separates the nasal cavities and is composed of cartilage covered by mucous membrane. (Eubanks, p 162; Kacmarek, p 39)

21. List the names of the paranasal sinuses. (Eubanks, p 162; Kacmarek, p 39)

    a. _____

    b. _____

    c. _____

    d. _____

22. Label the anatomic structures depicted in Figure 2-4. (Kacmarek, p 39)

    a. _____   d. _____

    b. _____   e. _____

    c. _____   f. _____

23. Label the anatomic subdivisions of the pharynx depicted in Figure 2-5. (Eubanks, p 162; Kacmarek, p 39)

    a. _____

    b. _____

    c. _____

24. Describe the epiglottis. (DesJardins, p 11; Eubanks, p 164)

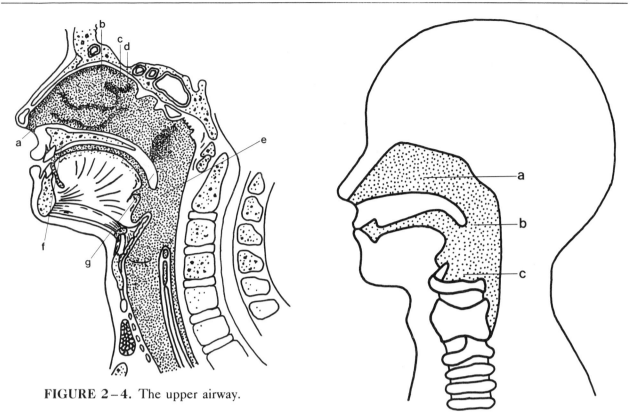

FIGURE 2–4. The upper airway.

FIGURE 2–5. The pharynx.

_____

_____

25. List two functions of the larynx. (DesJardins, p 11; Eubanks, p 163; Kacmarek, p 47)

 a. _____

 b. _____

26. How many cartilages make up the larynx?

_____

27. Label the anatomic structures depicted in Figure 2–6. (DesJardins, p 12; Eubanks, p 164; Kacmarek, p 48)

 a. _____ d. _____

 b. _____ e. _____

 c. _____

28. Describe the trachea. (DesJardins, p 23; Eubanks, p 164; Kacmarek, p 48)

_____

_____

_____

29. What gives the trachea its shape and support? (DesJardins, p 23; Eubanks, p 164; Kacmarek, p 53)

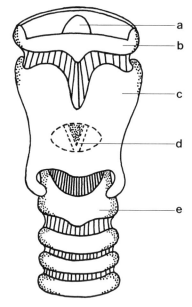

FIGURE 2-6. The larynx.

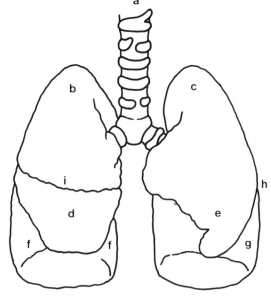

FIGURE 2-7. The lower airway.

_____

_____

30. The point at which the trachea divides to form the right and left main stem bronchus is called the _____ . (DesJardins, p 23; Eubanks, p 164; Kacmarek, p 53)

31. The lining of the conducting airways is composed to what type of cells? (Kacmarek, p 55)

_____

32. The right lung has _____ lobes. The left lung has _____ lobes. (DesJardins, p 38; Eubanks, p 166; Kacmarek, p 63).

33. Label the anatomic structures depicted in Figure 2-7. (DesJardins, p 36; Kacmarek, p 64)

    a. _____   f. _____

    b. _____   g. _____

    c. _____   h. _____

    d. _____   i. _____

    e. _____

34. The left lung is divided into _____ segments. List the segments and the location in the lobe. (DesJardins, p 38; Eubanks, p 166)

_____

_____

_____

35. The right lobe is divided into _____ segments. List the segments and the position in the right lobe. (DesJardins, 38; Eubanks, p 166)

_____

_____

_____

36. List in the correct anatomic order the bronchiolar divisions occurring from the trachea to the alveoli. (DesJardins, p 17; Eubanks, p 158; Kacmarek, p 53)

_____

_____

_____

37. At what generation of the bronchi is there no cartilage within the walls? (DesJardins, p 17; Eubanks, p 158; Kacmarek, p 56)

_____

38. Name the generations of the tracheobronchial tree that make up the conducting zone. (DesJardins, p 17; Eubanks, p 158; Kacmarek, p 57)

_____

39. What is the function of the conducting zone? (DesJardins, p 17; Eubanks, p 158; Kacmarek, p 58)

_____

40. What are generations 17 to 23 of the tracheobronchial tree termed? (DesJardins, p 17; Eubanks, p 158; Kacmarek, p 58)

_____

41. List the names of the generations of the tracheobronchial tree that compose the respiratory zone. (DesJardins, p 17; Eubanks, p 160; Kacmarek, p 58)

    a. _____

    b. _____

    c. _____

42. The unit of gas exchange is called the _____ . (Eubanks, p 160)

43. Define the following terms: (DesJardins, p 28; Eubanks, p 160)
    a. clara cells:

    _____

    b. Type I cells:

    _____

    c. Type II cells:

    _____

    d. Type III cells:

    _____

44. The vascular supply to the lungs is made up of what two systems? (DesJardins, p 29; Eubanks, p 161)

a. _____

b. _____

45. Unoxygenated blood is delivered to the lungs via? (DesJardins, p 29; Eubanks, p 161, Kacmarek, p 113)

_____

46. What is the function of the bronchial arteries? (Eubanks, p 161)

_____

47. What are the two most important muscles of ventilation? (Eubanks, p 51; Kacmarek, p 68)

_____

_____

48. Label the muscles of ventilation in Figure 2–8. (Kacmarek, p 69)

a. _____   f. _____

b. _____   g. _____

c. _____   h. _____

d. _____   i. _____

e. _____   j. _____

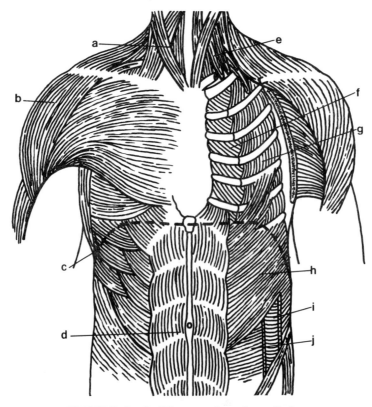

FIGURE 2–8. The muscles of ventilation.

ANSWERS TO STUDY QUESTIONS

1. a. clavicles
   b. costal cartilage
   c. rib
   d. manubrium
   e. body of sternum
   f. xiphoid process

2. a, b, and c

3. a. houses vital organs of cardiopulmonary system
   b. protects vital organs of the cardiopulmonary system
   c. gives support to shoulder girdle
   d. provides attachment for muscles.

4. a. manubrium
   b. body
   c. xiphoid process

5. a. 12
   b. 7
   c. 3
   d. 2

6. twelve

7. a. shock absorber
   b. protection of nerves

8. a. true ribs
   b. false ribs
   c. floating ribs

9. a. parietal
   b. visceral

10. parietal

11. the visceral pleura

12. pleural space

13. The fluid functions to permit the layers to move on each other with minimal pain and friction.

14. pericardial sac

15. a. right atrium
    b. right ventricle
    c. left atrium
    d. left ventricle

16. False, False, False, True, False

17. a. inferior vena cava
    b. right ventricle
    c. tricuspid
    d. right atrium
    e. pulmonic valve

f. superior vena cava
g. right pulmonary artery
h. aorta
i. left pulmonary artery
j. left atrium
k. pulmonary veins
l. aortic valve
m. bicuspid
n. left ventricle
o. interventricular septum
p. left ventricular muscle mass

18. coronary

19. nasal conchae

20. nasal septum

21. a. ethmoid
    b. sphenoid
    c. frontal
    d. maxillary

22. a. vestibule
    b. inferior conchae
    c. middle conchae
    d. superior conchae
    e. pharynx
    f. hard palate
    g. soft palate

23. a. hypopharynx
    b. oropharynx
    c. nasopharynx

24. The epiglottis is a plate-like structure that extends from the base of the tongue backward and upward

25. a. sound production
    b. protection
    c. passageway for food/air

26. nine

27. a. epiglottis
    b. hyoid bone
    c. thyroid cartilage
    d. vocal cords
    e. cricoid cartilage

28. The trachea is a tubular structure that begins at the neck below the cricoid cartilage at the level of C-6. It ends in the thorax at the sternal angle, where it divides into the right and left main stem bronchi at the carina. It is 11 to 13 cm long in the adult and supported by 15 to 20 C-shaped cartilages.

29. The cartilage rings (15 to 20) that are C-shaped and the muscle between the rings give the trachea its shape and support.

30. carina

31. pseudostratified columnar epithelium

32. three lobes on the right and two lobes on the left

33. a. trachea
    b. right upper lobe
    c. left upper lobe
    d. right middle lobe
    e. lingula
    f. right lower lobe
    g. left lower lobe
    h. horizontal fissure
    i. oblique fissure

34. 8, upper lobe: (upper division) apical/posterior and anterior (lower division) superior lingula and inferior lingula
    lower lobe: superior, anterior medial, lateral basal, and posterior basal

35. 10, upper lobe: apical, posterior, and anterior
    middle lobe: lateral and medial
    lower lobe: superior, medial basal, anterior basal, lateral basal, and posterior basal

36. trachea, main stem bronchi, lobar bronchi, segmental bronchi subsegmental bronchi, bronchi, terminal bronchi, bronchioles, terminal bronchioles, respiratory bronchioles, alveolar ducts and sacs, and the alveoli

37. the bronchioles

38. This zone is made up of the generations 1 through 19.

39. The conducting zone functions to condition and conduct gas to the respiratory zone

40. transitional and respiratory zones

41. a. the respiratory bronchioles
    b. the alveolar sacs and ducts
    c. the alveoli

42. alveoli

43. a. columnar cells found in the terminal bronchioles, responsible for mucous production and/or surfactant, true function, controversial at this time
    b. squamous pneumocytes found as part of the make-up of the alveolar epithelium
    c. granular pneumocytes, responsible for the production of surfactant
    d. alveolar macrophages, free moving cells, responsible for ingestion and removal of foreign materials

44. a. pulmonary vasculature
    b. bronchial vasculature

45. the pulmonary artery

46. The bronchial arteries function to provide oxygenated blood for the metabolism of lung tissues

47. The diaphragm and the intercostals are considered the two main muscles of ventilation

48. a. sternocleidomastoid
    b. pectoralis major
    c. diaphragm
    d. rectus abdominis
    e. the scalenus
    f. internal intercostals
    g. external intercostals
    h. external oblique
    i. internal oblique
    j. transverse abdominis

PRACTICE QUIZ

1. How many pairs of ribs are there in the normal patient?
    a. 6
    b. 7
    c. 8
    d. 10
    e. 12

2. What is the bifurcation of the trachea termed?
    a. carina

b. angle of Louis
c. eye of Murphy
d. mediastinum
e. hilar region

3. The pleura covering the surface of the lung is termed:
   a. respiratory pleura
   b. ventilatory pleura
   c. visceral pleura
   d. parietal pleura
   e. periosteum

4. Which of the following comprises the respiratory unit?
   I. alveoli
   II. terminal bronchioles
   III. respiratory bronchioles
   IV. alveolar ducts and sacs
   a. I, II, III, IV, V
   b. I, II, IV
   c. II, III, V
   d. I, III, IV
   e. I, II, V

5. Which of the following are not sections of the sternum?
   I. scapula
   II. body
   III. clavicle
   IV. manubrium
   V. xiphoid process
   a. I, III, V
   b. II, IV, V
   c. I, II, III
   d. I, II
   e. I, III

6. What point in the tracheobronchial tree represents the end of the conducting zone?
   a. terminal bronchiole
   b. respiratory bronchiole
   c. right main stem
   d. carina
   e. alveolar duct

7. The tracheobronchial tree divides into how many generations?
   a. 5
   b. 10
   c. 17
   d. 23
   e. 28

8. The serous sac that surrounds the heart is called the:
   a. endocardium
   b. pericardium
   c. exocardium
   d. mediastinum
   e. hilar sac

9. Which of the following is a function of the thorax?
    I. provide points of attachment
    II. give support
    III. protect vital organs
    IV. house vital organs
    V. supply nutrition
    a. I, II, III, IV, V
    b. I, II, III, IV
    c. II, III, V
    d. I, III, IV
    e. III only

10. Which of the following are true?
    I. There are seven pairs of true ribs.
    II. There are two pairs of true ribs.
    III. There are two pairs of floating ribs.
    IV. There are twelve pairs of ribs.
    V. There are five pairs of true ribs.
    a. I, III, IV,
    b. I, II, V
    c. II, III, IV, V
    d. I, III, IV, V
    e. I, III, V

11. Blood leaves the pulmonary vein and enters which of the following structures?
    a. right atrium
    b. right ventricle
    c. left atrium
    d. left ventricle
    e. the lungs

12. Blood leaves the tricuspid valve and enters which of the following structures?
    a. right atrium
    b. right ventricle
    c. left atrium
    d. left ventricle
    e. the lungs

13. Which of the sinuses listed below are nasal sinuses?
    I. maxillary
    II. ethmoid
    III. sphenoid
    IV. septal
    V. frontal
    a. I, II, III, IV, V
    b. I, II, III
    c. I, II, III, V
    d. I, II, IV, V
    e. I, II

14. Which of the following are segments of the right upper lobe?
    I. apical
    II. lateral
    III. medial
    IV. posterior
    V. anterior

a. I, II, III, IV, V
b. I, IV, V
c. I, II, IV
d. I, IV
e. II, III, IV

15. Which of the following are the two most important muscles of ventilation?
    I. scalene
    II. transverse abdominis
    III. pectoralis major
    IV. diaphragm
    V. intercostals
    a. I, III
    b. II, III
    c. II, IV
    d. IV, V
    e. III, V

16. The alveolar cells responsible for ingestion and removal of cellular debris are termed?
    a. Type I cells
    b. Type II cells
    c. Type III cells
    d. macrophages
    e. c and d

17. The pharynx is divided into what divisions?
    I. nasopharynx
    II. oropharynx
    III. tracheopharynx
    IV. laryngopharynx
    V. hypopharynx
    a. I, II, III, IV, V
    b. I, II, III
    c. II, III, IV
    d. I, II, V
    e. I, IV, V

18. The thyroid cartilage is located in what portion of the respiratory system?
    a. nasal conchae
    b. pharynx
    c. larynx
    d. trachea
    e. bronchus

19. What portion of the respiratory system is composed of 16 to 20 C-shaped rings?
    a. hypopharynx
    b. larynx
    c. carina
    d. respiratory unit
    e. trachea

20. The only cartilage ring in the larynx to form a complete circle is which of the following?
    a. thyroid
    b. arytenoid
    c. cricoid
    d. hyoid
    e. sphenoid

ANSWERS TO THE PRACTICE QUIZ

1. e		11. c	
2. a		12. b	
3. c		13. c	
4. d		14. b	
5. e		15. d	
6. a		16. e	
7. d		17. d	
8. b		18. c	
9. b		19. e	
10. a		20. c	

CARDIOPULMONARY RESUSCITATION

LEARNING OBJECTIVES

Upon completion of this unit, the individual will:

1. Distinquish between respiratory arrest and respiratory insufficiency.
2. Define the following terms:
   a. atherosclerosis
   b. angina pectoris
   c. myocardial infarction
   d. sudden death
   e. EMS system
   f. clinical death
   g. biologic death
   h. fibrillation and defibrillation
   i. stroke

3. List the correct procedures for each of the following:
   a. one-person CPR
   b. two-person CPR
   c. child and infant CPR
   d. conscious and unconscious adult
   e. conscious and unconscious child and infant
   f. rescue breathing for adult, child, and infant
4. Explain the compression rates and ratios for the adult, child, and infant.
5. Explain the proper ways of opening the airway.
6. Describe preventive measures for airway obstruction, coronary artery disease, and stroke.
7. Explain the EMS system.

REFERENCES

Barnes, TA: Respiratory Care Practice. Year Book Medical Publishers, Chicago, 1988.

"Basic Life Support." In cooperation with American Heart Association. JAMA 225(21):2915, 1986.

Thomas, CL (ed): Taber's Cyclopedic Medical Dictionary, ed 15. FA Davis, Philadelphia 1985.

STUDY QUESTIONS

1. Distinguish between respiratory arrest and respiratory insufficiency. (Basic Life Support, American Heart Association [BLS], p 18)

   _____

   _____

2. Define central respiratory arrest, according to the Journal of American Medical Association. (BLS, p 18)

   _____

3. List the possible causes of central respiratory arrest. (BLS, p 18)

   a. _____

   b. _____

   c. _____

   d. _____

   e. _____

   f. _____

4. Define atherosclerosis. (BLS, p 18; Taber's, p 149)

   _____

   _____

5. Many risks factors are associated with coronary artery disease. List as many factors as you can. (BLS, p 19)

   _____

   _____

6. Explain prudent heart living. (BLS, p 21)

   _____

   _____

   _____

7. Define angina pectoris. (BLS, p 25; Taber's, p 90)

   _____

   _____

8. List the most common symptoms associated with angina pectoris. (BLS, p 25)

   a. _____

   b. _____

   c. _____

9. Angina pectoris can be relieved by _____. (BLS, p 25)

10. Define myocardial infarction. (BLS, p 25, Taber's, p 1087) _____

    _____

11. What signs and symptoms are associated with myocardial infarction? (BLS, p 26)

    _____

    _____

    _____

    _____

12. Describe the procedure(s) you would follow in the initial treatment of an acute myocardial infarction in a patient in whom the cardiac condition is known versus that in a patient in whom the cardiac condition is unknown. (BLS, p 26)

    _____

    _____

    _____

    _____

    _____

    _____

    _____

    _____

13. Define sudden death, according to the Journal of American Medical Association. (BLS, p 27)

    _____

14. Describe how each of the following can cause the cessation of breathing: (BLS, p 27)

    a. blocked airway: _____

    _____

    b. brain injury: _____

    _____

    c. drug overdose: _____

    _____

    d. electrocution: _____

    _____

    e. drowning: _____

    _____

15. The major cause of cardiac arrest is _____. (BLS, p 27)

16. Describe ventricular fibrillation. (BLS, p 28; Barnes, pp 268–270)

17. The application of an electrical shock that momentarily stops all electrical activity and allows spontaneous coordinated electrical function to return is called _____ . (BLS, p 28; Tabers, p 430)

18. Significant brain damage will occur within _____ minutes after cardiac arrest. (BLS, p 29)

19. Distinguish between clinical and biologic death. (BLS, pp 29–30, Taber's, p 423)

20. List the physiologic causes of stroke (cerebral vascular accident). (BLS, p 33; Taber's, p 1640)

    a. _____

    b. _____

    c. _____

21. What are the ABC's of cardiopulmonary resuscitation? (BLS, p 39)

22. Describe the emergency medical system. (BLS, p 40)

23. What information should be supplied to the emergency medical system from the caller? (BLS, p 40)

    a. _____

    b. _____

    c. _____

    d. _____

    e. _____

    f. _____

24. What method is employed to determine unresponsiveness in an adult? (BLS, p 41; Barnes, p 250)

25. For cardiopulmonary resuscitation to be effective, how should the patient be positioned? (BLS, p 41; Barnes, pp 253–254)

26. What are the two major methods of opening the airway? (BLS, pp 42–44; Barnes, pp 250–251)

27. In the adult patient where do you check for pulselessness, and for how long? (BLS, p 47; Barnes, p 253)

_____

28. In an adult, if a pulse is present but breathing is absent, rescue breathing should be repeated every _____ seconds, or _____ times per minute. (BLS, p 47; Barnes, p 251)

29. Explain proper hand positioning when doing external cardiac message on an adult. (BLS, pp 49–50; Barnes, pp 254–255)

_____

_____

_____

30. The sternum should be depressed _____ inches when doing external cardiac message on an adult. (BLS, p 50; Barnes, p 254)

31. From Figure 3–1, identify the proper landmarks, by filling in the blanks. (BLS, p 49; Barnes, p 255)

a. _____   e. _____

b. _____   f. _____

c. _____   g. _____

d. _____   h. _____

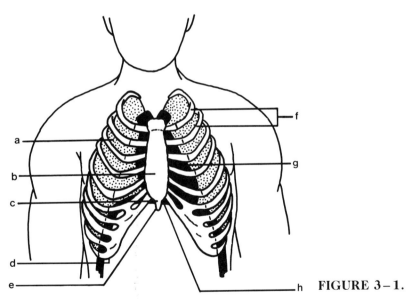

FIGURE 3–1.

32. The compression-to-breathing ratio for one-person CPR is _____. (BLS, p 54; Barnes, p 254)

33. At what point during cardiopulmonary resuscitation should you re-evaluate the patient? (BLS, p 54)

_____

34. Evaluation of the effectiveness of cardiopulmonary resuscitation can be accomplished by what methods? (Barnes, pp 277–278)

_____

_____

_____

_____

_____

35. Discuss the method of entry for a second rescuer to perform two-person CPR. (BLS, p 57)

_____

_____

_____

_____

_____

36. Compression ratio for two-person CPR _____. (BLS, p 59; Barnes, p 254)

37. Since foreign body obstruction usually happens during eating, what precautions can be taken to prevent this from occurring? (BLS, p 65; Barnes, p 270)

_____

_____

_____

_____

_____

38. Describe Figure 3–2. _____

_____ (BLS, p 65)

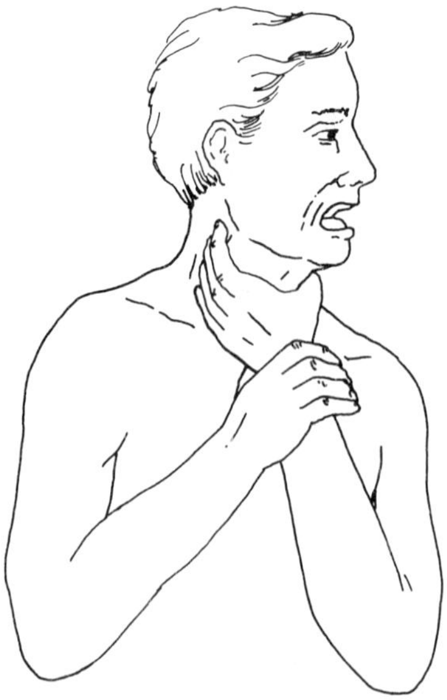

FIGURE 3–2.

39. The manuever to relieve an obstructed airway is termed the _____

_____. (Barnes, p 270)

40. The most common cause of upper airway obstruction in an unconscious person is the _____ _____. (BLS, p 65)

41. Describe the sequence to relieve an obstructed airway in an adult. (Barnes, p 271)

_____

_____

_____

42. What adjustments are made to relieve an obstructed airway in the person who is either pregnant or obese? (BLS, p 68; Barnes, p 270)

_____

43. List the steps necessary for beginning ventilations and relieving the airway obstruction in an unconscious person. (BLS, pp 70–71)

_____

_____

_____

_____

44. What is/are the major cause(s) of cardiopulmonary arrest in infants and small children? (BLS, p 73)

_____

_____

45. What changes in CPR, if any, are needed for a child? (BLS, p 74; Barnes, pp 254–255)

_____

_____

_____

46. What is the major difference between relieving a foreign body obstruction in an unconscious child and in an unconscious adult? (BLS, pp 76–77; Barnes, p 271)

_____

47. What is the proper procedure for opening the infant airway? (BLS, p 76)

_____

48. When ventilating an infant, a tight seal is made over the infant's _____ and _____. (BLS, p 76)

49. Describe what the rescuer is doing in Figure 3–3. (BLS, p 78)

_____

50. How is correct hand position determined for compressions in an infant? (BLS, p 78–79)

_____

_____

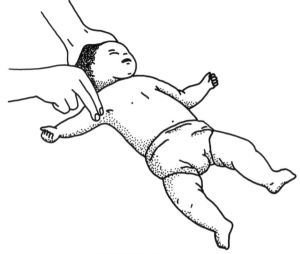

FIGURE 3–3.

51. The sternum should be depressed _____ inches when doing external cardiac message on an infant. (BLS, p 79; Barnes, p 255)

52. The ratio of compressions to ventilations in an infant is _____. (BLS, p 79; Barnes, p 255)

53. The compression rate for an infant is _____ per minute. (BLS, p 79; Barnes, p 255)

54. In an infant, if a pulse is present but breathing is absent, rescue breathing should be repeated every _____ seconds, or _____ times per minute. (BLS, pp 76–77)

55. Give the procedure to relieve an airway obstruction on an infant. (BLS, pp 76–77; Barnes, p 271)

_____

_____

_____

56. After CPR has been initiated, it may be terminated only when: (BLS, p 185)

    a. _____

    b. _____

    c. _____

    d. _____

ANSWERS TO STUDY QUESTIONS

1. respiratory arrest—absence of breathing
   respiratory insufficiency—inability to maintain normal carbon dioxide and oxygen levels

2. any condition that depresses or destroys the respiratory center

3. a. shock
   b. cardiac arrest
   c. stroke
   d. drug overdose
   e. barbiturates
   f. head trauma

4. deposition of fatty deposits (cholesterol, lipids), fibrin, and eventually calcium resulting in a gradual narrowing of the lumen of the arterial wall

5. heredity, gender, race, age, cigarette smoking, increase blood pressure, blood cholesterol, diabetes, obesity, lack of exercise, and stress

6. that lifestyle that minimizes the risk of future heart disease; should include, but is not limited to, weight control, physical fitness, proper diet, no smoking, decreased blood fats, and control of blood pressure

7. pain and discomfort due to decreased blood to the myocardium; may be brought on by excercise, stress, or exertion

8. a. retrosternal pain—crushing, pressing, constricting, a heavy feeling
   b. radiating pain—usually left arm, shoulder, neck, back, epigastrium, and jaw
   c. nausea

9. rest and/or nitroglycerin and the administration of oxygen

10. death of heart tissue

11. Most common symptoms include uncomfortable pressure in the chest (squeezing; fullness and tightness; crushing, heavy sensation) retrosternal pain (shoulders, arm, jaw, back). The feeling will last longer than 2 minutes and will not be relieved by rest or nitroglycerin. Other symnptoms are sweating; nausea; shortness of breath; feeling of weakness; cold, clammy skin.

12. a. Have the person rest quietly and calmly (allow person to assume the most comfortable position).
    b. If the person is a known heart patient:
       1. Administer nitroglycerin.
       2. Repeat administration of nitroglycerin every 3 to 5 minutes, up to three tablets.
       3. Call the emergency medical system (usually 911).
    c. If the person is unknown as a heart patient:
       1. If pain persists for 2 minutes or more, call the emergency medical system.

13. the unexpected cessation of breathing and circulation

14. a. blocked airway—cessation of breathing because of lack of oxygen
    b. brain injury—interference with the nerve impulses to the muscles of ventilation
    c. drug overdose—interference with the nerve impulses to the muscles of ventilation
    d. electrocution—interference with the electrical activity of the brain and the nerve impulses to the muscles of ventilation

   e. drowning—cessation of breathing resulting from lack of oxygen

15. coronary artery disease

16. chaotic, uncoordinated quivering of the myocardium (ventricles)

17. defibrillation

18. 4 to 6 minutes

19. Clinical death—cessation of the cardiovascular and pulmonary systems; fully reversible if person is resuscitated
    Biologic death—permanent, irreversible brain death

20. a. thrombosis
    b. embolism
    c. hemorrhage due to hypertension or an aneurysm

21. *a*irway, *b*reathing, and *c*irculation

22. a community-wide, coordinating means of responding to a sudden illness or injury

23. a. where the emergency is
    b. phone number of where the call is made
    c. what happened
    d. how many persons are involved and need assistance
    e. condition of victim(s)
    f. what aid, if any, is being given

24. Shake and shout; if an infant is involved you may want to flick or pinch the foot.

25. For cardiopulmonary resuscitation to be effective, the victim must be horizontal, supine, and on a firm surface.

26. modified head tilt/chin lift, or jaw thrust

27. carotid artery located in the neck; for 5 full seconds

28. 5 seconds, 12 times per minute

29. Find the lower margin of the ribs, move fingers up the rib cage to the sternal notch, heal of one hand next to the index finger, and then place the other hand on top of the first hand. Lock fingers to keep them off the chest.

30. $1\frac{1}{2}$ to 2 inches

31. a. lungs
    b. sternum
    c. sternal notch
    d. lower rib margin
    e. xiphoid process
    f. ribs

g. heart
h. diaphragm

32. 15:2

33. after four full cycles of 15 compressions to two ventilations or 1 minute

34. a. determining the adequacy of ventilation by inspection, auscultation, inflation pressures
    b. checking arterial blood gases to determine oxygenation
    c. checking for pulse during each compression
    d. observing the reactivity of the pupils to check cerebral blood flow

35. a. Identify self and qualify to help.
    b. First rescuer stops after two ventilations.
    c. One rescuer checks pulse for 5 seconds.
    d. Second rescuer locates proper hand position, while first rescuer checks pulse. If no pulse, one breath is given.
    e. Second rescuer starts compressions at the rate of 80 to 100/minute.

36. 5:1

37. a. Cut food into small pieces and chew slowly and thoroughly.
    b. Avoid laughing and talking while chewing.
    c. Avoid excessive alcohol intake before and during meals.
    d. Restrict children from walking and running with food in their mouth.
    e. Keep small objects away from small children and infants.

38. the universal sign for choking

39. Heimlich maneuver

40. tongue

41. Stand behind victim, wrap arms around victim, make fist with one hand with thumb side against victim's abdomen midline between belly button and xiphoid process. Press fist into abdomen with quick upward thrusts, and repeat 6 to 10 times. If obstruction unrelieved, repeat procedure.

42. Chest thrusts are used.

43. The same steps are used as in CPR until you get to the ventilations.
    Reposition the head and try ventilations again.
    Give 6 to 10 abdominal thrusts.
    Perform finger sweep and then attempt to ventilate.

44. accidents—motor vehicle, fire, drowning, falls, choking from foreign objects, suffocation, and poisoning

45. Compress chest 1 to $1\frac{1}{2}$ inches.
    Size of child determines one-handed or two-handed compressions.
    5:1 ratio

46. You should not perform a blind finger sweep in an infant or child.

47. neutral position—hand under the shoulder blades

48. nose and mouth

49. feeling for a brachial pulse in an infant

50. locate mid-nipple line and place fingers one fingerwidth below, 2 to 3 fingers on sternum for compressions

51. $\frac{1}{2}$ to 1 inch

52. 5:1

53. 100 to 120/minute

54. 3 seconds, 20 times per minute

55. Assess the infant
    Give four back blows with head down.
    Give four abdominal thrusts with head down.

56. a. rescuer is too tired to continue
    b. person who is being resuscitated is declared dead
    c. rescuer gets relief
    d. person who is being resuscitated revives

PRACTICE QUIZ

1. The most common cause of an airway obstruction in an unconscious person is:
   a. food
   b. mucous
   c. dentures

d. tongue

e. foreign bodies

2. The pulse of an adult victim suspected of having a myocardial infarction should be checked at which of the following locations.

a. brachial artery

b. carotid artery

c. femoral artery

d. temporal artery

e. all of the above

3. An infant's chest should be depressed:

a. $\frac{1}{2}$ to 1 inch

b. $\frac{3}{4}$ to $1\frac{1}{2}$ inches

c. $1\frac{1}{2}$ to 2 inches

d. 2 to 3 inches

e. none of the above

4. Other than mouth-to-mouth ventilations, which of the following can be utilized?

    I. Mouth to stoma

    II. Nose to nose

    III. Mouth to nose

    IV. Hand resuscitator to mouth

a. I only

b. I, II, III, IV

c. II and IV

d. I, III, IV

e. I and III

5. The most common cause of cardiac arrest in a child is

a. coronary artery disease

b. electrocution

c. cigarette smoking

d. foreign bodies

e. accidents

6. Atherosclerosis means

a. hardening of the arteries

b. gradual narrowing of the lumen of an artery

c. inadequate oxygenation of the blood vessel

d. no hemoglobin

e. none of the above

7. Which of the following risk factors can not be controlled by conventional methods?

    I. Heredity

    II. Smoking

    III. Obesity

    IV. Stress

    V. Blood cholesterol

a. I, II, III, IV, V

b. II, III, IV, V

c. II, IV, V

d. V only

e. I only

8. The proper ratio of compressions to ventilations for one-person CPR on an adult is:
   a. 5:1
   b. 5:2
   c. 15:1
   d. 15:2
   e. 15:5

9. The proper rate of rescue breathing in an infant is:
   a. 10/minute
   b. 20/minute
   c. 15/minute
   d. 5/minute
   e. 30/minute

10. To open an airway of a victim suspected of a neck fracture, which of the following methods can be employed?
    a. perform head tilt
    b. perform a tracheostomy
    c. do not touch the person
    d. perform jaw thrust maneuver
    e. use a hand resuscitator bag and mask

11. Brain damage will occur within _____ minutes without oxygen?
    a. 1 to 2 mintues
    b. 3 to 4 minutes
    c. 4 to 6 minutes
    d. 8 to 10 minutes
    e. greater than 10 minutes

12. List the correct sequence of events in assessing, initiating, and performing CPR:
    _____   a. Position victim.
    _____   b. Open airway.
    _____   c. Determine unresponsiveness.
    _____   d. Determine breathlessness.
    _____   e. Call for help.
    _____   f. Give two slow deep breaths.
    _____   g. Activate the emergency medical system.
    _____   h. Perform external cardiac massage.
    _____   i. Determine pulselessness.

13. How many ventilations are given initially to a patient who has had a cardiac arrest?
    a. two slow deep breaths
    b. four slow deep breaths
    c. four quick breaths
    d. four "stairstep" breaths
    e. two quick breaths

14. What is the CPR compression rate to use for a child?
    a. 60/minute
    b. 80/minute
    c. 100/minute
    d. 130/minute
    e. 150/minute

15. Where do you check for the pulse on an infant?
    a. carotid artery

b. brachial artery
c. femoral artery
d. dorsal artery
e. radial artery

16. The proper ratio of compressions to ventilations, on an infant is:
    a. 5:2
    b. 10:1
    c. 20:1
    d. 5:1
    e. 30:2

17. The heart lies between:
    a. the clavicle and the scapula
    b. the sternum and the ribs
    c. the clavicle and the spine
    d. the sternum and the spine
    e. the sternum and the xiphoid process

18. Complications that may result from chest compressions include which of the following:
    I. Punctured lungs
    II. Punctured heart
    III. Laceration of the liver
    IV. Fractured ribs
    V. Fractured sternum
    a. I, II, IV
    b. II, IV
    c. I, III, IV, V
    d. II, III, IV, V
    e. I, II, III, IV, V

19. After determining that an unconscious patient has an obstructed airway, the next step is to:
    a. check pulse
    b. call for help
    c. activate the emergency medical system
    d. reposition the head and try to ventilate again
    e. start compressions

20. Which of the following pieces of information is/are not given to the emergency medical system:
    I. Where the emergency is located
    II. Your name
    III. What happened
    IV. How many persons were involved
    V. Your home telephone number
    a. I, III, IV
    b. II only
    c. I, II, III, IV
    d. IV and V
    e. II and V

ANSWERS TO THE PRACTICE QUIZ

1. d
2. b
3. a
4. d
5. e
6. b
7. e
8. d
9. b
10. d

11. c
12. c, e, a, b, d, f, i, g, h
13. a
14. c
15. b
16. d
17. d
18. e
19. d
20. e

PATIENT ASSESSMENT

LEARNING OBJECTIVES

Upon completion of this unit, the individual will:

1. Define and explain the techniques involved in:
   a. observation
   b. palpation
   c. percussion
   d. auscultation
2. Define the following body positions:
   a. Fowler's
   b. Trendelenburg
   c. prone
   d. supine
3. Define and list normal and abnormal findings involved in tactile fremitus.

4. Label and describe the functional components of the stethoscope.
5. List the auscultation uses of the stethoscope.
6. List and define descriptive terminology with regard to breath sounds.
7. List the acceptable sites and method for evaluation of the pulse.
8. Define systolic, diastolic, pulse, and normal blood pressure.
9. Define cyanosis and cough.
10. List the points of evaluation of cough and sputum production.

REFERENCES

Barnes, TA: Respiratory Care Practice. Year Book Medical Publishers, Chicago, 1988.

Deshpande, VM, Pilbean, SP, and Dixon, RJ: A Comprehensive Review in Respiratory Care. Appleton and Lange, Norwalk, CT, 1988.

Shapiro, BA, Harrison, RA, and Kacmarek, RM: Clinical Application of Respiratory Care, ed 3. Year Book Medical Publishers, Chicago, 1985.

Thomas, CL (ed): Taber's Cyclopedic Medical Dictionary, ed 15. FA Davis, Philadelphia, 1985.

Wilkins, RL, Sheldon, RL, and Krider, SJ: Clinical Assessment in Respiratory Care. CV Mosby, St Louis, 1985.

STUDY QUESTIONS

1. Define the following terms: (Barnes, p 472)

   a. observation: _____

   b. palpation: _____

   c. percussion: _____

   d. auscultation: _____

2. List some aspects of the patient's condition that are evaluated with observation techniques. (Barnes, p 472)

   a. _____

   b. _____

   c. _____

   d. _____

3. Define the following body positions: (Taber's, pp 642, 1388, 1658, 1767)

   a. Fowler's: _____

   b. Trendelenburg: _____

   c. prone: _____

   d. supine: _____

4. The process of using the hands and sense of touch to detect physical signs of the patient's condition is known as _____. (Barnes, p 472)

5. List four aspects of the patient's condition that may be detected via the use of palpation techniques. (Barnes, p 472)

   a. _____

   b. _____

   c. _____

   d. _____

6. The term tactile fremitus refers to what? (Barnes, p 472)

_____

7. Mark the following as True or False, with regard to the technique used for determination of tactile fremitus. (Barnes, p 472)

_____ a. The patient should repeat a phrase such as 99.

_____ b. The hands are moved about the chest, comparing the transmission of sound.

_____ c. The examiner uses the fingertips only.

_____ d. The key is to recognize areas of increased transmission of sound only.

_____ e. The hand should be pressed lightly on the patient's chest.

8. List four abnormal occurrences that will decrease tactile fremitus. (Barnes, p 473)

a. _____

b. _____

c. _____

d. _____

9. Differentiate between immediate and mediate percussion. (Taber's, p 1257)

_____

_____

10. Tissue that is well aerated will produce what type of sound when percussed? (Barnes, p 474)

_____

11. Match each of the five basic percussion notes on the left with its appropriate description given on the right. (Barnes, p 474)

_____ flatness   a. short dead sound, solid material

_____ dullness   b. drum-like sound, air-filled tissue

_____ resonance   c. produced in the normal lung

_____ hyper-resonance   d. soft, higher pitched, a thud

_____ tympany   e. lower pitch, booming sound

12. What three aspects of the sounds heard in percussion should be noted? (Barnes, p 474)

a. _____

b. _____

c. _____

13. How is the patient positioned to achieve the best results for percussion? (Barnes, p 472)

_____

14. Label the components of the stethoscope in Figure 4–1. (Wilkins, p 66)

a. _____   d. _____

b. _____   e. _____

c. _____   f. _____

15. Differentiate between those sounds picked up by the bell and by the diaphragm of the stethoscope. (Wilkins, p 65) _____

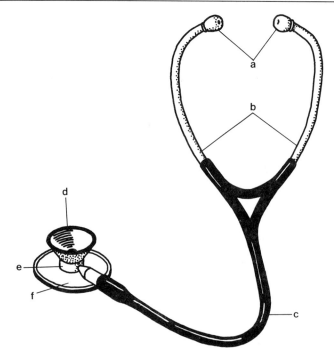

FIGURE 4–1. The stethoscope.

16. How should the patient be instructed to breathe during auscultation of the chest? (Wilkins, p 65)

17. List three descriptive terms used to describe normal breath sounds. (Wilkins, p 67)

    a. _____

    b. _____

    c. _____

18. Define the following abnormal auscultation findings. (Wilkins, p 68)

    a. wheeze: _____

    b. rhonchi: _____

    c. crackles: _____

19. Sensorium is a term used to describe what aspect of the patient's condition? (Wilkins, p 44)

20. List four acceptable sites where pulse can be evaluated. (Wilkins, p 46)

    a. _____

    b. _____

    c. _____

    d. _____

21. The pulse should be counted for ———— seconds and the result multiplied by ————, if it is regular. (Wilkins, p 46)

22. Why should the thumb never be used by an individual to palpate a pulse of a patient? (Wilkins, p 47)

——

23. What is the quickest noninvasive method of measuring the effectiveness of the cardiovascular system? (Wilkins, p 47) ————————————————————————————

——

24. Define the following: (Wilkins, p 47)

    a. systolic pressure: ——————————————————————————————

    b. diastolic pressure: —————————————————————————————

    c. pulse pressure: ————————————————————————————————

25. Blood pressure is recorded in what units? (Wilkins, p 47)

——

26. Define cyanosis. (Wilkins, p 78)

——

27. Normal urinary output is: (Wilkins, p 233)

    a. ——————————————— in an adult.

    b. ——————————————— in a child.

28. Define cough. (Wilkins, p 24)

——

29. When evaluating the patient's history of cough, what questions should be asked? (Wilkins, p 25)

——

30. List four important characteristics of sputum that need to be assessed. (Wilkins, p 28)

    a. ——————————————————————————————————————

    b. ——————————————————————————————————————

    c. ——————————————————————————————————————

    d. ——————————————————————————————————————

31. Match the color of sputum with the appropriate description on the right. (Wilkins, p 28)

    ———— gray, thick sputum   a. pulmonary edema

    ———— pink, frothy   b. pneumococcal pneumonia

    ———— blood in sputum   c. infection present

    ———— brown sputum   d. old blood

    ———— yellow or green   e. cigarette smoker

32. Describe the following: (Taber's, p 482, 407, 303)

   a. Dittrich's plugs: _____

   b. Curshmann's spirals: _____

   c. Charcot-Leyden crystals: _____

ANSWERS TO STUDY QUESTIONS

1. a. visual inspection
   b. process of applying the hands or fingers to the external surface of the body to detect abnormalities.
   c. tapping upon the surface to evaluate underlying structures.
   d. process of listening

2. a. ability to ventilate
   b. chest configuration
   c. respiratory pattern
   d. use of accessory muscles

3. a. semi-sitting position
   b. head lower than feet, legs, and body
   c. lying horizontal, face downward
   d. lying on back, face upward

4. palpation

5. a. vocal fremitus
   b. expansion
   c. surface condition
   d. tracheal and bony structure position

6. sense of vibration in the hand when it is laid upon the chest and the patient speaks

7. True, True, False, False, True

8. a. obesity
   b. pneumothorax
   c. emphysema
   d. large chest wall

9. mediate—striking a finger placed against the chest wall
   immediate—directly striking the chest wall with a finger

10. low-pitched, resonant sound

11. a, d, c, e, b

12. a. intensity
    b. pitch
    c. loudness

13. upright, relaxed muscles, on side if unable to sit

14. a. earpieces

   b. biaurals
   c. conducting tube
   d. bell
   e. chest piece
   f. diaphragm

15. bell—very low-pitched, heart diaphragm—low-pitched and high pitched chest sounds

16. deeply through the mouth

17. a. vesicular
    b. bronchovesicular
    c. bronchial

18. a. high-pitched continuous lung sounds
    b. low-pitched, continuous lung sound
    c. discontinuous lung sounds

19. the state of the patient with regard to mental awareness and or level of consciousness

20. a. radial
    b. brachial
    c. femoral
    d. carotid

21. 15 seconds, and multiplied by 4

22. Your own pulse is felt through the thumb and this may be confusing.

23. blood pressure

24. a. peak force exerted during left ventricular contraction
    b. resting pressure
    c. systolic minus diastolic

25. d. mmHg

26. bluish discoloration of the nailbeds, skin, lips, and mucous membranes, decrease of 5 g Hgb.

27. a. 0.5 ml/kg/hr in an adult
    b. 1 ml/kg/hr in a child

28. a forced expiratory effort against an initially closed glottis

29. quality, time, and setting

30. a. consistency
    b. quantity
    c. color
    d. time of production

31. a, d, b, e, c

32. a. small particles of fetid sputum made up of pus, fat, and bacteria
    b. coiled spirals of mucus
    c. colorless, hexagonal, needle-like crystals found in sputum of patients with asthma

---

PRACTICE QUIZ

1. Which of the following may be detected via the use of palpation techniques?
   I. Skin temperature
   II. Chest motion
   III. Points of tenderness
   IV. Quality of vibrations
   V. Crepitus
   a. I, II, III, IV, V
   b. I, III, V
   c. I, II, III
   d. II, IV, V
   e. I, III, IV

2. Which of the following involves the evaluation of breath sounds with a stethoscope?
   a. observation
   b. palpation
   c. percussion
   d. auscultation
   e. vibration

3. Which of the disease states listed below will *not* decrease tactile fremitus?
   a. pneumothorax
   b. fluid
   c. atelectasis
   d. masses within the lung
   e. none of the above

4. Of the anatomic positions listed below, which will be noted when using palpation techniques?
   I. Position of the mediastinum
   II. Position of the aorta
   III. Position of the trachea
   IV. Position of the diaphragm
   V. Point of maximal pulse
   a. I, II, III, IV, V
   b. I, II, V
   c. I, III, IV, V
   d. III, IV, V
   e. III only

5. Of the five basic percussion notes, which is produced in the normal lung?
   a. flatness
   b. dullness
   c. resonance
   d. hyper-resonance
   e. tympany

6. Which of the following lung sounds is defined as a "cavernous" sound, like air moving over the top of a bottle?
   a. adventitious
   b. amphori
   c. rhonchi
   d. rub
   e. stridor

7. You have a patient in the ER who has an elevated arterial carbon dioxide tension. How might that patient's sensorium evaluation read?
   a. confused
   b. disoriented
   c. somnolent
   d. drowsy
   e. all of the above

8. You walk into the patient's room and note the patient is breathing deeper than usual and is also breathing at a rate of 32 breaths a minute. You would describe this as:
   a. Cheyne-Stokes respirations
   b. bradypnea
   c. tachypnea
   d. hyperpnea
   e. hypopnea

9. The pattern of respiration that is most often associated with diabetic ketoacidosis is:
   a. Kussmaul's breathing
   b. Biot's respirations
   c. Cheyne-Stokes respirations
   d. eupnea
   e. none of the above

10. Which of the following terms describes normal mucous?
    I. Thick
    II. Thin
    III. Clear
    IV. White
    V. Odorless
    a. I, II, IV, V
    b. II, III, IV, V
    c. I, II, III, IV, V
    d. III, IV, V
    e. III only

11. A breathing pattern that is noted to have an increased respiratory rate and depth with irregular periods of apnea may be classified as:
    a. eupnea
    b. Kussmaul's
    c. apnea
    d. Biot's
    e. Cheyne-Stokes

12. You note that your patient has normal breath sounds on the physical examination. What is the correct terminology for this condition?
    a. eupnea
    b. wheezes

    c. apnea
    d. vesicular
    e. adventitious

13. When assessing the temperature of the newborn, you should use which site to obtain an accurate measurement?
    a. rectal
    b. axillary
    c. oral
    d. it doesn't matter

14. Pointed, needle-like, formed crystals found in the sputum of asthmatic patients are termed:
    a. Dittrich's plugs
    b. Curshmann's spirals
    c. mucous plugs
    d. Charcot-Leyden crystals
    e. asthmatic crystals

15. When assessing the breath sounds of a patient, which of the following conditions should be met?
    I. A quiet room
    II. A dark room
    III. The patient should be sitting upright if possible
    IV. The bell of the stethoscope should be used
    V. The anterior portion of the chest need only be auscultated.
    a. I, II, III, IV, V
    b. I, II, V
    c. I, III
    d. III, IV, V
    e. III, V

16. You enter the room and find the patient lying face down on the bed. How would you describe this position?
    a. supine
    b. Trendelenburg
    c. prone
    d. Fowler's
    e. semi-Fowler's

17. During chest auscultation the patient should be instructed to breath in what manner?
    I. with deep breaths
    II. through the mouth
    III. through the nose
    IV. slowly
    V. with a pause at end inspiration
    a. I, II, III, IV, V
    b. I, III, IV, V
    c. I, II, IV, V
    d. II, IV
    e. I, III, IV

18. When evaluating the pulse, which of the following should be noted:
    I. Rate
    II. Rhythm
    III. Volume
    IV. Irregularities

V. Pressure
a. I, II, III, IV, V
b. I, II, III, IV
c. I, II, IV
d. III, IV, V
e. I and II only

19. Which of the following is/are acceptable sites from which to take a pulse:
     I. Radial
     II. Brachial
     III. Carotid
     IV. Femoral
     V. Pedal
   a. I, II, III, IV, V
   b. I, II, III, IV
   c. I, III, IV
   d. I, II, V
   e. I only

20. "Funnel chest" is another term used to describe which configuration of the chest?
   a. kyphosis
   b. pectus carinatum
   c. kyphoscoliosis
   d. pectus excavatum
   e. scoliosis

ANSWERS TO THE PRACTICE QUIZ

1. a		11. d	
2. d		12. d	
3. e		13. a	
4. c		14. d	
5. c		15. c	
6. b		16. c	
7. e		17. c	
8. d		18. c	
9. a		19. b	
10. b		20. d	

Chapter 5

MEDICAL GAS THERAPY

Outline

MEDICAL GASES
Physical Properties
Production
STORAGE SYSTEMS
Cylinders
    Manufacturing
    Identification
    Sizes and colors
    Safety systems
    Storage
    Duration of flow

Piping Systems
    Maintenance
    Valve systems
REDUCING SYSTEMS
Operation
Stages
FLOWMETERS
Function
Classification
PRACTICE QUIZ

Learning Objectives

Upon completion of this unit, the individual will:

1. Classify any given gas as medical, therapy, or laboratory.
2. Identify any given gas as flammable, nonflammable, or supporting combustion.
3. Identify all shoulder markings on any given cylinder.
4. List five or six specifications for cylinders and their construction and the agency that enforces these regulations.
5. Given any cylinder size and its gas, list the following:
   a. color
   b. cubic feet of gas
   c. pressure

   d. connection system to pressure-reducing regulators
6. Describe the methods of testing cylinders, to include retest dates and pressures involved in testing.
7. State the method of measuring the contents of any cylinder.
8. Calculate the duration of cylinder flow for any size cylinder, given the appropriate information.
9. List at least four regulations dealing with cylinder storage.
10. List/discuss the steps involved in fractional distillation

11. Define the following in terms of their function in the hospital:
    a. zone valves
    b. riser valve
    c. station outlet
    d. main supply valve
12. Differentiate among the three safety-indexed connector systems:
    a. DISS
    b. PISS
    c. ASSS
13. Describe the structure and function of a Thorpe tube flowmeter.
14. Differentiate between pressure-compensated and -noncompensated flowmeter.

REFERENCES

Barnes, TA: Respiratory Care Practice. Year Book Medical Publishers, Chicago, 1988.

Burton, G, and Hodgkin, J: Respiratory Care: A Guide to Clinical Practice, ed 2. JB Lippincott, Philadelphia, 1984

Deshpande, VM, Pilbeam, SP, and Dixon, RJ: A Comprehensive Review in Respiratory Care. Appleton and Lange, Norwalk, CT, 1988.

Egan, DF, Sheldon, RL, and Spearman, CB: Egan's Fundamentals of Respiratory Therapy, ed 4. CV Mosby, St Louis, 1982

Eubanks, D, and Bone, R: Comprehensive Respiratory Care. CV Mosby, St Louis, 1985.

Kacmarek, RM, Mack, CW, and Dimas, S: The Essentials of Respiratory Therapy, ed 2. Year Book Medical Publishers, Chicago, 1985.

McPherson, SP: Respiratory Therapy Equipment, ed 3. CV Mosby, St Louis, 1985

Shapiro, BA, Harrison, RA, Kacmarek, RM, and Cane, RD: Clinical Application of Respiratory Care, ed 3. Year Book Medical Publishers, Chicago, 1985.

STUDY QUESTIONS

1. Match the following medical gases with the appropriate chemical symbols: (Eubanks, p 128; Kacmarek, p 358)

   _____ cyclopropane   a. C_2H_4

   _____ carbon dioxide   b. N_2O

   _____ helium   c. $(CH_2)_3$

   _____ nitrogen   d. O_2

   _____ ethylene   e. CO_2

   _____ nitrous oxide   f. N_2

   _____ oxygen   g. He

2. Which of the gases listed in question 1 is/are flammable? (Kacmarek, p 358)

   _____

3. Which of the gases listed in question 1 is/are able to support combustion? (Barnes, p 287; Deshpande, p 198; Kacmarek, p 358)

   _____

4. Which of the gases listed in question 1 is/are nonflammable? (Barnes, p 287; Deshpande, p 198; Kacmarek, p 358)

   _____

5. How is air produced for commercial use? (Eubanks, p 118; Kacmarek, p 368)

   _____

6. Most medical gases are produced by the process of _____
   _____. (Eubanks, p 118; Kacmarek, p 368)

7. Describe the process by which oxygen is manufactured. (Eubanks, p 118)

   _____

   _____

   _____

   _____

8. List three medical gases produced by fractional distillation of liquified air. (Eubanks, p 118)

   a. _____

   b. _____

   c. _____

9. Circle the letters of the statements that correctly describe oxygen. (Barnes, p 287; Eubanks, p 119)
   a. density of 1.43 g/l at 0 degrees Centigrade and 760 mmHg
   b. atomic number is 10
   c. colorless, odorless, and tasteless
   d. boils at −183 degrees Centigrade
   e. makes up 78.08 percent of earth's atmosphere

10. List three widely accepted methods of production of medical gas cylinders. (Barnes, p 291; Eubanks, p 121)

    a. _____

    b. _____

    c. _____

11. The FDA regulates what three aspects of cylinder production and storage? (Barnes, p 291; Eubanks, p 121)

    a. _____

    b. _____

    c. _____

12. The Department of Transportation regulates cylinder: (Barnes, p 294; Eubanks, p 121, Kacmarek, p 368)

    a. _____

    b. _____

    c. _____

    d. _____

13. What aspects of cylinder regulation are the function of the Compressed Gas Association (CGA)? (Barnes, p 294; Eubanks, p 121; Kacmarek, p 368)

    a. _____

    b. _____

    c. _____

14. What aspects of liquid systems are regulated by the American Society of Mechanical Engineers? (Barnes, p 293; Eubanks, p 121)

    a. _____

    b. _____

    c. _____

    d. _____

15. What agency is responsible for codes covering gas storage and delivery? (Barnes, p 299; Deshpande, p 197; Eubanks, p 122; Kacmarek, p 368)

    _____

16. Identify the cylinder markings in Figure 5–1. (Barnes, p 299; Deshpande, p 196; Eubanks, p 126; Kacmarek, p 359)

    a. _____   e. _____

    b. _____   f. _____

    c. _____   g. _____

    d. _____   h. _____

17. What information about the cylinder is provided by listing the maximum working pressure? (Barnes, p 299; Eubanks, p 125; Kacmarek, p 359)

    _____

    _____

18. By what means is cylinder integrity tested?

    _____

19. Explain the Water-Jacket volumetric expansion test. (Barnes, p 301; Kacmarek, p 361)

    _____

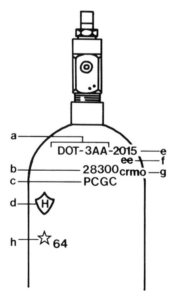

FIGURE 5–1. E cylinder for oxygen.

_____

_____

_____

20. Cylinders made to the specifications of 3AA or 3A are to be retested every _____ to _____ years. (Barnes, p 299; Eubanks, p 125; Kacmarek, p 359)

21. A five-point star on the cylinder indicates what information? (Barnes, p 299; Eubanks, p 125; Kacmarek, p 359)

_____

22. Fill in the blanks with the appropriate information. (Barnes, p 302; Eubanks, p 137; Kacmarek, p 360)

Size	Capacity	Tank Factor
D	_____ cu ft	_____ l/psi
E	_____ cu ft	_____ l/psi
G	_____ cu ft	_____ l/psi
H/K	_____ cu ft	_____ l/psi

23. How many liters are in a cubic foot of gas? (Barnes, p 301; Kacmarek, p 360)

_____

24. Provide the formula to determine the volume of a gas in liters in a full cylinder. (Barnes, p 301; Kacmarek, p 360)

_____

25. Provide the formula needed to provide the tank factor used in calculating duration of flow. (Barnes, p 301; Eubanks, p 137, Kacmarek, p 360)

_____

26. Provide the formula used to calculate duration of flow in minutes. (Barnes, p 301; Deshpande, p 197; Kacmarek, p 360)

_____

27. Provide the color code for E cylinders filled with the gases listed below. (Barnes, p 301; Eubanks, p 128; Kacmarek, p 361)

a. oxygen: _____

b. carbon dioxide: _____

c. helium: _____

d. air: _____

e. cyclopropane: _____

f. nitrous oxide: _____

g. ethylene: _____

h. helium and oxygen: _____

i. carbon dioxide and oxygen: _____

28. Mark the following as True or False with regard to general safe practices with oxygen cylinders. (Barnes, p 287; Eubanks, p 126)

    _____ Petroleum-based products should not be used.

    _____ Alcohol vapors might ignite in the presence of high concentrations of oxygen.

    _____ Oxygen will burn.

    _____ Oxygen administered in a croup tent needs no special precautions while in use.

    _____ Electrical toys and equipment are not permitted in a croup tent.

29. Large cylinders (G, H, K) use a _____ _____, which will rupture within 5 percent of the pressure at which the cylinder would burst. (Barnes, p 302; Deshpande, p 197)

30. Small cylinders use a _____ _____, which will melt at a temperature of _____ to _____ degrees Fahrenheit. (Barnes, p 302; Deshpande, p 197).

31. Differentiate between the Pin Index Safety System and the American Standard Safety System. (Barnes, p 303; Eubanks, p 122; Kacmarek, p 366)

    _____

    _____

    _____

    _____

32. Provide the Pin locations for the following gases. (Barnes, p 304; Eubanks, p 123; Kacmarek, p 366)

    a. oxygen   _____ and _____

    b. nitrous oxide   _____ and _____

    c. cyclopropane   _____ and _____

    d. compressed air   _____ and _____

    e. ethylene   _____ and _____

    f. CO_2/O_2 (CO_2 <7%)   _____ and _____

    g. He/O_2 (He >80%)   _____ and _____

33. Explain the precautions instituted via usage of the diameter index safety system (DISS). (Barnes, p 303; Eubanks, p 123; Kacmarek, p 367)

    _____

    _____

    _____

34. Give the American Standard Safety System connection number for oxygen and explain each component. (Deshpande, p 200; Eubanks, p 124; Kacmarek, p 367)

    _____

    _____

35. Give the DISS connection for oxygen. (Eubanks, p 124; Kacmarek, p 367)

    _____

36. List four general rules of safe storage of cylinders. (Barnes, p 299; Eubanks, p 127)

    a. _____

    b. _____

    c. _____

    d. _____

37. Hospital piping systems provide a psi of _____ (Barnes, p 296; Eubanks, p 143)

38. Give the function of the valves listed below as they are used in hospital piping systems. (Barnes, p 298; Eubanks, p 143).

    a. station outlet: _____

    b. zone valve: _____

    c. riser valve: _____

    d. main supply valve: _____

39. Piping material used in the hospital must be of what type? (Barnes, p 296; Eubanks, p 144)

    _____

40. List two functions of the reducing valve. (Barnes, p 303; Eubanks, p 132; Kacmarek, p 361)

    a. _____

    b. _____

41. List three functions of the flowmeter. (Barnes, p 309; Eubanks, p 132)

    a. _____

    b. _____

    c. _____

42. Mechanical flowmeters are classified as the following: (Eubanks, p 136)

    a. _____

    b. _____

43. The Bourdon gauge measures _____ and indicates _____. (Barnes, p 309; Eubanks, p 136)

44. If back pressure is applied to the Bourdon gauge, it will indicate a flow _____ than that being delivered. (Barnes, p 309; Eubanks, p 136).

45. Differentiate between a compensated and uncompensated flowmeter when back pressure is applied distal to the needle valve. (Barnes, p 314; Eubanks, p 134).

    _____

    _____

    _____

ANSWERS TO STUDY QUESTIONS

1. c, e, g, f, a, b, d

2. cyclopropane and ethylene

3. oxygen, nitrous oxide, and admixtures with either component included

4. helium, nitrogen, carbon dioxide

5. collection, filtering, and compressing air using an H_2O-sealed compressor

6. fractional distillation

7. Air is compressed to 100 atm and heat is removed. Air is then compressed to 200 atm and cooled with salt water. Air is passed into a liquifier and heat is absorbed. Each quantity of air that escapes is colder and colder and is liquified. Gases are warmed. As air is warmed, products rise off at different points and are separated.

8. a. helium
   b. oxygen
   c. carbon dioxide

9. a, c, d

10. a. spun
    b. circular steel disks
    c. steel billet

11. a. purity
    b. identifying labels
    c. precautionary statement

12. a. shipping
    b. filling
    c. marking
    d. labeling

13. a. handling and storage of cylinders
    b. piping and fittings
    c. cylinder markings

14. a. construction
    b. operating limits
    c. maintenance
    d. safety valves

15. National Fire Protection Agency (NFPA)

16. a. DOT specifications
    b. serial number
    c. ownership mark
    d. manufacturer's mark
    e. service pressure
    f. elastic expansion
    g. chrome-molybdenum steel used
    h. original hydrostatic test

17. This tells the cylinder pressure that may not be exceeded by 10 percent. (For example: 2015 mwp (PSI) = allowable pressure of 2200).

18. hydrostatic testing

19. The cylinder is placed in H_2O vessel. Pressure is applied to the interior of the cylinder, causing a volume of H_2O to be displaced. The interior pressure is released and some of the original displaced volume returns. The original volume displaced is equal to total expansion. Total expansion minus permanent expansion equals elastic expansion.

20. 5 to 10 years

21. The cylinder is to be retested in 10 years.

22. D = 12.7 cu ft. and 0.16 l/psi
    E = 22 cu ft. and 0.28 l/psi
    G = 187 cu ft. and 2.41 l/psi
    H/K = 244 cu ft. and 3.14 l/psi

23. There are 28.3 liters in a cubic foot of gas.

24. Cubic foot volume × 28.3 l/cu ft

25. Factor for duration of flow = (cu ft) (28.3 l/cu ft) divided by maximum filling pressure (2200 PSI).

26. Duration of flow = (gauge pressure) (duration of flow factor) divided by flow in l/minute.

27. a. green (white)
    b. gray
    c. brown
    d. black, yellow (varies)
    e. orange
    f. light blue
    g. red
    h. brown shoulder and light green body
    i. gray shoulder and light green body

28. True, True, False, False, True

29. frangible disk

30. fusible plug, melts at 150 to 170 degrees Fahrenheit

31. The Pin Index Safety System provides a method of preventing accidental attachment of reducing valves for a specific type of gas to a cylinder with the wrong connector. It is used for small cylinders and has pin placement ports. The American Standard Safety System is for the same type of protection for large

cylinders using a threaded connection system of protection.

32. a. 2 and 5   e. 1 and 3
    b. 3 and 5   f. 2 and 6
    c. 3 and 6   g. 4 and 6
    d. 1 and 5

33. The DISS is used on all connections distal to the regulator when maximum working pressure is below 200 PSIG. It ensures the connection of equipment to oxygen and air delivery systems by matching male and female connectors.

34. No. 540, .903-14, NGO-RH, ext. The connection is CGA No. 540, the outlet has a thread diameter of 0.903 inch, there are 14 threads per inch, and the threads are right-handed and external.

35. No. 1240, 0.5625 inch diameter, 18 threads per inch

36. a. Store in dry, cool, well-ventilated room.
    b. Place cylinders against the wall, secured to prevent movement.
    c. Do not store flammable gases with oxgyen.
    d. No smoking signs should be posted.

37. fifty

38. a. shut off to individual outlets at patient station
    b. isolate branches or wings of hospital
    c. isolates floor or floor sections
    d. isolates hospital from the gas supply

39. K seamless copper

40. a. to reduce cylinder pressure to service pressure
    b. to provide steady, even flow of gas to therapy equipment.

41. a. to receive gas at 50 PSIG
    b. to control gas to patient to safe levels of flow
    c. to measure gas leaving the system in l/minute

42. a. Thorpe type
    b. Bourdon type

43. pressure, flow

44. higher

45. In the compensated tube, back pressure applied will cause no change in the reading of the float; the patient is getting what the float indicates. In the uncompensated tube, the float will be forced downward and will read lower than the actual amount being delivered to the patient.

PRACTICE QUIZ

1. Which of the following gases is/are nonflammable?
    I. Oxygen
    II. Carbon Dioxide
    III. Cyclopropane
    IV. Nitrogen
    V. Helium
    a. I, II, III, IV, V
    b. I, II, IV, V
    c. II, IV, V
    d. I, III, IV
    e. I, II, V

2. Which of the following is/are methods accepted for production of medical gas cylinders?
    I. Spun
    II. Fractional distillation
    III. Steel billet
    IV. Circular steel disks
    V. Metal compression

    a. I, II, III, IV, V
    b. I, III, IV, V
    c. I, III, IV
    d. II, IV
    e. I only

3. The Department of Transportation regulates cylinder:
    I. Handling
    II. Shipping
    III. Labeling
    IV. Marking
    V. Filling
    a. I, II, III, IV, V
    b. I, II, V
    c. III, IV, V
    d. II, III, IV, V
    e. III, V

4. Which agency is responsible for regulating cylinder purity?
    a. ASME
    b. FDA
    c. DOT
    d. NFPA
    e. CGA

5. At STP, 1 cu ft of a gas is equal to how many liters?
    a. 12.7
    b. 22
    c. 187
    d. 28.3
    e. 24.4

6. The color code for E cylinders filled with helium is:
    a. brown
    b. orange
    c. gray
    d. white
    e. black

7. The color code for a E cylinder filled with cyclopropane is:
    a. brown
    b. orange
    c. gray
    d. white
    e. black

8. The pin locations for oxygen are:
    a. 2 and 6
    b. 2 and 5
    c. 1 and 4
    d. 1 and 6
    e. 3 and 5

9. Which of the following is/are a method(s) of determining the contents of a cylinder?
    I. Analyze the gas
    II. Read the label

III. Check the cylinder color
IV. Check the pin locations
V. Check the safety systems
  a. I, II, III, IV, V
  b. II, III, IV, V
  c. I, III, V
  d. III, IV, V
  e. II, IV

10. Which of the following functions as a shut-off valve to individual outlets at the patient station?
  a. main supply valve
  b. riser valve
  c. zone valve
  d. station outlet valve
  e. unit valve

11. The Bourdon gauge measures
  a. flow
  b. pressure
  c. percent oxygen
  d. cylinder content
  e. none of the above

12. The star insignia on a medical gas cylinder indicates:
    I. Cylinder has been tested
    II. Cylinder has passed inspection
    III. Cylinder needs to be retested in 10 years
    IV. Cylinder needs to be retested every 5 years
    V. Cylinder failed inspection
  a. I, II, IV
  b. II, III, IV
  c. I, II, III
  d. I, III, V
  e. I, II, IV, V

13. Your patient has a nasal cannula running at 2 LPM. He is on an E cylinder with 1600 PSIG tank reading. How long will this tank last?
  a. 3 hours and 42 minutes
  b. 4 hours and 15 minutes
  c. 3 hours and 20 minutes
  d. 4 hours and 48 minutes
  e. 4 hours and 13 minutes

14. What is the tank factor for a D cylinder filled with oxygen?
  a. 3.14
  b. 2.41
  c. 0.28
  d. 0.16
  e. 0.12

15. If back pressure is applied distal to the Bourdon gauge, it will indicate a flow _____ the actual flow being delivered.
  a. the same as
  b. higher than
  c. lower than

  d. equal to
  e. unrelated to

16. Which of the following is/are true about regulators?
    I. They limit pressure only to 50 PSI or less.
    II. A single-stage regulator has 2 pop-off valves.
    III. A multistage regulator has a final pressure pop-off valve set at 200 PSI.
    IV. One can tell how many stages a regulator has by counting the number of pop off valves.
    V. Regulators should be cleaned with vinegar regularly.
  a. I, II, III, IV, V
  b. I, II, III
  c. II, IV, V
  d. I, IV
  e. IV

17. Which of the following is/are flammable?
  a. cyclopropane
  b. oxygen
  c. carbon dioxide
  d. helium
  e. nitrogen

18. Which of the following is/are produced for medical use via fractional distillation?
  a. nitrous oxide
  b. oxygen
  c. carbon dioxide
  d. helium
  e. b, c, and d

19. The frangible disk is used as a safety system for:
  a. pressure
  b. temperature
  c. oxygen concentrations
  d. high flow systems
  e. E cylinders

20. If the cylinder fails inspection, it is:
  a. patched and retested
  b. destroyed
  c. respun
  d. resealed
  e. used only half-filled

ANSWERS TO PRACTICE QUIZ

1. b	11. b
2. c	12. c
3. d	13. a
4. b	14. d
5. d	15. b
6. a	16. e
7. b	17. a
8. b	18. e
9. a	19. a
10. d	20. b

OXYGEN THERAPY

OUTLINE

LEARNING OBJECTIVES

Upon completion of this unit, the individual will:

1. Describe the physical properties of oxygen.
2. List the indications for oxygen therapy.
3. Define the four types of hypoxia.
4. List the three clinical goals of oxygen therapy.
5. Describe the two phases of oxygen toxicity.
6. On the following oxygen delivering devices, describe the operation, clinical uses, flow rates, and oxygen concentrations obtainable:
   a. nasal catheter
   b. nasal cannula
   c. simple oxygen mask
   d. partial rebreathing mask and bag
   e. nonrebreathing mask and bag
   f. air-dilution masks
   g. oxygen hood
   h. aerosol delivering equipment (i.e., aerosol mask, T-piece, tracheostomy mask)
   i. incubators
   j. manual resuscitators
7. List the clinical criteria for administering oxygen by low-flow devices.
8. List four factors that will influence the deliv-

ered oxygen concentrations in a low-flow device.

9. Define and give examples of high- and low-flow devices.

10. Describe the two types of hyperbaric chambers.

11. Describe the positive and negative effects of hyperbaric therapy.

12. Give an example of each type of oxygen analyzer.

13. Describe the principle of operation of the paramagnetic analyzer.

14. Describe the Pauling principle.

15. Describe the principle of operation of the Wheatstone bridge.

16. Describe the operation of the galvanic fuel cell and the polarographic electrode.

17. List the three factors that distinguish the galvanic fuel cell from the polarographic electrodes.

REFERENCES

Barnes, TA: Respiratory Care Practice. Year Book Medical Publishers, Chicago, 1988.

Burton, G, and Hodgkin, J: Respiratory Care: A Guide to Clinical Practice, ed 2. JB Lippincott, Philadelphia, 1984.

Deshpande, WM, Pilbeam, SP, and Dixon, RJ: A Comprehensive Review in Respiratory Care. Appleton and Lange, Norwalk, CT, 1988.

Egan, DF, Sheldon, RL, and Spearman, CB: Egan's Fundamentals of Respiratory Therapy, ed 4. CV Mosby, St Louis, 1982

Eubanks, D, and Bone, R: Comprehensive Respiratory Care. CV Mosby, St Louis, 1985

Kacmarek, RM, Mack, CW, and Dimas, S: The Essentials of Respiratory Therapy, ed 2. Year Book Medical Publishers, 1985

McPherson, SP: Respiratory Therapy Equipment, ed 3. CV Mosby, St Louis, 1985

Shapiro, BA, Harrison, RA, Kacmarek, RM, and Cane, RD: Clinical Application of Respiratory Care, ed 3. Year Book Medical Publishers, Chicago, 1985

STUDY QUESTIONS

1. Fill in the blanks. (Barnes, p 288; Deshpande, p 200; Eubanks, p 118)

   a. Oxygen has the molecular weight of _____ g.

   b. Oxygen has the density of _____ g/l at STP.

   c. The partial pressure of oxygen at sea level is _____ mmHg.

   d. Oxygen makes up _____ percent of the atmosphere.

   e. Oxygen is produced naturally by the process of _____.

2. List five factors to be reviewed to determine the need for oxygen therapy. (Barnes, p 142; Deshpande, p 201; Shapiro, p 188)

   a. _____

   b. _____

   c. _____

   d. _____

   e. _____

3. List three desired effects of supplemental oxygen use. (Barnes, p 142, Shapiro, p 176)

   a. _____

   b. _____

   c. _____

4. Define the following terms: (Burton, p 404; Kacmarek, p 370)

   a. anemic hypoxia: _____

   b. stagnant hypoxia: _____

   c. histotoxic hypoxia: _____

   d. hypoxemic hypoxia: _____

   e. hypoxemia: _____

5. Which types of hypoxemia are responsive to oxygen therapy? (Burton, p 404; Kacmarek, p 370)

   a. _____

   b. _____

6. List five factors that affect the toxic response to oxygen. (Barnes, p 158; Egan, p 452)

   a. _____

   b. _____

   c. _____

   d. _____

   e. _____

7. The pathology of oxygen toxicity is nonspecific and consists of a variety of manifestations. List some of these. (Barnes, p 158; Egan, p 452)

   a. _____

   b. _____

   c. _____

   d. _____

   e. _____

   f. _____

8. Describe the two phases of the oxygen toxic response. (Barnes, p 158; Deshpande, p 202; Egan, p 452)

   a. exudative phase: _____

   _____

   b. proliferation phase: _____

   _____

9. List five hazards of oxygen therapy. (Deshpande, p 201; Egan, p 449)

   a. _____

   b. _____

   c. _____

   d. _____

   e. _____

10. Oxygen toxicity occurs in patients who receive oxygen at _____ percent or above for _____ hours. (Kacmarek, p 374)

11. List below the clinical symptoms associated with oxygen toxicity. (Barnes, p 159; Deshpande, p 202; Egan, p 449)

    a. _____

    b. _____

    c. _____

    d. _____

    e. _____

    f. _____

    g. _____

12. Describe the basic clinical management principle for oxygen usage. (Barnes, p 159)

    _____

13. Oxygen-delivery devices are commonly grouped into two classifications. Describe the difference between the two. (Barnes, p 323; Deshpande, p 202; Shapiro, p 180)

    a. low-flow: _____

    _____

    _____

    b. high-flow: _____

    _____

    _____

14. What variables affect the F_{IO_2} delivered with the usage of a low-flow oxygen delivery device? (Barnes, p 328; Shapiro, p 183)

    a. _____

    b. _____

    c. _____

    d. _____

    e. _____

15. Classify the following as high-flow (HF) or low-flow (LF). (Barnes, 324; Deshpande, p 203)

    a. _____ Briggs adapter   e. _____ simple mask

    b. _____ Venturi mask   f. _____ mist tent

    c. _____ partial rebreather   g. _____ nonrebreather

    d. _____ cannula   h. _____ nasal catheter

16. Provide the correct information about the nasal catheter. (Barnes, p 324; Shapiro, p 182)

    a. placement techniques:_____

    b. maintenance: _____

    c. complications: _____

    d. performance: _____

17. List four advantages and disadvantages incurred with the use of the nasal catheter. (Barnes, p 325)

Advantages	Disadvantages
a. _____	a. _____
b. _____	b. _____
c. _____	c. _____
d. _____	d. _____

18. Provide the correct information about the nasal cannula. (Barnes, p 329; Deshpande, p 203; Eubanks, p 257)

   a. placement technique: _____

   b. maintenance: _____
   _____

   c. complications: _____
   _____

   d. performance: _____
   _____
   _____

19. List four advantages and disadvantages of the usage of the nasal cannula for oxygen therapy. (Barnes, p 329; Eubanks, p 258)

Advantages	Disadvantages
a. _____	a. _____
b. _____	b. _____
c. _____	c. _____
d. _____	d. _____

20. Provide the correct information concerning the simple mask. (Barnes, p 332; Deshpande, p 203; Eubanks, p 263)

   a. placement techniques: _____
   _____

   b. maintenance: _____
   _____

   c. complications: _____
   _____

   d. performance: _____
   _____

21. List four advantages and disadvantages of the simple mask. (Barnes, p 334; Deshpande, p 203; Eubanks, p 263; McPherson, p 90)

Advantages	Disadvantages
a. _____	a. _____
b. _____	b. _____
c. _____	c. _____
d. _____	d. _____

22. Provide the correct information for the use of the reservoir mask for oxygen delivery. (Barnes, p 334; Eubanks, p 332)

    a. placement techniques: _____

    _____

    b. maintenance: _____

    _____

    c. complications: _____

    _____

    d. performance: _____

    _____

23. List four advantages and disadvantages of the reservoir mask for oxygen delivery. (Barnes, p 337; Eubanks, p 362)

    Advantages   Disadvantages

    a. _____   a. _____

    b. _____   b. _____

    c. _____   c. _____

    d. _____   d. _____

24. Provide the correct information for the air-entrainment Venturi mask for use in oxygen delivery. (Barnes, p 337; Eubanks, p 261)

    a. placement techniques: _____

    _____

    b. maintenance: _____

    _____

    c. complications: _____

    _____

    d. performance: _____

    _____

25. List four advantages and disadvantages of use of the air-entrainment Venturi mask for oxygen delivery. (Barnes, p 339; Deshpande, p 204; Eubanks, p 262)

    Advantages   Disadvantages

    a. _____   a. _____

    b. _____   b. _____

    c. _____   c. _____

    d. _____   d. _____

26. Provide the correct information about the use of the air-entrainment nebulizer. (Barnes, p 340)

    a. types: _____

    _____

    b. placement techniques: _____

    _____

c. maintenance: _____

_____

d. complications: _____

_____

e. performance: _____

_____

27. Complete the following chart. (Barnes, p 340; Deshpande, p 202)

Device	F_{IO_2} Range
a. nasal cannula	_____
b. simple mask	_____
c. partial rebreathing mask	_____
d. nonrebreathing mask	_____
e. Venturi mask	_____
f. air-entrainment nebulizer	_____

28. Given a large-volume nebulizer set at 0.40 F_{IO_2} and driven by an oxygen flow rate of 15 LPM, what is the total flow to the patient? (McPherson, p 107)

_____

29. Provide the correct information about the use of the oxygen hood for the delivery of oxygen. (Barnes, p 342; McPherson, p 97)

a. placement: _____

_____

b. maintenance: _____

_____

c. complications: _____

_____

d. performance: _____

_____

30. Provide the correct information concerning the use of the oxygen tent and aerosol enclosures. (Barnes, p 344; McPherson, p 97)

a. placement: _____

b. maintenance: _____

_____

_____

c. complications: _____

d. performance: _____

31. Isolettes have the capability to provide control of what four aspects of the neonate's environment? (Barnes, p 334; McPherson, p 102)

a. _____

b. _____

c. _____

d. _____

32. Complete the following about the use of an incubator: (Barnes, p 344; McPherson, p 102)

    a. The temperature should be maintained at _____ .

    b. Clean the humidifier every _____ hours.

    c. Humidity chamber is filled with _____ and _____ _____ (20 ml) to restrict growth.

    d. A _____ type humidifier is used.

33. List the five standard components of manual resuscitators. (Barnes, p 263)

    a. _____

    b. _____

    c. _____

    d. _____

    e. _____

34. List four standards for manual resuscitators recommended by the American Society for Testing and Materials. (Barnes, p 265)

    a. _____

    _____

    b. _____

    _____

    c. _____

    d. _____

35. Give the type of patient valve used in the following manual resuscitators: (McPherson, p 180)

    a. Hope: _____

    b. Hope II: _____

    c. AMBU E-2: _____

    d. Laerdal: _____

    e. PMR: _____

    f. Hudson Life Saver II Pediatric: _____

36. List the indications for hyperbaric oxygen therapy. (Barnes, p 344; Egan, p 479)

    a. _____   f. _____

    b. _____   g. _____

    c. _____   h. _____

    d. _____   i. _____

    e. _____   j. _____

37. Describe the two types of chambers used most often in hyperbaric oxygen therapy. (Barnes, p 344; McPherson; 479)

_____

_____

38. List common problems associated with hyperbaric therapy. (Barnes, p 345; McPherson, p 479)

    a. _____

    b. _____

    c. _____

    d. _____

    e. _____

    f. _____

39. List three methods commonly used to measure oxygen concentrations. (Barnes, p 348; Egan, p 476; McPherson, p 205)

    a. _____

    b. _____

    c. _____

40. Describe the design of the Beckman Model D-2 oxygen analyzer and its operation. (Barnes, p 348; Egan, p 477)

_____

_____

_____

_____

_____

41. The only paramagnetic analyzer manufactured in the United States today is the _____. (Barnes, p 348)

42. The paramagnetic analyzers are designed based on the Pauling principle. Describe that principle. (Barnes, p 348; Egan, p 477)

_____

_____

_____

43. The Beckman analyzer responds to _____ _____ of oxygen and reads out in _____ of oxygen. (Barnes, p 348)

44. Indicate which of the following are True or False about the paramagnetic analyzer. (Barnes, p 348; Egan, p 477; McPherson, p 207)

    a. _____ It must be corrected for water vapor.

    b. _____ It is safe for operating room use.

c. _____ It can only make static spot analysis.

d. _____ It must be calibrated for altitude.

45. What is the basic principle of operation of the thermoconductive analyzer. (Barnes, p 348; Egan, p 478; McPherson, p 208)

_____

_____

_____

_____

_____

46. Thermoconductive analyzers actually measure the oxygen _____. (Barnes, p 349; Egan, p 478; McPherson, p 208)

47. List two types of thermoconductive analyzers. (Barnes, p 349; Egan, p 477; McPherson, p 208)

a. _____

b. _____

48. List two disadvantages of using the thermoconductive units. (Barnes, p 349)

a. _____

b. _____

49. List the two types of electrochemical cells or electrodes used as analyzers. (Barnes, p 348)

a. _____

b. _____

50. List the similarities between the polarographic analyzer and the galvanic fuel cell. (Barnes, p 349; Egan, p 476; McPherson, p 209)

a. _____

b. _____

c. _____

d. _____

51. Describe the functioning of the polarographic analyzer. (McPherson, p 208)

_____

_____

_____

_____

52. Describe the functioning of the galvanic fuel cell. (McPherson, p 208)

_____

_____

_____

_____

53. List three concerns about the maintenance of the polarographic analyzer. (Barnes, p 350)

    a. _____

    b. _____

    c. _____

54. The electrode used in transcutaneous oxygen monitoring is a _____ electrode that operates on the _____ principle. (Deshpande, p 221)

55. How are transcutaneous monitoring devices used? (Deshpande, p 222)

    _____

    _____

56. List three hazards of $TcPo_2$ monitoring. (Deshpande, p 224)

    a. _____

    b. _____

    c. _____

57. List three advantages of $TcPo_2$ monitoring. (Deshpande, p 224)

    a. _____

    b. _____

    c. _____

58. Explain the operation of the pulse oximeter. (Deshpande, p 226)

    _____

    _____

    _____

ANSWERS TO THE STUDY QUESTIONS

1. a. 32
   b. 1.43
   c. 149.37
   d. 20.95
   e. photosynthesis

2. a. arterial Po_2
   b. hemoglobin saturation
   c. oxygen transport
   d. cardiovascular status
   e. work of breathing

3. a. increase PAo_2
   b. decrease work of breathing
   c. decrease work of myocardium

4. a. decreased carrying capacity of blood for oxygen
   b. decreased circulation – cardiac output
   c. inability of the tissue to utilize available oxygen
   d. decreased diffusion of oxygen across alveolar capillary membrane
   e. inadequate quantity of oxygen in the blood

5. a. hypoxemic hypoxia
   b. anemic hypoxemia

6. a. concentration of oxygen administered
   b. previous exposure to oxygen
   c. length of exposure
   d. age
   e. nutritional status

7. a. atelectasis
   b. pulmonary edema

c. alveolar hemorrhage
d. inflammation
e. fibrin deposition
f. thickening and hyalinization of the alveolar membranes

8. exudative: early phase, 24 to 72 hours, changes in alveolar Type II cells, destruction of pulmonary capillary endothelial cells, necrosis of type I cells, interstitial and intra-alveolar edema, hemorrhage, and hyaline membrane formation.
proliferation: late phase, after 72 hours, hyperplasia of alveolar type II cells, thickening of alveolar septa, hyperplasia of pulmonary capillaries, and fibroblastic proliferation.

9. a. oxygen toxicity
b. absorption atelectasis
c. oxygen-induced hypoventilation
d. retrolental fibroplasia (RLF)
e. bronchopulmonary dysplasia

10. forty percent or above, 12 to 24 hours

11. a. nausea
b. vomiting
c. dyspnea
d. tachypnea
e. cough
f. fatigue
g. anxiety
h. substernal pain
i. paresthesia

12. improve oxygenation at the lowest possible F_{IO_2}

13. a. These devices supply oxygen at a fixed flow. They do not provide the patient's total needed minute ventilation. The oxygen concentration delivered varies depending on the change in patient demand, the liter flow rate, and the patient's ventilatory pattern.
b. These devices supply all the patient's inspiratory requirements. They provide a flow that exceeds the patient's demand. Generally oxygen concentration delivered is not affected by a change in patient ventilatory need.

14. a. respiratory rate
b. ventilatory pattern
c. equipment reservoir
d. patient's anatomic reservoir
e. tidal volume

15. a. HF
b. HF

c. LF
d. LF
e. LF
f. HF
g. LF
h. LF

16. a. inserted into the nares to lie just behind the uvula in the oropharynx.
b. changed every 8 hours
c. mainly insertion and removal, nosebleeds, mucosal surface damage, poor placement
d. low F_{IO_2}, variable with V_T, respiratory rate, and ventilatory pattern

17. Advantages
a. patient may eat and speak without obstruction
b. less subject to patient manipulation
c. nonclaustrophobic
d. used in unconscious obtunded children and adults

Disadvantages
a. insertion and removal may be traumatic
b. frequent changes needed
c. variable F_{IO_2}
d. nasal trauma

18. a. elastic headband adjusts to hold prongs in the nares
b. watch flowmeter accuracy, twisted cannula, humidifier seal, and water in the tubing
c. variable F_{IO_2} with ventilatory changes, pressure point sores, nasal mucosa drying
d. variable F_{IO_2} with change in patient ventilatory pattern; comfortable, lightweight, and inexpensive; fairly reliable for patients with stable ventilatory patterns

19. Advantages
a. easy placement and maintenance
b. comfortable and lightweight
c. unobtrusive
d. inexpensive

Disadvantages
a. variable F_{IO_2}
b. nasal mucosa drying
c. pressure sores
d. limited to low to moderate F_{IO_2}

20. a. fastened via adjustable elastic headband; has malleable metal band for adjustment to bridge of the nose
b. maintain a minimum flow of above 5 LPM to aid in ventilation and prevent build-up of CO_2
c. pressure sores on facial skin, risk of aspiration of vomitus, possible CO_2 build-up

d. FIO delivered dependent upon a stable ventilatory pattern, mask volume, and oxygen flow to the device

21. Advantages
   a. inexpensive
   b. easy to apply
   c. may apply humidification
   d. increased flows possible without nasal mucosa drying

   Disadvantages
   a. risk of aspiration of vomitus
   b. may cause claustrophobic reactions
   c. minimum flow must be strictly maintained
   d. difficult to determine exact FIO_2 being delivered

22. a. elastic headband to fit to patient's head, needs a good seal, malleable metal piece to adjust across bridge of nose
   b. watch for tight seal, careful adjustment of flow levels to ensure patient's ventilatory demand is met with this device and air entrainment
   c. risk of aspiration of vomitus, CO_2 build-up possible, poor fit common, facial pressure sores, leaks will decrease FIO_2
   d. may be too large (poor fit hampers ability to produce desired results, as will large reservoirs)

23. Advantages
   a. moderate to high concentrations of oxygen are available
   b. disposable
   c. easy to use
   d. high flows available

   Disadvantages
   a. warm
   b. risk of aspiration of vomitus
   c. uncomfortable
   d. poor seal may produce variable delivery of FIO_2

24. a. mask attached to jet device, elastic headband to fit to patient's head, malleable metal piece fits to bridge of nose
   b. flow rates must be maintained to meet patient's needs; watch for obstruction of entrainment ports
   c. some patients find claustrophobic, risk of aspiration of vomitus, increased FIO_2 with obstruction of flow, condensation may occur
   d. very accurate FIO_2, FIO_2 dependent on air-oxygen entrainment ratio

25. Advantages
   a. accurate FIO_2
   b. high flows and FIO_2 possible
   c. disposable
   d. additional humidity possible

   Disadvantages
   a. uncomfortable
   b. high flows bother some patients
   c. may block entrainment ports
   d. high flows may produce bubbling noise

26. a. aerosol face mask, face tent, tracheostomy collar, Briggs adapter (T-piece)
   b. dependent upon type used; all use large-bore tubing to connect to nebulizer unit
   c. rainout in tubing should be cleared often, supply adequate FIO_2 with adequate flow, watch mist at end-inspiration
   d. swelling of secretions, change in flow, watch increased humidity level, not good for all patients
   e. highest input flow should be used; patients with rapid RR may not get specific FIO_2 desired

27. a. 0.21 to 0.44
   b. 0.40 to 0.60
   c. 0.60 to 0.80
   d. 0.80 to 1.00
   e. 0.24 to 0.40 (0.60 dependent upon unit)
   f. 0.24 to 1.0 dependent upon unit

28. total flow = flow of air + flow of oxygen
   total flow = (3.17 × 15) + 15 = 63 LPM

29. a. cover only head of infant, connected to source through large-bore tubing, thermometer in place, and sound-reducing sponge used on preference, analyze at patient's face
   b. keep rainout clear in large-bore tubing, ensure correct-size hood, temperature, and flow
   c. cold O_2, increased FIO_2, noise from the hood, fogging of the hood
   d. fairly reliable, flows of 10 to 15 LPM adequate for most

30. a. units completely enclose patient
   b. no electrical items or sparks in the tent, analyze at patient's face, watch water level and rainout, vent-off body heat
   c. biggest hazard is fire
   d. variable FIO_2 and flows

31. a. temperature
   b. oxygen concentration
   c. humidity

   d. filtered gas environment

32. a. between 31 and 32 degrees centigrade
    b. 12 hours
    c. water and acetic acid
    d. wick

33. a. self-inflating bag
    b. air intake valve
    c. nonrebreathing valve
    d. oxygen-inlet valve
    e. high oxygen concentration reservoir attachment

34. a. oxygen capabilities to 85 to 100 percent at 15 LPM flow
    b. designed to prevent valve malfunction at flows of 30 LPM
    c. air intake valve should be able to disassemble and reassemble in 20 seconds
    d. adapter—15 mm female and 22 mm male

35. a. spring disk
    b. spring ball
    c. diaphragm
    d. diaphragm and duckbill
    e. diaphragm and duckbill
    f. duckbill

36. a. gas gangrene
    b. cyanide poisoning
    c. air embolism
    d. ischemic tissue transplant
    e. chronic osteomyelitis
    f. carbon monoxide poisoning
    g. severe acute anemia
    h. facilitation of heart surgery in cyanotic heart disease
    i. body surface and inhalation burns
    j. decompression sickness

37. fixed multiplate unit—enclosed rooms, multiple subjects, simple decompression
    single or monoplate unit—somewhat portable, one patient only, or patient and attendant

38. a. poor patient access in some units
    b. can cause claustrophobic reaction
    c. electrical fire hazard
    d. tympanic membrane rupture
    e. air-filled cavity rupture
    f. air volume variances in endotracheal tube cuffs

39. a. paramagnetic
    b. thermoconductivity
    c. electrochemical cells

40. It contains a glass dumbell filled with nitrogen that is suspended on a quartz fiber. Magnets hold the dumbbell in a specific position. When oxygen is attracted to the magnetic field, it alters the position of the nitrogen-filled spheres. This alteration allows the dumbbell to rotate. A mirror attached to the dumbbell reflects a light focused on a translucent scale. Changes in the dumbbell position are shown as a change in partial pressure.

41. Beckman D-2

42. It is a physical principle that oxygen's electron shell configuration causes it to exhibit magnetic qualities. Increasing the oxygen level intensifies the magnetic field around a permanent magnet.

43. partial pressure, percent

44. False, True, True, True

45. The Wheatstone bridge is used to compare the resistance to current flow through two wires. The reference wire is exposed to room air; the sample wire is in the gas chamber. When the sample wire is exposed to oxygen, it is cooled. This allows the wire to accept more current flow. The change in current is compared with the reference wire. The difference between the two readouts is read as oxygen percent.

46. concentration

47. a. MIRA
    b. OEM

48. a. only analyze static samples
    b. some older models unsafe in the operating room

49. a. polarographic
    b. galvanic fuel cell

50. a. both utilize the principle that increases in partial pressure of oxygen cause increases in a chemical reaction that result in electrical activity
    b. both can measure gas samples continuously
    c. both use a probe that can be placed in the gas environment
    d. both readout percent or FIO_2 and measure partial pressure

51. It uses a battery to polarize the electrodes to improve response time. The oxygen molecule passes through a semipermeable membrane into an electrolyte solution. Oxygen moves to a charged cathode; this generates an increased number of electrons. The electron current is measured as oxygen percent.

52. Oxygen passes through a semipermeable membrane to a hydroxide bath. A gold electrode and a lead electrode are in the bath. Oxygen combines with water in the bath to form hydroxyl ions. These travel to the gold electrode and then to the lead electrode. Here they form lead oxide and electrons. The electron current is measured on a scale as oxygen percent.

53. a. battery integrity
    b. KCl solution integrity
    c. membrane integrity

54. Clark, polarographic

55. They are used during childbirth and to monitor high-risk neonates and infants, and also in the ICU to correlate PaO_2 and $TcPO_2$ and mechanical ventilation.

56. a. burns
    b. erythematous circles
    c. variable accuracy

57. a. avoids arterial sampling
    b. provides a continual reading
    c. may be used in a variety of settings

58. An oximeter transmits a light beam through a perfused area of the ear lobe, pinna, or finger. This light beam is picked up by a photosensor. The amount of light absorbed by the blood is compared with a reference.

PRACTICE QUIZ

1. What is the density of oxygen?
   a. 1.43 g/l
   b. 1.59 g/l
   c. 2.09 g/l
   d. 3.24 g/l
   e. 5.60 g/l

2. Which of the following is/are a desired effect of supplemental oxygen therapy?
   a. increased PaO_2
   b. increased PAO_2
   c. decreased work of breathing
   d. decreased myocardial work
   e. all of the above

3. Which of the following types of hypoxia is/are responsive to oxygen therapy?
   a. hypoxemic hypoxia
   b. stagnant hypoxia
   c. histotoxic hypoxia
   d. a and c
   e. b and c

4. Which of the following affect the FIO_2 delivered with the use of a low-flow oxygen delivery device?
   I. Respiratory rate
   II. Ventilatory pattern
   III. Tidal volume
   IV. Patient's anatomic reservoir
   V. Equipment reservoir
   a. I, II, III, IV, V
   b. I, II, III, IV
   c. I, II, III
   d. I, II, IV
   e. II, III, V

5. Which of the following statements are not true about the Beckman D-2 oxygen analyzer?

I. Under room air conditions, the dumbbell is stationary.
II. The rotation is proportional to the partial pressure of oxygen.
III. The gas analyzed must be humidified.
IV. The Beckman D-2 is safe for operating room use.
V. The Beckman D-2 is not affected by changes in altitude.
a. I, II, III, IV, V
b. III, IV, V
c. I, II
d. III, IV
e. I, III

6. A Briggs adapter setup is set at 0.60 oxygen delivered. The oxygen flow meter is set at 12 LPM. What is the total flow being delivered to the patient?
a. 12 LPM
b. 20 LPM
c. 24 LPM
d. 30 LPM
e. 36 LPM

7. Which of the following is/are true about low-flow variable performance devices?
I. They supply oxygen at a fixed flow rate.
II. They deliver only a portion of the inspired gas.
III. Changes in patient demand will change the F_{IO_2}.
IV. An example is the Venturi mask.
V. The F_{IO_2} delivered is consistent.
a. I, II, III, IV, V
b. I, II, III, IV
c. I, II, III
d. I, III, V
e. I, II, IV

8. Which of the following devices must be changed every 8 hours?
a. nasal cannula
b. nasal catheter
c. Briggs adapter
d. Venturi mask
e. partial rebreather

9. Which of the following is a disadvantage of using a reservoir mask for oxygen therapy?
I. A loose seal will decrease the percent delivered.
II. It may not deliver enough flow to the patient.
III. It is uncomfortable for long periods.
IV. It may cause a claustrophobic reaction.
V. It has a variable performance with deep ventilatory pattern.
a. I, II, III, IV, V
b. I, III, IV, V
c. I, II, V
d. III, IV, V
e. II, III, IV

10. Your patient has a variable respiratory rate of 20. She exhibits a change in ventilatory pattern often and has a variable tidal volume. Which device would you recommend, based on a need for 28 percent delivered?
a. nasal cannula
b. partial rebreathing mask

    c. nonrebreathing mask
    d. Venturi mask
    e. simple mask

11. Which of the following is/are types of chambers used in hyperbaric oxygen therapy?
    a. fixed multiplace unit
    b. monoplace unit
    c. hypoxic unit
    d. a and b
    e. none of the above

12. Identify the common problems associated with hyperbaric oxygen therapy.
      I. It may cause claustrophobia.
      II. It is an electrical fire hazard.
      III. Air-filled cavities may rupture.
      IV. Soft tissue pressure sores may develop.
      V. Pupils may rupture.
    a. I, II, III
    b. I, II, IV
    c. II, IV, V
    d. II, V
    e. III only

13. Which of the following statements accurately describes the electrochemical cell analyzer?
      I. Polarographic and galvanic fuel cell are examples.
      II. Both measure partial pressure of oxygen.
      III. Neither is safe for operating room use.
      IV. Both readout percent oxygen.
      V. Both measure a continuous gas sample.
    a. I, II, III, IV, V
    b. I, II, III, IV
    c. I, II, IV, V
    d. II, III, IV
    e. I, IV, V

14. Which of the oxygen analyzers should not be taken into the operating room?
    a. Teledyne
    b. OEM
    c. Ohio
    d. Beckman D-2
    e. IMI

15. The cathode of the Clark electrode is commonly made of which material?
    a. platinum
    b. silver
    c. bronze
    d. lead
    e. gold

16. A type of hypoxia that occurs when there is an inability of the tissues to utilize available oxygen is _____.
    a. anemic
    b. stagnant
    c. histotoxic
    d. hypoxemic
    e. chloride

17. If the oxygen tubing pops off the humidifier connected to a nasal cannula, the most common cause is:
    a. flow too high on the meter
    b. obstructed cannula
    c. patient is breathing back on the cannula
    d. humidifier is not sealed
    e. the cannula is broken

18. Which of the following is not a hazard of oxygen therapy?
    a. oxygen toxicity
    b. retrolental fibroplasia
    c. bronchopulmonary dysplasia
    d. atelectasis
    e. pneumothorax

19. The exudative phase of an oxygen toxic response is manifested in which of the following ways?
    I. Onset is from 24 to 48 hours.
    II. Thickening of the alveolar septa occurs.
    III. Hyperplasia of the pulmonary capillaries occurs.
    IV. Changes occur in the alveolar type II cells.
    V. Fibroblastic proliferation occurs.
    a. I, IV
    b. I, II, IV
    c. II, III
    d. IV, V
    e. I

20. Which of the following incorporates gas-analyzing principles?
    a. polarographic units
    b. oximeters
    c. electrochemical units
    d. transcutaneous oxygen monitors
    e. all of the above

ANSWERS TO THE PRACTICE QUIZ

1. a	11. d
2. e	12. a
3. a	13. c
4. a	14. b
5. d	15. a
6. c	16. c
7. c	17. b
8. b	18. e
9. a	19. a
10. d	20. e

HUMIDITY AND AEROSOL THERAPY

OUTLINE

LEARNING OBJECTIVES

Upon completion of this unit, the individual will:

1. Be able to define the following:
   a. humidity
   b. relative humidity
   c. absolute humidity
   d. water vapor pressure
   e. percent body humidity
   f. humidity deficit
2. Being given the temperature of a gas and either the partial pressure of water vapor or the absolute humidity, calculate the relative humidity.
3. List/describe the anatomical structures responsible for the body's normal humidification process and each structure's role in humidifying the inspired gas.
4. Explain the goals and hazards in administering humidity therapy
5. Describe four factors that could increase the efficiency of a humidifier.
6. Identify six types of humidifiers and explain the principle of operation of each.
7. Be able to define the following:
   a. aerosol
   b. stability
   c. instability
8. List/describe five factors that influence aerosol penetration and deposition.
9. Construct a chart illustrating the micron size of aerosol particles and where the particles would deposit within the respiratory system.
10. Explain the mechanism of clearance involved in the upper airways as well as in the pulmonary tissues.
11. Compare/contrast atomization and nebulization in reference to aerosol particles.
12. List/describe the goals and hazards of aerosol therapy.
13. Identify/explain the various types of intermittent nebulizers.
14. Identify/describe six types of continuous nebulizing units.
15. Explain the operation of the ultrasonic nebulizer.
16. Identify/describe the components of the ultrasonic nebulizer.
17. Describe factors that influence the output and the particle size of an ultrasonic nebulizer.

REFERENCES

Barnes, TA: Respiratory Care Practice. Year Book Medical Publishers, Chicago, 1988.

Burton, G, and Hodgkin, J: Respiratory Care: A Guide to Clinical Practice, ed 2. JB Lippincott, Philadelphia, 1984

Egan, DF, Sheldon, RL, and Spearman, CB: Egan's Fundamentals of Respiratory Therapy, ed 4. CV Mosby, St Louis, 1982

Eubanks, D, and Bone, R: Comprehensive Respiratory Care. CV Mosby, St Louis, 1988.

Kacmarek, RM, Mack, CW, and Dimas, S: The Essentials of Respiratory Therapy, ed 2. Year Book Medical Publishers, Chicago, 1985

McPherson, SP: Respiratory Therapy Equipment, ed 3. CV Mosby, St Louis, 1985.

Shapiro, BA, Harrison, RA, Kacmarek, RM, and Cane, RD: Clinical Application of Respiratory Care, ed 3. Year Book Medical Publishers, Chicago, 1985

STUDY QUESTIONS

1. Define humidity. (Shapiro, p 90; Kacmarek, p 21)

2. Define absolute humidity. (Shapiro, p 90; Kacmarek, p 21)

_____

3. Describe/define relative humidity in equation form. (Shapiro, p 91; Kacmarek, p 22)

_____

_____

_____

4. At 28°C the absolute humidity is 20.5 mg/l, the capacity at 28°C is 27.2 mg/l. What is the relative humidity? (Shapiro, p 91; Kacmarek, p 22)

_____

5. At 10°C room air holds 9.40 mg/l at 100% saturation. If the relative humidity is 85%, what is the absolute humidity? (Shapiro, p 91; Kacmarek, p 22)

_____

_____

6. Define water vapor pressure. (Kacmarek, p 21; Barnes, p 164)

_____

7. What is the capacity of water vapor in mg/l at 37°C? (Kacmarek, p 21; Barnes, p 165; Shapiro, p 91)

_____

8. What is the water vapor pressure at 37°C and 100% saturation? (Kacmarek, p 21; Barnes, p 165; Shapiro, p 91)

_____

9. Define percent body humidity. (McPherson, p 123)

_____

_____

10. If the absolute humidity is 8 mg/l, what is the percent body humidity? (McPherson, p 123)

_____

11. Define humidity deficit. (Shapiro, p 91; Barnes, p 166)

_____

12. If a person was breathing room air at 25°C, with the capacity at 23.0 mg/l and the relative humidity at 40%, what would this person's humidity deficit be? (Shapiro, p 91; Barnes, p 167)

_____

_____

13. According to the anatomic structures listed below, discuss their role in the normal humidification process and the approximate relative humidity at each point. (Shapiro, p 91)

   a. nose: _____

   b. oropharynx: _____

   c. carina: _____

14. Clinical indications for humidity therapy include: (Shapiro, p 91; Barnes, pp 167–169)

    a. _____

    b. _____

    c. _____

15. Three major goals of humidity therapy are: (Shapiro, p 92)

    a. _____

    b. _____

    c. _____

16. Several factors relate to the efficiency of any humidifier. List four factors that increase a humidifier's efficiency, and give an example of each by listing a device which uses that principle. (Burton, pp 383–384; McPherson, p 123)

    a. _____

    b. _____

    c. _____

    d. _____

17. Identify each type of humidifier in Figures 7–1 through 7–7 by name. (McPherson, p 125–135; Eubanks, pp 284–289; Barnes, pp 385–389)

    a. Fig. 7–1: _____   e. Fig. 7–5: _____

    b. Fig. 7–2: _____   f. Fig. 7–6: _____

    c. Fig. 7–3: _____   g. Fig. 7–7: _____

    d. Fig. 7–4: _____

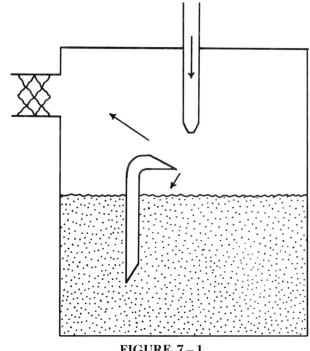

FIGURE 7–1.

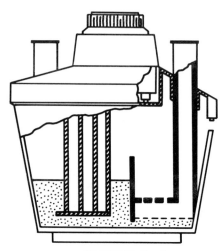

FIGURE 7–2.

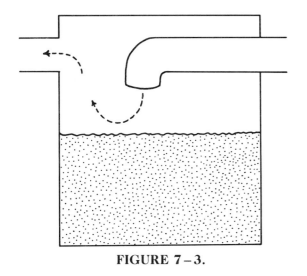

FIGURE 7–3.

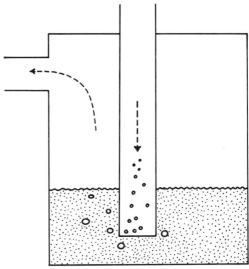

FIGURE 7–4.

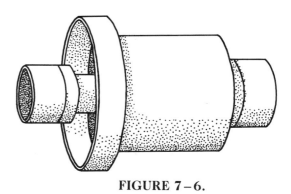

FIGURE 7–6.

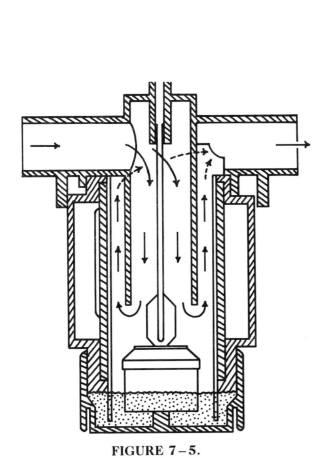

FIGURE 7–5.

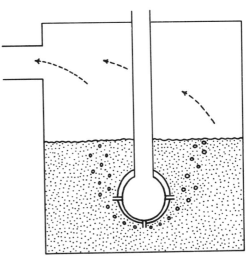

FIGURE 7–7.

18. Describe the operation of each unit as labeled in question 17. (McPherson, pp 125–135; Eubanks, pp 284–289; Barnes, pp 385–389)

    a. _____

    _____

    b. _____

    _____

    _____

    _____

    _____

    _____

    c. _____

    _____

    d. _____

    _____

    _____

    e. _____

    _____

    _____

    _____

    _____

    _____

    _____

    f. _____

    _____

    _____

    _____

    _____

    g. _____

    _____

    _____

    _____

19. List two major clinical applications for using humidifiers. (Shapiro, p 94)

    a. _____

    b. _____

20. In the event of an obstruction most humidity generators incorporate a pressure relief using a pop-off valve set at approximately _____. (McPherson, p 127; Barnes, pp 385–389)

21. An instrument that can be used to measure absolute and relative humidity is known as a _____. (Eubanks, pp 290–291)

22. Define aerosol and give three examples. (Shapiro, p 95; McPherson, p 137)

_____

_____

23. Particle size is expressed as _____. (McPherson, p 137; Kacmarek, p 392)

24. Aerosol stability and instability refer to _____ (stability) and _____. (instability). (Shapiro, p 95; Kacmarek, p 391)

25. List the characteristics that affect the stability of a particle. (Egan, p 347; Kacmarek, p 391)

    a. _____

    b. _____

    c. _____

    d. _____

    e. _____

26. Optimum stability occurs when the particle diameter is between _____ and _____ microns. (Shapiro, p 95; Barnes, pp 169–172)

27. Define deposition and penetration. (Shapiro, p 96; Kacmarek, p 391)

_____

_____

_____

28. Match the particle size with its approximate deposition in the respiratory tract. (Egan, p 353; McPherson, pp 138–143)

    _____ trapped in the nose   a. 100 microns

    _____ alveoli   b. 5–100 microns

    _____ do not enter respiratory tract c. 2–5 microns

    _____ minimal settling   d. 1–2 microns

    _____ bronchi   e. 1–0.25 microns

29. List the factors that influence particle penetration and deposition. Give a brief explanation of each. (Shapiro, p 96; McPherson, p 137)

    a. _____

    _____

    b. _____

    _____

    c. _____

    _____

    d. _____

    _____

e. _____

_____

f. _____

_____

30. Explain the type of ventilatory pattern that will produce maximum deposition. (Shapiro, p 98; McPherson, p 142)

_____

_____

31. Optimal particle size for maximal aerosol deposition is between _____ and _____ microns. (McPherson, p 142; Barnes, pp 172–174)

32. Describe what happens to the particles in the respiratory tract if the particle composition is: (McPherson, p 140)

a. hypotonic saline: _____

b. hypertonic saline: _____

c. isotonic saline: _____

33. What effect does an aerosol have on airway resistance? (Shapiro, p 99)

_____

34. Define clearance. (Shapiro, p 100; Kacmarek, p 392)

_____

35. List the three major goals of aerosol therapy. (Shapiro, p 106; Kacmarek, p 393)

a. _____

_____

b. _____

c. _____

36. Hazards associated with the administration of aerosol therapy are: (Shapiro, p 108; Kacmarek, p 393)

a. _____

b. _____

c. _____

d. _____

37. The principle employed by a jet nebulizer is known as: (McPherson, p 143; Burton, p 387)

_____

38. Distinguish between the two diagrams in Figure 7–8.

_____

_____

39. Intermittent nebulizers are used to deliver medication. Using the diagrams in Figures 7–9, 7–10, and

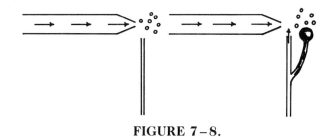

FIGURE 7–8.

7–11, label each and briefly describe their operation. What is the advantage of each? (McPherson, p 146; Eubanks, p 302)

a. Fig. 7–9: _____

_____

b. Fig. 7–10: _____

_____

c. Fig. 7–11: _____

_____

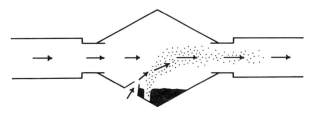

FIGURE 7–9.

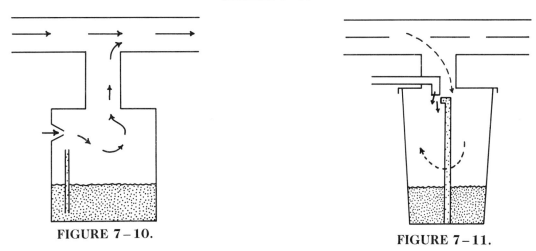

FIGURE 7–10.   **FIGURE 7–11.**

40. Identify the intermittent nebulizers pictured in Figures 7–12 and 7–13. (Eubanks, p 301)

    a. Fig. 7–12: _____

    b. Fig. 7–13: _____

41. Label the diagram in Figure 7–14. (McPherson, p 151)

    a. _____   d. _____

    b. _____   e. _____

    c. _____   f. _____

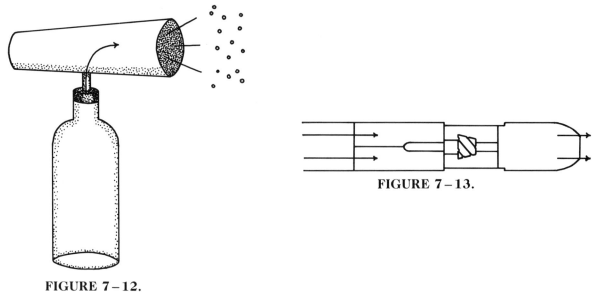

FIGURE 7-12.

FIGURE 7-13.

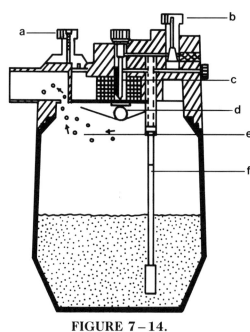

FIGURE 7-14.

42. Discuss the operation of the labeled diagram in question 41 in terms of: (Eubanks, p 303; Shapiro, pp 101–102; Barnes, pp 367–369)

    a. principle of operation: _____

    b. indication for clinical use: _____

    c. output: _____

43. Label the diagram in Figure 7–15. (Eubanks, p 304)

    a. _____   d. _____

    b. _____   e. _____

    c. _____

44. Discuss the operation of the labeled diagram in question 43 in terms of the following: (Eubanks, p 304; McPherson, p 155)

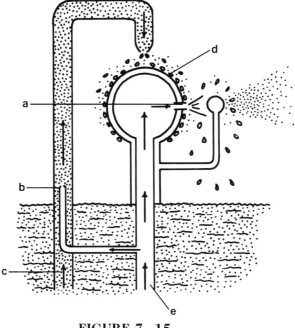

FIGURE 7–15.

a. principle of operation: _____

b. indications for clinical use: _____

c. output: _____

45. Label the diagram in Figure 7–16. (McPherson, p 156)

a. _____

b. _____

c. _____

d. _____

46. Discuss the operation of the labeled diagram in question 45 in terms of the following: (McPherson, p 155; Burton, pp 389–390)

a. principle of operation: _____

b. indications for clinical use: _____

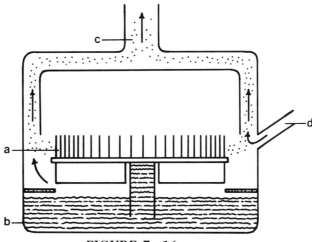

FIGURE 7–16.

47. Describe the principle of operation for the ultrasonic nebulizer. (McPherson, p 156; Shapiro, pp 104–105)

_____

_____

_____

_____

_____

_____

_____

48. What are the two most common output ranges using the ultrasonic nebulizer aerosol generator? (McPherson, p 157; Barnes, pp 374–381)

_____

49. Label the diagram in Figure 7–17. (Eubanks, p 306; Barnes, pp 374–381)

a. _____   f. _____

b. _____   g. _____

c. _____   h. _____

e. _____   i. _____

50. What is the purpose of using tap water in the couplant chamber? (McPherson, p 157; Barnes, pp 374–381)

_____

51. Frequency determines _____, while amplitude dictates

_____. (McPherson, p 157; Barnes, pp 374–381)

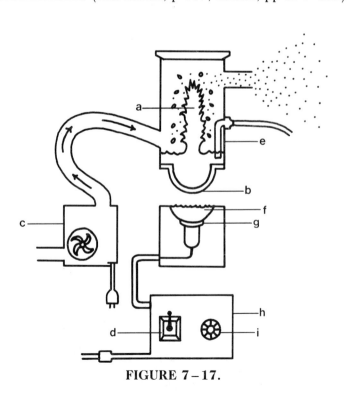

FIGURE 7–17.

52. Particle size ranges between _____ and _____ on the ultrasonic nebulizer. (McPherson, p 157; Kacmarek, p 395)

53. In a jet nebulizer, what effect does changing the air-entrainment ratio have on aerosol output? (Kacmarek, p 36)

54. In a jet nebulizer, what effect does changing air-entrainment ratio have on aerosol density? (Barnes, p 371)

55. Indicate which apparatus you would use in the following situations (e.g., humidifier/heated humidifier, intermittent nebulizer, large reservoir nebulizer, heated nebulizer):

    a. A patient who is on a mechanical ventilator.

    b. A patient who was ordered aerosol with 0.3 cc alupent and 2.5 cc normal saline.

    c. A patient receiving oxygen via nasal cannula at 2 l/min.

    d. A pediatric patient with croup.

    e. A patient who has just recently been weaned from a mechanical ventilator and still has an endotracheal tube in place.

ANSWERS TO STUDY QUESTIONS

1. water in gaseous (vapor) or molecular form; increasing temperature increases the amount of water vapor a gas can hold.

2. actual weight of water in a gas at a given temperature; measured in mg/l, g/cubic meter

3. ratio of actual water vapor content compared with the maximum (potential) the gas could hold at that temperature
   relative humidity = actual/potential × 100% or content/capacity × 100%

4. $\dfrac{20.5 \text{ mg/l}}{27.2 \text{ mg/l}} \times 100\% = 75\%$

5. content/capacity × 100% = RH, RH × content = absolute humidity 85% × 9.40 mg/l = 7.99 mg/l

6. pressure exerted by water vapor molecules in relation to temperature.

7. 43.8 mg/l or 44 mg/l

8. 47 mmHg

9. relative humidity of water vapor present (absolute) compared with water vapor at body temperature × 100%

10. body humidity = $\dfrac{8 \text{ mg/l}}{44 \text{ mgl/l}} \times 100\% = 18\%$

11. the difference (mathematical) between water vapor content in alveolar air and inspired air

12. RH × capacity = content, 0.40 × 23.0 mg/l = 9.2 mg/l
    44 mg/l − 9.2 mg/l = 34.8 mg/l

13. a. warms, filters, humidifies inspired gas; RH = 80%
    b. humidifies and warms inspired gas; RH = 90%

c. warms inspired gas to 37°C; RH = 100% (theoretically)

14. a. decrease the humidity deficit
    b. prevent drying of the tracheal bronchial tree
    c. for patient comfort

15. a. decrease the humidity deficit
    b. breathing a dry gas
    c. mucosal crusting

16. a. temperature: e.g., incubator, isolette, cascade, and wick
    b. increase surface area: e.g., diffuser, cascade, and jet
    c. agitation (increase kinetic activity): e.g., cascade
    d. time: e.g., cascade, jet, and underwater jet

17. a. jet
    b. cascade
    c. pass-over
    d. underwater jet
    e. wick
    f. condensing
    g. bubble diffuser

18. a. jet: Production of aerosol; employing a baffle system, whereby particles are removed or evaporated before leaving unit; increases time and gas/water surface area.
    b. cascade: Gas travels down a tower and passes through a grid. From the tower gas enters at a chamber below the grid, and water in the chamber is displaced by the gas raising the water level in the reservoir allowing water to enter above grid through a port. Water forms a film over grid that becomes a froth. One-way valve in tower acts to retard the drift of humidity back toward apparatus. Sensing port in tower allows gas communication with ventilator inlet so patient effort can be sensed. Employs heater.
    c. pass-over: Gas passes over water surface and pick up evaporated water which then flows to the patient.
    d. underwater jet: incorporates principles from bubble-jet. Gas conducted below surface of water to jet using Bernoulli's principle. As gas bubbles float to surface of water, gas/water contact and time of exposure are increased.
    e. wick: Heater surrounds wick (absorbant blotting type paper), saturated with water absorbed form a reservoir. Gas enters and is directed downward and into chamber containing wick. As gas flows past the wet,

heated paper, water evaporates and gas leaves the unit saturated and heated. Constant water level is maintained by a reservoir feed system. Float allows water to enter periodically to replace the water that has evaporated.
    f. condensing: Device placed between patient and breathing circuit. During exhalation gases at body humidity enter unit which heats the hygroscopic filter medium and condenses water into it. During next inhalation inspiration gas is warmed and humidified as it passes through the heat-moisture exchanger.
    g. bubble-diffuser: Gas is conducted below surface of water and allowed to bubble back to the top of water. Time and surface area contact have been increased. Some units employ diffusers to break up the gas into smaller bubbles, increasing gas/water surface area.

19. a. oxygen therapy
    b. by-pass the body's normal humidification process.

20. 2 psi

21. hygrometer

22. very fine particles (liquid or solid) suspended in a gas (examples: dust, aerosolized medication, fog, spray paint)

23. microns

24. the ability to remain in suspension for a significant period of time (stability); the tendency for particles to be removed from suspension (instability)

25. a. size
    b. nature of the particle
    c. density (concentration of the particle)
    d. ambient humidity
    e. mobility of carrier gas

26. 0.2, 0.7 microns

27. deposition: the settling out (rain out) of particles related to aerosol instability
    penetration: maximum depth the suspended particle can be carried into the respiratory tract.

28. b, d, a, e, c

29. a. gravity: Stokes' law (the heavier the particle, the greater the effect gravity will have on the particle)
    b. kinetic activity of the gas molecule: Brown-

ian movement (collision of molecules results in deposition of particles); effects particles 1 micron or less

   c. particle inertia: the larger the mass the greater the tendency to travel in a straight line (since airways have a lot of curves, the larger particles are more likely to be deposited)

   d. physical nature of the particle: hypotonic (particle tends to decrease in size as it enters the airway); hypertonic (particle tends to increase in size as it enters the airway); isotonic (particle stays the same size when it enters airway)

   e. temperature and humidity: an increase in temperature and humidity cause coalescence as gas cools, which increases the size of particles, causing them to deposit.

   f. ventilatory pattern: depth and rate of breathing will affect particle deposition and penetration

30. slow (200 to 300 ml/sec flowrate), deep breath (tidal volume 1200 to 1400 cc or $1\frac{1}{2}$ to 2 ml times the tidal volume), with a breath hold (10 to 15 seconds)

31. 0.5, 3 microns

32. a. hypotonic saline: particle decreases in size as it penetrates the airway
   b. hypertonic saline: particle increases in size as it penetrates the airway
   c. isotonic saline: particle remains stable as it penetrates the airway

33. increases the airway resistance

34. removal of particle from the respiratory tract once they have deposited

35. a. aid to bronchial hygiene (maintain mucus blanket, restore mucus (hydrate dried secretions), promote expectoration, and improve cough
   b. humidification of inspired gas
   c. deliver medication

36. a. swelling of retained secretions
   b. precipitation of bronchospasm
   c. fluid overload (especially in infants and older adults)
   d. cross-contamination

37. Bernoulli's principle

38. atomizer: no baffle; produces larger particles
   nebulizer: baffle; produces smaller particles

39. a. mainstream: aerosol created within the main flow of gas

(advantages—increases particle size, increases output, and increases humidity)

   b. slipstream: main flow of gas is diverted down to where the aerosol is being produced
   (advantages—increases output and increases humidity)

   c. sidestream: aerosol drifts up into the main flow of gas. (advantage—decreases particle size)

40. a. metered dose inhaler
   b. spinhaler

41. a. air-entrainment
   b. source gas
   c. jet
   d. baffle
   e. aerosol
   f. capillary tube

42. a. Bernoulli's law
   b. any situation that warrants the use of an aerosol; can be heated
   c. 1 to 2 ml/min

43. a. small orifice (jet)
   b. Venturi
   c. solution being drawn up capillary tube
   d. liquid film
   e. gas inlet

44. a. Babbington
   b. any situation that warrants the use of an aerosol; can be heated
   c. 1 to 7 ml/min

45. a. breaker combs
   b. water
   c. aerosol
   d. air inlet

46. a. impeller or centrifugal
   b. to add humidity to the room

47. Electrical current produces sound waves which break up the solution into aerosol particles. An electrical charge is applied intermittently (at high frequency of vibrations) to a substance that has a piezoelectric quality (ability to change shape when a charge is applied to it). Electrical current causes vibrations at the same frequency as the electrical charge applied to the piezoelectric transducer. These vibrations travel through water to the surface of the solution to produce an aerosol.

48. 0 to 3 ml/min and 0 to 6 ml/min

49. a. aerosol (geyser)
   b. membrane

   c. blower
   d. on/off switch
   e. nebulizer chamber
   f. couplant chamber
   g. piezoelectric transducer
   h. electrical module
   i. output control

50. help absorb mechanical heat and acts as a transfer medium

51. particle size, output

52. 1, 10 microns

53. As you increase air-entrainment, you increase output.

54. As you increase air-entrainment, you decrease density.

55. a. heated humidifier
   b. intermittant nebulizer
   c. humidifier
   d. large reservoir nebulizer
   e. heated large reservoir nebulizer

PRACTICE QUIZ

1. A patient in the ICU has been complaining of thick, productive sputum for the last two days. Upon examination of the humidity level and temperature of the room, it was found that the relative humidity was 40%, and at 100% saturation at that temperature the capacity was found to be 25 mg/l. What is this person's humidity deficit?
   a. 19.0 mg/l
   b. 24.0 mg/l
   c. 34.0 mg/l
   d. 40.0 mg/l
   e. 47.0 mg/l

2. The percent body humidity in the patient in question 1 is:
   a. 22.7%
   b. 56.8%
   c. 40.0%
   d. 45.0%
   e. 47.0%

3. Which of the following is *not* a hazard of aerosol therapy?
   a. cross-contamination
   b. salt retention
   c. swelling of hydroscopic sputum
   d. fluid overload
   e. increased urine output

4. A sidestream nebulizer is characterized as:
   a. diverting the main gas flow through the nebulizer
   b. diverting part of the main gas flow through the nebulizer
   c. contributing the aerosol to the carrier gas independent of the main gas flow
   d. producing the aerosol in the main flow of gas
   e. none of the above

5. Which of the following devices produces the highest relative humidity?
   a. cool jet nebulizer
   b. bubble type humidifier
   c. heated jet nebulizer
   d. vaporizer
   e. atomizer

6. Which of the following is *not* a cause of an inadequate mucus blanket?
   a. dehydration
   b. inadequate cough
   c. glandular abnormality
   d. mucosal hyperemia
   e. ciliary abnormality

7. Which of the following has no effect on aerosol particle size?
   a. orifice size
   b. number and placement of baffles
   c. jet pressure
   d. oxygen concentration
   e. none of the above

8. A piezoelectric transducer can be described as a:
   a. device that transforms electrical energy into kinetic energy
   b. device that transforms vibrational energy into electrical energy
   c. device that transforms acoustic energy into electrical energy
   d. device that transforms electrical energy into vibrational energy
   e. device that changes its shape when amperage is applied to it

9. With reference to an aerosol, the word "stability" refers to:
   a. the ability of particles to rain out
   b. the maximum depth particles penetrate
   c. the ability of particles to remain suspended
   d. how rapidly particles are exhaled
   e. the tendency of particles to coalesce

10. On a Purtain all-purpose nebulizer, at which setting can you achieve the highest percent relative humidity output to the patient?
    a. 40%
    b. 70%
    c. 100%
    d. depends on the wall pressure
    e. none of the above

11. The little opening just above the grid in the cascade tower:
    a. functions as a water inlet for the grid
    b. functions as a gas inlet for the grid
    c. functions as a port allowing gas to flow during the final portion of inspiration
    d. functions as one-way valve
    e. allows patient effort to be sensed by the machine

12. The amount of moisture present in normal alveolar air is:
    a. 40 mg/l
    b. 44 torr
    c. 44 mg/l
    d. 47 torr
    e. 47 mg/l

13. If the temperature of the room is raised and no humidity is added:
    a. the relative humidity will increase
    b. the relative humidity will not be affected
    c. the absolute humidity will decrease
    d. the relative humidity will decrease
    e. none of the above

14. Medical aerosols are believed to have optimal stability when the particle diameter is:
    a. less than 0.25 microns
    b. 4 to 5 microns
    c. 2 to 3 microns
    d. more than 5 microns
    e. 0.2 to 0.7 microns

15. An aerosol particle that is influenced by inertial impaction has which of the following forces acting upon it?
    a. particle position in the gas stream
    b. inertial forces
    c. air friction
    c. level of turbulence
    e. all of the above

16. The ideal breathing pattern for maximal aerosol deposition and retention is:
    a. rapid, shallow inspiration
    b. slow, deep inspiration with an apneustic hold followed by a passive exhalation
    c. rapid, deep inspiration with a prolonged expiration
    d. slow, deep inspiration with a fast expiration
    e. none of the above

17. Ciliary activity is usually impaired in the patient who has undergone a tracheostomy because:
    I. Inadequate humidification of inspired air
    II. Inadequate warming of inspired air.
    III. Medications are usually given to help reduce secretions as these interfere with ciliary activity
    IV. Air flow through the trachea is usually diminished
    a. I only
    b. II only
    c. I and II only
    d. III and IV
    e. I, II, IV

18. In heated nebulizers, reservoir temperatures should be maintained from:
    a. 27 to 32 degrees centigrade
    b. 34 to 39 degrees centigrade
    c. 42 to 49 degrees centigrade
    d. 54 to 60 degrees centigrade
    e. 63 to 68 degrees centigrade

19. A physician asks a respiratory care practitioner how particle size from an ultrasonic nebulizer can be permanently adjusted. Which of the following would be the practitioner's most appropriate response?
    a. Baffles should be used.
    b. The amplitude of the nebulizer should be changed.
    c. The flow rate and breathing pattern of the patient should be altered.
    d. Filters should be used.
    e. It is impossible because the frequency is preset at the factory.

20. What is the predicted outflow from a nebulizer setup given the following information: oxygen flow 10 l/min and FiO_2 0.40?
    a. 20 l/min
    b. 25 l/min
    c. 30 l/min
    d. 35 l/min
    e. 40 l/min

ANSWERS TO THE PRACTICE QUIZ

1. c
2. a
3. e
4. c
5. c
6. d
7. d
8. d
9. c
10. a

11. e
12. c
13. d
14. e
15. e
16. b
17. c
18. b
19. e
20. e

Chapter 8

THERAPEUTIC MODALITIES

OUTLINE

LEARNING OBJECTIVES

Upon completion of this unit, the individual will:

1. Define intermittant positive pressure breathing.
2. List/describe the physiologic effects of IPPB therapy.
3. List the hazards associated with IPPB therapy.
4. List the clinical goals of IPPB therapy.
5. Explain the effectiveness of an IPPB treatment.

6. List the contraindications of IPPB therapy.
7. Troubleshoot an IPPB treatment and take corrective action.
8. Differentiate between the Bird Mark 7, 8, 10, and 14.
9. Differentiate between the PR-1 and PR-2 Bennett series.
10. Identify the parts of the Bird Mark 7.
11. Identify/explain the Bennett valve and the Diluter regulator.
12. Define sustained maximal inspiration and incentive spirometry.
13. List/describe the clinical goals of sustained maximal inspiration.
14. Explain the criteria for appropriate administration of sustained maximal inspiration.
15. Identify/name the lobes and segments of each lung.
16. Define the following:
    a. chest physical therapy
    b. postural drainage
    c. percussion
    d. vibration
17. Describe the different positions for each of the 18 lung segments.
18. Describe the hazards and contraindications for chest physical therapy.
19. Explain the procedure used in splinting and coughing a patient.

REFERENCES

Barnes, TA: Respiratory Care Practice. Year Book Medical Publishers, Chicago, 1988.

Burton, G, and Hodgkin, J: Respiratory Care: A Guide to Clinical Practice, ed 2. JB Lippincott, Philadelphia, 1984.

Eubanks, D, and Bone, R: Comprehensive Respiratory Care. CV Mosby, St Louis, 1985.

Kacmarek, RM, Mack, CW, and Dimas, S: The Essentials of Respiratory Therapy, ed 2. Year Book Medical Publishers, Chicago, 1985.

McPherson, SP: Respiratory Therapy Equipment, ed 3. CV Mosby, St Louis, 1985.

Shapiro, BA, Harrison, RA, Kacmarek, RM, and Cane, RD. Clinical Application of Respiratory Care, ed 3. Year Book Medical Publishers, Chicago, 1985.

STUDY QUESTIONS

1. Define intermittent positive pressure breathing. (Burton, p 530; Shapiro, p 123)

2. Indicate by writing "up" or "down" the effect of positive airway pressure on the following: (Kacmarek, p 406; Burton, p 531; Burton, p 124)

   a. intrathoracic pressure _____

   b. right atrial filling _____

   c. intrapleural pressure _____

   d. cardiac output _____

   e. work of breathing _____

   f. intracranial pressure _____

   g. tidal volume _____

3. List three indications for intermittent positive pressure breathing. (Kacmarek, p 408; Burton, p 535; Shapiro, pp 124–125)

   a. _____

b. _____

c. _____

4. List three goals for intermittent positive pressure breathing. (Kacmarek, p 408; Shapiro, pp 124–125)

a. _____

b. _____

c. _____

5. There are many hazards associated with the administration of IPPB therapy. List at least seven. (Kacmarek, p 409; Shapiro, pp 128–131; Burton, pp 546–548)

a. _____   e. _____

b. _____   f. _____

c. _____   g. _____

d. _____

6. _____ is an absolute contraindication for IPPB therapy. (Burton, p 548; Kacmarek, p 411)

7. During IPPB therapy, what precautions should you take or look for? (Burton, pp 551–554)

_____

_____

8. On the Bird Mark 7 ventilator, identify the components from Figure 8–1. (Eubanks, p 445)

a. _____   h. _____

b. _____   i. _____

c. _____   j. _____

d. _____   k. _____

e. _____   l. _____

f. _____   m. _____

g. _____

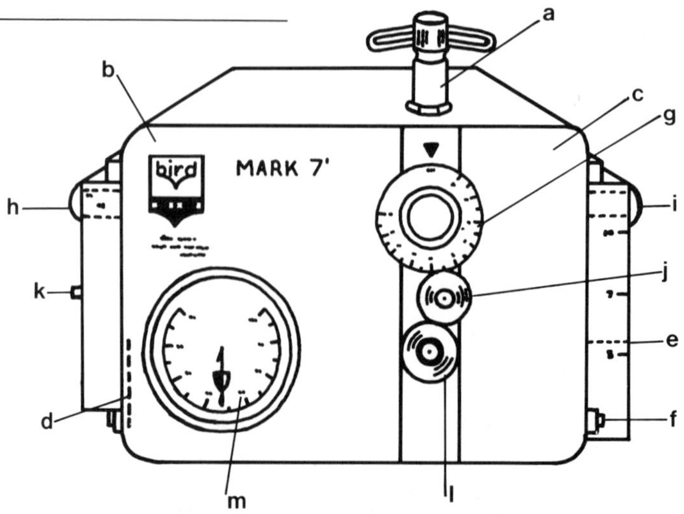

FIGURE 8–1. Bird Mark 7.

9. What gas source pressure is required to power the Bird Mark 7? (McPherson, p 271)

_____

10. What is the primary principle of Bird respirators? (McPherson, p 269)

_____

11. What is the primary difference between the Bird Mark 7 and the Bird Mark 8? What is this change in the Bird Mark 8 used for? (McPherson, p 283; Barnes, p 412)

_____

_____

12. How do the Birk Mark 10 and Mark 14 differ from the Bird Mark 7? (McPherson, pp 287–289; Barnes, pp 412–413)

_____

_____

_____

13. Second-generation Bird 7A and 8A differ from the first generation in what ways? (Barnes, pp 412–413; McPherson, pp 305–312)

_____

14. According to McPherson, the diluter regulator on the Bennett respirators is actually a(n) _____. (McPherson, p 317)

15. Identify Figure 8–2. (McPherson, p 318)

_____

16. What power source is required to operate the Bennett AP seris? PR seris? (McPherson, pp 325–343; Barnes, pp 406–408)

_____

17. Identify from Figure 8–3 which manometer measures machine pressure (control) and which manometer measures patient pressure (system)? (McPherson, p 320)

_____

_____

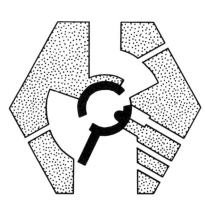

FIGURE 8–2.

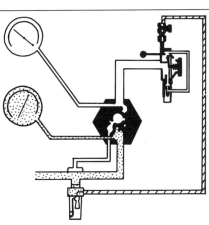

FIGURE 8–3.

18. What modifications differ between the PR-1 and PR-2? (McPherson, p 340; Barnes, pp 408–409)

_____

_____

19. The accumulators located atop of the PR seris ventilators are numbered 1, 2, and 3, respectively. Describe the function of each accumulator. (McPherson, p 332)

_____

_____

20. In each of the following situations describe what you would do to remedy the problem: (Eubanks, pp 449–450)

    a. machine won't cycle into exhalation: _____

    _____

    b. machine rapidly cycles on and off: _____

    _____

    c. machine won't cycle on: _____

    _____

21. Define sustained maximal inspiraton (SMI) and incentive spirometry. (Shapiro, p 145; Barnes, pp 208–215)

_____

_____

_____

22. How does incentive spirometry differ, in terms of physiology and advantages, from IPPB? (Shapiro, pp 145–146; Barnes, pp 208–215)

_____

_____

23. List the major goals for sustained maximal breathing? (Shapiro, p 146; Barnes, pp 208–215)

    a. _____

    b. _____

    c. _____

24. For performing adequately on an SMI maneuver using an incentive spirometer, the criteria should include the following: (Shapiro, p 146; Barnes, pp 212–213)

_____

_____

25. Adequate breathing instruction to a patient by a respiratory care practitioner should include the following: (Shapiro, p 147; Barnes, pp 212–213; Eubanks, p 453)

_____

_____

_____

26. What are two possible complications from incentive spirometry? (Barnes, p 213; Kacmarek, p 412)

    a. _____

    b. _____

27. What are two major device designs of incentive spirometry? (Kacmarek, p 411; Barnes, pp 418–425)

    a. _____

    b. _____

28. Identify/name the lung segments in Figures 8–4 and 8–5. (Eubanks, p 465; Burton, p 666)

Right Lung	Left Lung
1. _____	1–2. _____
2. _____	3. _____
3. _____	4. _____
4. _____	5. _____
5. _____	6. _____
6. _____	8. _____
7. _____ (not pictured)	9. _____
8. _____	10. _____
9. _____	
10. _____	

29. Chest physical therapy is a general term composed of what therapies? (Kacmarek, p 397; Barnes, pp 181–182)

    a. _____

    b. _____

    c. _____

    d. _____

    e. _____

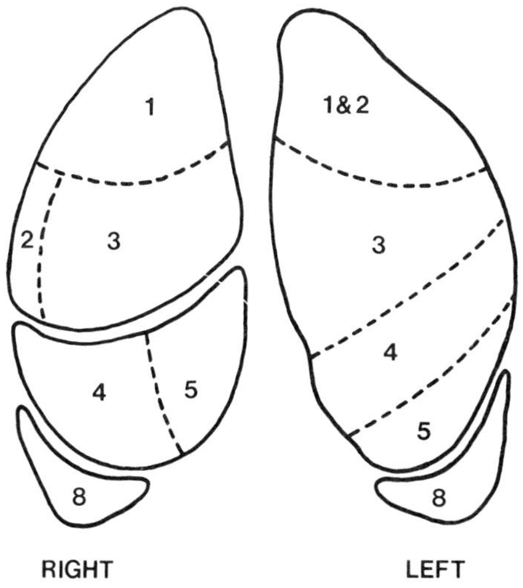

FIGURE 8–4. Anterior view of lungs.

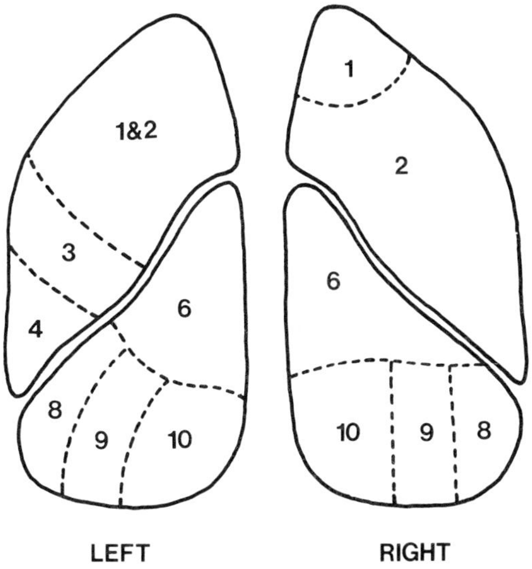

FIGURE 8–5. Posterior view of lungs.

30. According to Shapiro, what are the three goals of chest physical therapy? (Shapiro, p 134)

    a. _____

    b. _____

    c. _____

31. Two major indications for chest physical therapy are: (Barnes, p 183; Kacmarek, p 397)

    a. _____
    _____

    b. _____
    _____

32. Define postural drainage. (Barnes, p 85; Shapiro, p 134)

    _____
    _____

33. Identify from Figures 8–6 through 8–13 which lung segment(s) will be properly drained using postural drainage techniques. (Barnes, pp 186–187; Kacmarek, pp 398–403)

    a. Fig. 8–6: _____   e. Fig. 8–10: _____

    b. Fig. 8–7: _____   f. Fig. 8–11: _____

    c. Fig. 8–8: _____   g. Fig. 8–12: _____

    d. Fig. 8–9: _____   h. Fig. 8–13: _____

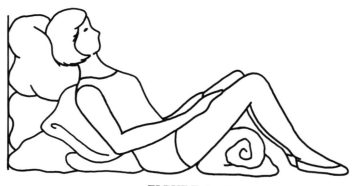

FIGURE 8–6.

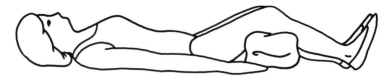

FIGURE 8–7.

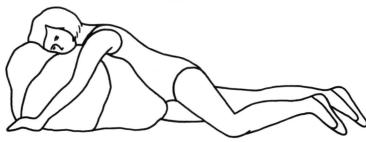

FIGURE 8–8.

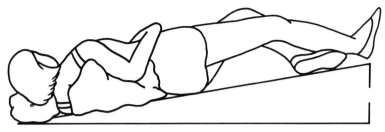

FIGURE 8-9.

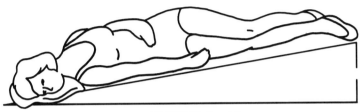

FIGURE 8-10.

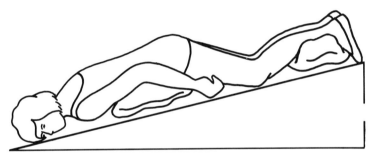

FIGURE 8-11.

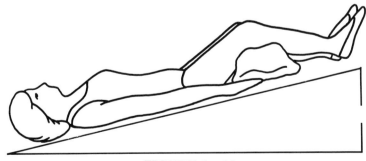

FIGURE 8-12.

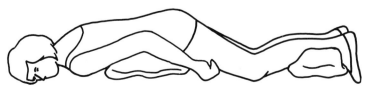

FIGURE 8-13.

34. List the conditions in which precautions should be taken during the postural drainage procedure. (Barnes, p 183; Kacmarek, p 399)

_____

_____

35. List the conditions that may be contraindicated in the head-down position. (Kacmarek, p 399; Barnes, pp 183–184)

_____

_____

_____

36. Define chest percussion. (Kacmarek, p 400; Barnes, p 185)

_____

37. List the contraindications for chest percussion, other than the complications listed for postural drainage. (Kacmarek, pp 400–401; Eubanks, p 471)

_____

_____

38. Define chest vibrations and describe the proper technique. (Kacmarek, p 401; Shapiro, p 140)

_____

_____

39. Describe the sequence of the normal cough. (Kacmarek, p 402; Shapiro, pp 140–141)

_____

_____

40. Explain how you would instruct a patient to cough. (Shapiro, p 141)

_____

_____

41. What modifications can be utilized with a patient following abdominal or thoracic surgery?

_____

42. In patients with an ineffective cough, such as those with spinal injury, what method can be employed to help increase cough effectiveness? (Shapiro, p 141)

_____

ANSWERS TO STUDY QUESTIONS

1. therapeutic application of inspiratory positive pressure to the airways

2. a. up
   b. down
   c. up
   d. down
   e. down
   f. up
   g. up

3. a. hypoventilation (inadequate V_T)

b. retained secretions (mucostasis)
c. prophylactic (after surgery adbominal or chest)

4. a. improve distribution of ventilation
b. deliver medication
c. improve and promote cough
d. decrease work of breathing
e. deeper breaths with better I : E ratios.

5. a. hyperventilation
b. excessive oxygenation
c. hyperinflation (air trapping)
d. decreased cardiac output
e. increased intracranial pressure
f. barotrauma
g. hemoptysis
h. gastric distenion
i. psychologic dependence

6. untreated pneumothorax

7. tiredness, breathing pattern, chest pain, color of patient, state of consciousness, check pulse, check blood pressure

8. a. gas inlet
b. ambient compartment
c. pressure compartment
d. metal filter
e. mainstream breathing hose connector
f. gas outlet to nebulization and exhalation port
g. flow rate control
h. sensitivity control
i. pressure control
j. air-mix control
k. hand timer rod
l. expiratory timer
m. pressure monometer

9. 50 psi

10. magnetism versus pressure

11. Mark 8 has expiratory flow switch that provides negative pressure to patient circuit. This negative pressure evacuates the gas in the patient circuit.

12. Mark 10: flow accelerator (adds flow to end of patient inspiratory cycle), no air-mix control
Mark 14: same as Mark 10 but larger pressure limit magnet to deliver higher pressures, finer sensitivity control (vernier)

13. no air-mix, PEEP and CPAP possibilities, time limiting is possible (apneustic hold)

14. adjustable reducing valve

15. Bennett valve

16. AP seris: electrical
PR seris: pneumatic

17. As you face the front of the PR series: right monometer—control; left monometer—patient
According to the picture: upper monometer—control pressure; lower monometer—patient pressure

18. PR-2: expiratory time control, peak flow control, negative pressure capabilities, terminal flow control, expiratory nebulization

19. Accumulator #1: exhalation
Accumulator #2: master (phases inspiration and expiration)
Accumulator #3: inhalation

20. a. check for leak, exhalation valve torn, Bennett valve or ceramic switch sticking
b. check sensitivity, pressure monometer, cycling control
c. check sensitivity, leak, gas source, manually cycle

21. Sustained maximal inspiration: deepest possible breath you can inspire with a breath hold at end inspiration
Incentive spirometry: device that allows a patient to perform SMI with an incentive goal

22. prophylactically, potentially more therapy, personnel time/cost minimized, negative inspiration versus positive inspiration

23. a. optimize lung inflation
b. optimize cough mechanism
c. allow early detection of acute pulmonary disease

24. alert, cooperative patient; preoperative teaching; no acute atelectasis pneumonia or retained secretions; FVC >15 ml/kg, IC >12 ml/kg, respiratory rate <25 BPM

25. patient education; explain device; proper positioning and technique; goal 2 times V_T, Q 1 hour $\times$ 6 to 10 breaths, 1 minute between breaths; slow, deep inspiration (5 to 15 sec) with a 3-second breath hold; evaluate patient goal and performance TID

26. a. hyperventilation (dizzyness, lightheadedness, tingling in extremities)
b. barotrauma (alveolar rupture)

27. a. flow-oriented
b. volume-oriented

28. Right Lung
1. apical

2. posterior
3. anterior
4. lateral
5. medial
6. superior
7. medial basal
8. anterior basal
9. lateral basal
10. posterior basal

   Left Lung
1–2. apical-posterior
   3. anterior
   4. superior
   5. inferior
   6. superior
   8. anterior basal
   9. lateral basal
   10. posterior basal

29. a. postural drainage
    b. chest percussion
    c. chest vibration
    d. cough training
    e. breathing retraining

30. a. prevent accumulation and improve mobilization of secretions
    b. improve efficiency and distribution of ventilation (decrease WOB)
    c. improve cardiopulmonary reserve using exercise techniques through reconditioning

31. prophylactic: preoperative high-risk, postoperative to mobilize secretions, neurologically damaged patient unable to cough, cystic fibrosis, bronchiectasis, and so on
    therapeutic: atelectasis due to secretions, retained secretions, musculoskeletal deformity (ineffective cough)

32. method of facilitating removal of secretions from tracheobronchial tree by proper positioning of the patient with the use of gravity

33. a. apical segments (upper lobes)
    b. anterior segment (upper lobes)
    c. posterior segment (left upper lobe)
    d. right middle lobe
    e. superior and inferior lingula (right middle lobes)
    f. posterior segment (lower lobes)
    g. anterior segment (lower lobes)
    h. superior segment (lower lobes)

34. empyema, pulmonary embolism, open wounds, untreated pneumothorax, flail chest, frank hemoptysis, orthopedic procedures, acute spinal cord injuries

35. unstable cardiac status, hypertension, head injuries, tracheoesophageal fistula, thoracic and abdominal surgery (some), COPD, recent meals and or tube feedings, diaphragmatic surgery

36. technique of rhythmically and alternately tapping the chest wall with cupped hands

37. cancer with known metastasis, anticoagulant therapy, active tuberculosis, osteoporotic changes, patient tolerance, chest tubes

38. shaking movement applied during exhalation; place one hand on top of the other and tense shoulders, keeping arms straight and apply vibration action

39. deep inspiration, closure of glottis, contraction of abdominal muscles, increase intrapulmonic pressure, open glottis, forceful and rapid exhalation

40. Have patient take a few deep breaths, then maximum inspiration with a breath hold; contract abdominal muscles, then cough twice in the same breath.

41. splint incision with towel or pillow, bend knees, or huff cough

42. Compress abdomen with an upward thrust under xiphoid process at end inspiration.

PRACTICE QUIZ

1. Which of the following statement(s) best describe the major therapeutic goals of IPPB?
   I. Decrease the respiratory rate.
   II. Maintain $Paco_2$ between 40 and 50 torr.
   III. Increase alveolar ventilation.
   IV. Decrease the mechanical and metabolic work of breathing.
   V. Prevent retention of tracheobronchial secretions.

    a. I, IV, V
    b. II, III, V
    c. I, III, IV, V
    d. III, IV, V
    e. I, II, III, IV, V

2. Bird ventilators function by means of which set of opposing forces?
    a. flow versus pressure
    b. time versus pressure
    c. magnetism versus pressure
    d. magnetism versus flow
    e. magnetism versus time

3. On the Bird Mark 10, the purpose of the flow accelerator cartridge is:
    a. to increase flow of gas for those who use a mask
    b. to prevent back-flow of gas through the ceramic switch
    c. to help close the Venturi gate at the end of inspiration
    d. to add an additional flow of gas into the patient circuit for leak compensation
    e. none of the above

4. The PR-2 cycles to expiration when:
    I. A set pressure is achieved.
    II. The rate control is set.
    III. The flow of gas to the patient is reduced to 1 to 3 l/min.
    a. I only
    b. II only
    c. III only
    d. I and III
    e. I, II, III

5. You receive an order to administer IPPB therapy to a postsurgical patient. You select an IPPB device and are checking its function prior to use. You find that the flow continues and cycling does not occur. Which of the following would be the probable cause?
    I. A sizeable leak in the circuit system
    II. The valve mechanism is stuck
    III. A dirty air entrainment filter
    IV. A hole in the Venturi system
    V. An internal leak in the machine
    a. I and III
    b. II, IV, V
    c. I, II, III, IV, V
    d. III and IV
    e. I, II, V

6. A patient receiving IPPB treatments via Bird with air-mix continually falls asleep and stops breathing during therapy. The therapist has to awaken the patient in order to continue therapy. Which statement best describes the situation?
    a. Respiratory alkalosis causes drowsiness.
    b. Respiratory acidosis causes drowsiness.
    c. Hypoxia is relieved and patient falls asleep.
    d. Cycling rhythm lulls the patient to sleep.
    e. IPPB causes cerebral hypoxia and the patient falls asleep.

7. As you treat a patient with IPPB, he complains of a tingling sensation in his fingertips and lightheadedness. Which of the following is the most likely cause?
    a. alveolar hyperventilation

    b. decreased cardiac output

    c. hyperoxygenation

    d. fatigue

    e. anxiety

8. Incentive spirometry, when used correctly and effectively, will change:
   - I. pH
   - II. Pa_{CO_2}
   - III. Pa_{O_2}
   a. II only
   b. III only
   c. I and II
   d. II and III
   e. I, II, III

9. Which of the following is *not* a goal of chest physical therapy?
   a. to improve effectiveness of a cough
   b. to relieve dyspnea
   c. to increase awareness of the muscle of respiration
   d. to improve blood gases
   e. to aid in the mobilization and removal of secretions

10. The physician orders chest physical therapy for a patient with an aspiration and subsequent pneumonia in his right middle lobe, how would the patient be positioned?
    a. head down 15 degrees supine
    b. head down 15 degrees rotated $\frac{1}{4}$ onto the left side
    c. head down 15 degrees rotated $\frac{1}{2}$ onto the right side
    d. head down 30 degrees lying on the left side
    e. none of the above

11. According to some authors, IPPB therapy is definitely contraindicated in patients presenting with which of the following?
    a. systemic hypertension
    b. pulmonary edema
    c. decreased intracranial pressure
    d. very recent myocardial infarction
    e. pneumothorax without chest tube in place

12. Which of the following statements best describes the difference betweeen IPPB and normal breathing?
    a. IPPB delivers greater volume during inspiration than normal breathing.
    b. During inspiration, the airway-alveolar pressure gradient is greater with IPPB than normal breathing.
    c. As compared with normal breathing, IPPB decreases both mechanical and metabolic work of breathing.
    d. At begin inspiration, intrapulmonic pressure is about -1 cmH_2O with IPPB as compared with -2 cmH_2O while breathing normally.
    e. none of the above

13. Which of the following would be inappropriate times for the application of postural drainage with chest percussion and vibration?
    - I. One half hour after a meal
    - II. One half hour after a tube feeding
    - III. One hour before administration of pain medication
    - IV. One hour before a meal
    a. I and III

b. II and IV
c. I, II, III
d. I, II, IV
e. II, III, IV

14. When the air-mix on a Bird Mark 7 is pushed in (to obtain 100% oxygen), with all other factors remaining the same, which of the following is most affected?
    a. inspiratory time
    b. medication nebulized
    c. pressure delivered
    d. sensitivity setting
    e. expiratory time

15. The tidal volume delivered by the Bird ventilator is determined by which of the following?
    I. Set pressure on the machine
    II. Patient's compliance
    III. Patient's airway pressure
    IV. Inspiratory flowrate
    V. Sensitivity setting
    a. I and II
    b. I, III, IV
    c. III, IV, V
    d. I, II, III, IV
    e. I, II, III, IV, V

16. The semi-Fowler's position best drains:
    a. apical segments
    b. middle lobes
    c. posterior basal segments
    d. lingular segments
    e. lower lobes

17. Which of the following is/are considered contraindications to incentive spirometry?
    I. Postoperative abdominal surgery
    II. Pneumonia
    III. Open heart surgery
    IV. Neuromuscular disorders
    V. Long-bone fractures
    a. I, II, III
    b. I and III
    c. II and IV
    d. IV only
    e. all of the above

18. What aspect(s) of the patient should be monitored during the administration of an IPPB treatment?
    I. The patient's respiratory rate before, during, and after the treatment
    II. The patient's sensorium
    III. The patient's pupil status
    IV. The patient's apical pulse
    V. The patient's chest should be auscultated
    a. I, II, V
    b. I, IV, V
    c. IV only
    d. I, II, IV, V
    e. I, II, III, IV, V

19. During an IPPB treatment, the I : E ratio that is most likely to decrease cardiac output the most would be:
    a. 1 : 1
    b. 1 : 7
    c. 1 : 3
    d. 0.5 : 1
    e. 1 : 4

20. In reference to "sensitivity" in the use of IPPB machines, the following is usually meant:
    a. the sensitivity of the device to gas flow
    b. the sensitivity of the device to pressure changes within the patient's lungs
    c. the effort required by the patient to stop the gas flow
    d. the effort required by the patient to start the gas flow
    e. none of the above

ANSWERS TO THE PRACTICE QUIZ

1. d	11. e
2. c	12. b
3. d	13. c
4. e	14. a
5. e	15. d
6. c	16. a
7. a	17. d
8. b	18. a
9. d	19. a
10. b	20. d

Chapter 9

AIRWAY MANAGEMENT

OUTLINE

TYPES OF AIRWAYS
Oropharyngeal
Nasopharyngeal
Oral Endotracheal
Nasal Endotracheal
Esophageal Obturator
Tracheostomy
AIRWAY CUFFS
Function
Pressures
Complications
Management
PROCEDURES
Intubation
Extubation

Cricothyroidotomy
Tracheostomy
SUCTIONING
Indications
Procedures
Complications
Adapters
INDICATIONS FOR ARTIFICIAL AIRWAYS
COMPLICATIONS OF ARTIFICIAL
    AIRWAYS
PRACTICE QUIZ

LEARNING OBJECTIVES

Upon completion of this unit, the individual will:

1. Be able to identify and label a variety of artificial airways.
2. Be able to discuss indications, management techniques, and complications of the airway cuffs.
3. Be able to describe the procedures for intubation, extubation, cricothyroidotomy, and tracheostomy.
4. Be able to recognize the indications and com-

plications of intubation, extubation, cricothyroidotomy, and tracheostomy.
5. Be able to describe indications, procedures, complications, and special equipment necessary for suctioning.
6. Be able to describe the indications of artificial airways.
7. Be able to describe the complications of artificial airways.

123

REFERENCES

Shapiro, BA, Harrison, RA, Kacmarek, RM, and Cane, RD: Clinical Application of Respiratory Care, ed 3. Year Book Medical Publishers, Chicago, 1985.

McPherson, SP: Respiratory Therapy Equipment, ed 3. CV Mosby, St Louis, 1985.

Eubanks, DH, and Bone, RC: Comprehensive Respiratory Care. CV Mosby, St Louis, 1985.

Harwood, R, McNeily, S, and Cline, A: Respiratory Therapy Review, ed 5. Kettering College of Medical Arts, School of Respiratory Care, Dayton, 1985.

Burton, G, and Hodgkin, J: Respiratory Care: A Guide to Clinical Practice, ed 2. JB Lippincott, Philadelphia, 1984

Roberts, JT: Fundamentals of Tracheal Intubation. Grune & Stratton, New York, 1983.

Kacmarek, RM, Mack, CW, and Dimas, S: The Essentials of Respiratory Therapy, ed 2. Year Book Medical Publishers, Chicago, 1985.

STUDY QUESTIONS

1. Identify the devices in Figures 9–1 and 9–2. (Eubanks, p 491; Shapiro, p 216)

   a. Fig. 9–1: _____

   b. Fig. 9–2: _____

2. Which of the airways depicted in question 1 is poorly tolerated by the alert or semicomatose patient? (Kacmarek, p 381; Shapiro, p 216)

   _____

3. Label the device in Figure 9–3. (Shapiro, p 213)

   _____

4. List four indications for use of the device depicted in Figure 9–3. (Kacmarek, p 385)

   a. _____

   b. _____

   c. _____

   d. _____

5. On what three assumptions is the use of the EOA based? (Kacmarek, p 385; Shapiro, p 230)

   a. _____

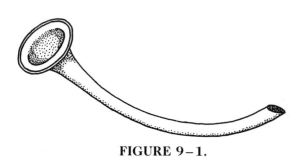

FIGURE 9–1.

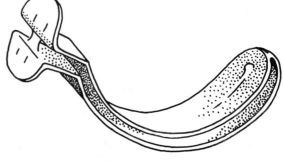

FIGURE 9–2.

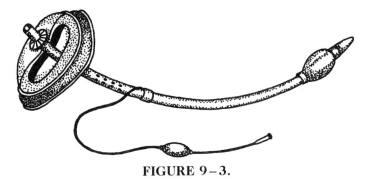

FIGURE 9–3.

b. _____

c. _____

_____

6. What precautions should be taken upon the removal of the esophageal obturator? (Kacmarek, p 381; Shapiro, p 233)

_____

7. List five reasons the oral endotracheal tube is not recommended for long-term use. (Kacmarek, p 381; Shapiro, p 233)

a. _____

b. _____

c. _____

d. _____

e. _____

8. Identify the devices in Figures 9–4, 9–5, and 9–6. (Eubanks, p 513)

a. Fig. 9–4: _____

b. Fig. 9–5: _____

c. Fig. 9–6: _____

9. Match the description of the tube on the left to the names listed on the right. (Kacmarek, p 387; Shapiro, p 261)

_____ double lumen endotracheal tube   a. fenestrated

_____ tube allows to instill solutions   b. Cole

_____ can assess ability to extubate   c. tracheostomy

_____ allows patient to verbalize   d. Pitt speaking

_____ airway of choice for long-term patient   e. Deane tube

_____ tube for jet ventilation   f. Carlens

_____ pediatric tube, tip smaller   g. Hi-Lo jet

10. How often should a tracheostomy tube be changed, and why? (Shapiro, p 283)

_____

_____

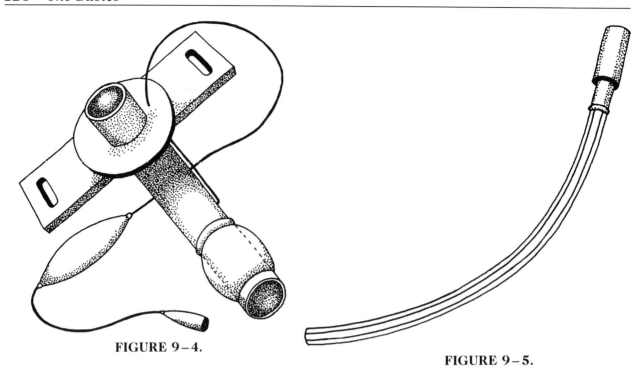

FIGURE 9–4.

FIGURE 9–5.

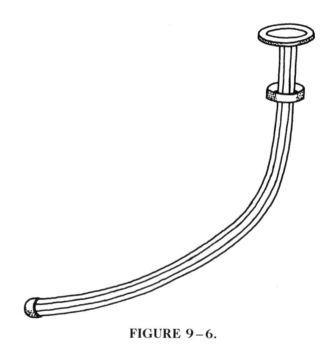

FIGURE 9–6.

11. List some common synthetic material used in the manufacturing of artificial airways. (Eubanks, p 505; Shapiro, p 240)

a. _____

b. _____

c. _____

d. _____

e. _____

12. What is the most widely used plastic for artificial airways? (Eubanks, p 505; Shapiro, p 240)

   _____

13. Identify the devices in Figures 9–7 through 9–10. (Kacmarek, p 385; Shapiro, p 261)

   a. Fig. 9–7: _____

   b. Fig. 9–8: _____

   c. Fig. 9–9: _____

   d. Fig. 9–10: _____

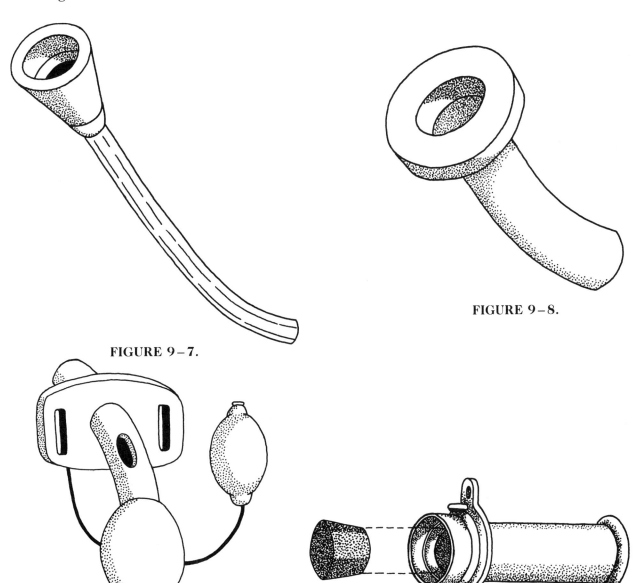

FIGURE 9–8.

FIGURE 9–7.

FIGURE 9–9.

FIGURE 9–10.

14. Identify the devices in Figures 9–11 through 9–14. (MacPherson, p 164)

    a. Fig. 9–11: _____

    b. Fig. 9–12: _____

    c. Fig. 9–13: _____

    d. Fig. 9–14: _____

15. List three advantages of tubes made of silicon. (Shapiro, p 240)

    a. _____

    b. _____

    c. _____

16. What must be considered prior to ETO sterilization of a tube composed of polyvinylchloride? (Shapiro, p 240)

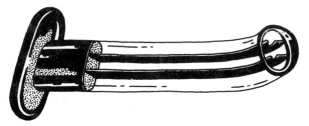

FIGURE 9–11.

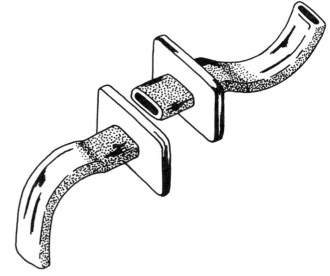

FIGURE 9–12.

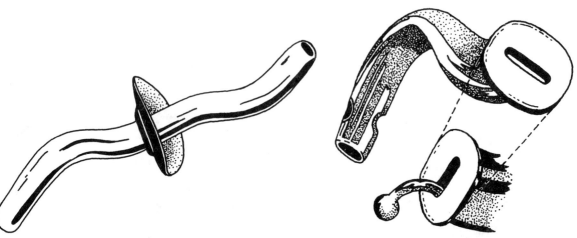

FIGURE 9–13.

FIGURE 9–14.

17. Which of the following describes the nasopharyngeal airway? Circle the correct letter. (Eubanks, p 496; Kacmarek, p 381)
    a. It is used as a bite block.
    b. Nasal necrosis is of no concern.
    c. It is better tolerated than the oral airway in alert patients.
    d. It should be moved from one nares to the other hourly.

18. List three steps to correctly prepare the fenestrated tracheostomy tube for patient use. (Kacmarek, p 383; Shapiro, p 261)

    a. _____

    b. _____

    c. _____

19. Fill in the blanks with the specific area of circulation that will be damaged by cuff pressures listed below. (Kacmarek, p 386; Shapiro, p 273)

    a. less than 5 mmHG: _____

    b. less than 18 mmHG: _____

    c. less than 30 mmHG: _____

20. The foam cuff brand name is _____. (Eubanks, p 502; Kacmarek, p 387)

21. Give considerations to keep in mind when inserting a tube with a foam cuff. (Eubanks, p 502; Kacmarek, p 387)

    _____

    _____

22. List two functions of the airway cuff. (Shapiro, p 273)

    a. _____

    b. _____

23. Cuff pressures should be kept below _____ mmHg to maintain tracheal capillary blood flow. (Shapiro, p 276)

24. List four effects of high lateral tracheal wall pressure in the order in which they would occur. (Kacmarek, p 386; Shapiro, p 274)

    a. _____

    b. _____

    c. _____

    d. _____

25. Explain the minimal leak technique. (Eubanks, p 503; Kacmarek, p 387)

    _____

    _____

26. Outside the surgical suite, only _____ residual volume _____ pressure cuffs are utilized. (Kacmarek, p 387; Shapiro, p 276)

27. What are the two most common types of laryngoscope blades? (Eubanks, p 508; Shapiro, p 221)

    a. _____

    b. _____

28. Give a description of the correct anatomic placement of the straight laryngoscope blade during endotracheal intubation. (Eubanks, p 508; Shapiro, p 221)

    _____

29. Describe the correct anatomic placement of the curved laryngoscope blade during endotracheal intubation. (Eubanks, p 508; Shapiro, p 221)

    _____

30. Describe the patient's position in Figure 9–15 and the use of the position in endotracheal intubation. (Eubanks, p 484; Shapiro, p 223)

    a. position: _____

    b. purpose: _____

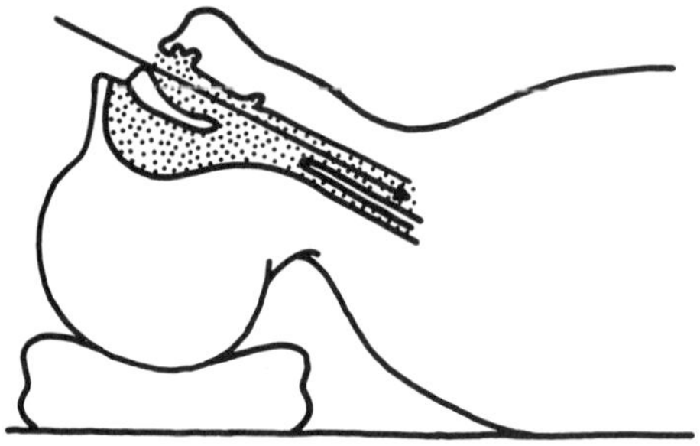

FIGURE 9–15.

31. In which hand is the standard laryngoscope made to be used? (Eubanks, p 508; Shapiro, p 224)

    _____

32. Label the devices in Figures 9–16 through 9–21 and provide a brief description of the function of each. (Eubanks, p 507)

    a. Fig. 9–16: _____

    b. Fig. 9–17: _____

    c. Fig. 9–18: _____

    d. Fig. 9–19: _____

    e. Fig. 9–20: _____

    f. Fig. 9–21: _____

33. The two primary landmarks for intubation are: (Eubanks, p 511; Shapiro, p 224)

    a. _____

    b. _____

34. List three methods to ensure correct endotracheal tube placement. (Shapiro, p 226)

    a. _____

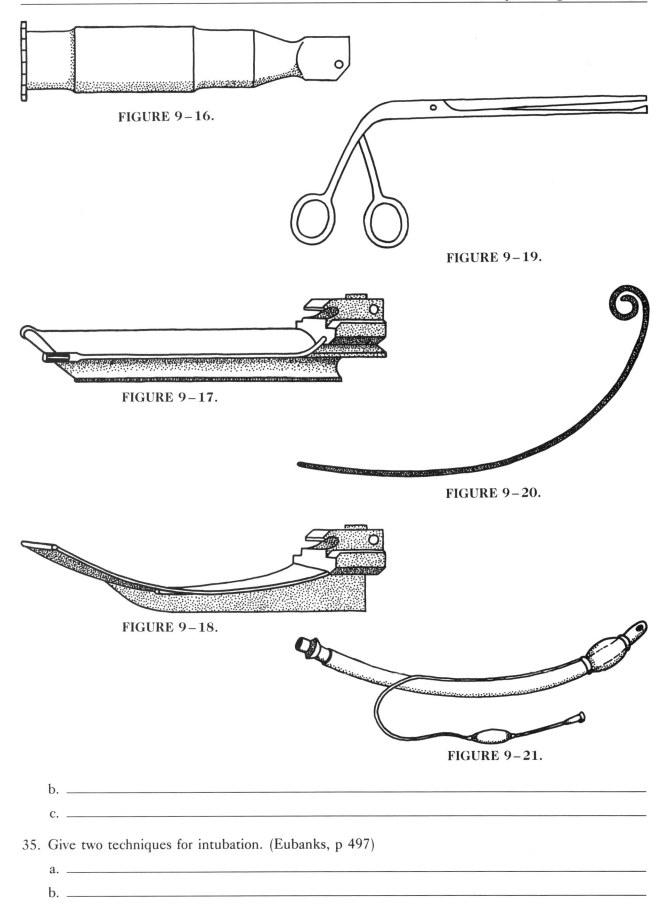

FIGURE 9–16.

FIGURE 9–19.

FIGURE 9–17.

FIGURE 9–20.

FIGURE 9–18.

FIGURE 9–21.

b. _____

c. _____

35. Give two techniques for intubation. (Eubanks, p 497)

   a. _____

   b. _____

36. List six complications associated with an attempted intubation. (Eubanks, p 503)

    a. _____   d. _____

    b. _____   e. _____

    c. _____   f. _____

37. Give four indications for intubation. (Eubanks, p 496)

    a. _____

    b. _____

    c. _____

    d. _____

38. Which complication of intubation is the most serious, and why? (Eubanks, p 496)

    _____

39. To maintain the artificial airway it is important to: (Shapiro, p 242)

    a. Provide _____ to avoid dehydration.

    b. _____ as needed to keep tube clear.

    c. Check _____ _____ often to ensure minimal tissue damage.

40. Give a description of correct extubation procedures. (Shapiro, p 261)

    _____

    _____

    _____

    _____

41. List three common complications of extubation. (Shapiro, p 261)

    a. _____

    b. _____

    c. _____

42. Give two reasons to reintubate postextubation. (Shapiro, p 261)

    a. _____

    b. _____

43. What pharmacologic agent may be given to decrease the severity of the complications in question 42? (Shapiro, p 260)

    _____

44. What is the emergency surgical procedure to enter the trachea? (Eubanks, p 484; Kacmarek, p 385; Shapiro, p 229)

    _____

45. Label the landmarks in Figure 9–22. (Shapiro, p 229)

    a. _____

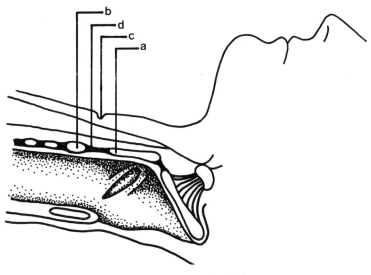

FIGURE 9–22.

b. _____

c. _____

d. _____

46. The incision is made at what anatomic location when performing the cricothyroidotomy? (Kacmarek, p 385)

_____

47. List three drugs that are often used during nasotracheal intubation, and give the reason(s) for using each of these drugs. (Shapiro, p 233)

a. _____

b. _____

c. _____

48. What is the most significant problem postextubation? (Shapiro, p 261)

_____

49. List three ways to treat the problem noted in question 48.

a. _____

b. _____

c. _____

50. List four complications of airway suctioning. (Kacmarek, p 388; Shapiro, p 249)

a. _____

b. _____

c. _____

d. _____

51. Give the way to prevent each complication listed in question 50. (Kacmarek, p 388; Shapiro, p 249)

a. _____

b. _____

c. _____

d. _____

52. A suction catheter should not occupy more than _____ of the internal diameter of the tube being suctioned. (Kacmarek, p 389)

53. Give the formula for converting mm to F (French) sizes. (Kacmarek, p 389; Shapiro, p 250)

_____

54. Give the formula for converting F sizes to mm. (Kacmarek, p 389)

_____

55. Most suction catheters are expressed in _____ sizes. (Kacmarek, p 389; Shapiro, p 249)

56. Most endotracheal tubes are expressed in _____ sizes. (Kacmarek, p 389; Shapiro, p 249)

57. List five characteristics of the ideal suction catheter. (Kacmarek, p 389; Shapiro, p 250)

a. _____

b. _____

c. _____

d. _____

e. _____

58. List three purposes of suctioning. (Shapiro, p 248)

a. _____

b. _____

c. _____

59. List three indications for suction and the clinical signs of each. (Eubanks, p 517)

Indications	Clinical Signs
a. _____	a. _____
b. _____	b. _____
c. _____	c. _____

60. Give acceptable pressure ranges for vacuum regulators. (Eubanks, p 517; Kacmarek, p 389)

a. Adult: _____ mmHg

b. Child: _____ mmHg

c. Infant: _____ mmHg

61. Circle the letter(s) of the statements that are true of the correct procedure for suctioning. (Eubanks, p 519; Kacmarek, p 389)

a. A sterile glove and catheter are used each time.
b. Suctioning should be done every 2 hours.
c. If secretions are too thick, raise the vacuum level.
d. Frequent suctioning may cause a hemorrhage.
e. You may instill 5 to 10 ml of saline to thin secretions.
f. The ideal suction catheter is 18 French reusable.

62. Label the suction adapter in Figure 9–23. (Shapiro, p 252)

   a. _____

   b. _____

   c. _____

63. What is the purpose of the device in Figure 9–23? (Shapiro, p 252)

   _____

   _____

64. Label the device in Figure 9–24. (Harwood, p G-14)

   a. _____

   b. _____

   c. _____

65. The device depicted in Figure 9–24 is a _____ . It is used
   to _____. (Harwood, p G-14)

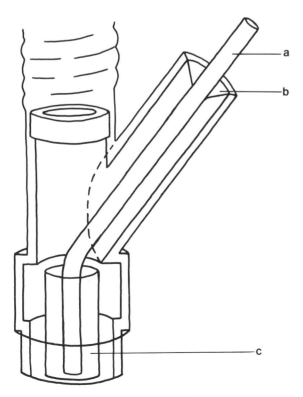

FIGURE 9–23.

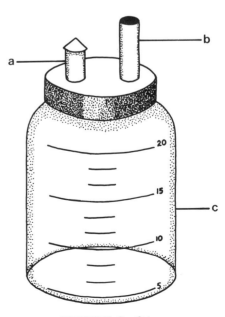

FIGURE 9–24.

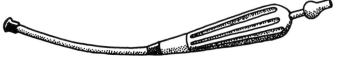

FIGURE 9–25

66. Consider Figure 9–25. (Eubanks, p 518)

    a. It is called: _____

    b. It is used to: _____

67. It is best to collect sputum specimens at what time of day? (Eubanks, p 735)

    _____

68. Convert the following: (Kacmarek, p 389)

    a. 10F = _____ mm

    b. 14F = _____ mm

    c. 18F = _____ mm

69. List two causes of obstruction in the upper airway. (Eubanks, p 483)

    a. _____

    b. _____

70. What is the cardinal sign of a partial airway obstruction? (Kacmarek, p 487)

    _____

71. List three signs of complete airway obstruction. (Eubanks, p 485; Kacmarek, p 487)

    a. _____

    b. _____

    c. _____

72. What is the treatment of a soft tissue obstruction? (Eubanks, p 485; Kacmarek, p 487)

    _____

73. What is the premier advantage the nasopharyngeal airway has over the oropharyngeal airway? (Eubanks, p 496; Kacmarek, p 487)

    _____

74. Define artificial airway. (Eubanks, p 492)

    _____

    _____

75. List four indications for the use of an artificial airway. (Eubanks, p 492; Kacmarek, p 381)

    a. _____

    b. _____

    c. _____

    d. _____

76. What are the four airway protective reflexes present in the correctly functioning respiratory system? (Shapiro, p 218)

    a. _____

    b. _____

    c. _____

    d. _____

77. What is the emergency airway of choice when there will be prolonged closed chest massage or other resuscitative efforts that may take a long period of time? (Shapiro, p 221)

    _____

78. When is nasotracheal intubation indicated? (Shapiro, p 233)

    _____

79. List four reasons why the nasotracheal intubation procedure is indicated for long-term intubation. (Shapiro, p 233)

    a. _____

    b. _____

    c. _____

    d. _____

80. List six limitations or hazards of long-term nasotracheal intubation. (Shapiro, p 234)

    a. _____   d. _____

    b. _____   e. _____

    c. _____   f. _____

81. What is considered to be the artificial airway of choice for the long-term compromised airway? (Eubanks, p 512; Shapiro, p 236)

    _____

82. Give six reasons why the device listed in question 81 is the airway of choice for the long-term patient. (Eubanks, p 512; Shapiro, p 236)

    a. _____   d. _____

    b. _____   e. _____

    c. _____   f. _____

83. List four significant concerns for establishment and maintenance of the artificial airway. (Kacmarek, p 382; Shapiro, p 220)

    a. _____

    b. _____

    c. _____

    d. _____

84. List the immediate complications of tracheostomy. (Eubanks, p 513; Kacmarek, p 382; Shapiro, p 237)

    a. _____

b. _____

c. _____

d. _____

85. List the late (post–24 hour) complications of the tracheostomy procedure. (Eubanks, p 512; Kacmarek, p 382; Shapiro, p 238)

a. _____

b. _____

c. _____

d. _____

86. Give two properties a gas should have while being delivered to a patient with an artificial airway. (Shapiro, p 253)

a. _____

b. _____

87. Why must we add the qualities listed in question 86? (Shapiro, p 253)

_____

88. List five common causes for artificial airway obstruction. (Shapiro, p 258)

a. _____

b. _____

c. _____

d. _____

e. _____

89. Give three steps to be taken to correct a possible obstruction in the artificial airway. (Shapiro, p 258)

a. _____

b. _____

c. _____

90. If you cannot pass a suction catheter through an artificial airway, you should _____. (Shapiro, p 258)

91. Give eight laryngotracheal complications of artificial airways. (Shapiro, p 266)

a. _____   e. _____

b. _____   f. _____

c. _____   g. _____

d. _____   h. _____

92. What is the cardinal sign of glottic edema? (Shapiro, p 266)

_____

93. Define tracheal stenosis. (Shapiro, p 270)

_____

_____

94. List six causes of tracheal stenosis. (Shapiro, p 272)

a. _____   d. _____

b. _____   e. _____

c. _____   f. _____

ANSWERS TO STUDY QUESTIONS

1. a. nasopharyngeal airway
    b. oral airway

2. the oropharyngeal airway

3. esophageal obturator airway (EOA)

4. a. emergency ventilation when intubation impossible
    b. untrained personnel
    c. short-term use
    d. better than bag-mask ventilation

5. a. esophagus easier to intubate than trachea
    b. adequate mask seal can be maintained
    c. seals off lower esophagus to avoid regurgitation and stomach inflation.

6. intubate prior to removal, prevents the aspiration of stomach contents

7. a. vagal stimulation
    b. difficulty stabilizing
    c. poor toleration in semiconscious or conscious
    d. may require bite block
    e. inadvertent extubation common

8. a. tracheostomy tube
    b. inner cannula
    c. obturator

9. f, e, a, d, c, g, b

10. Tracheostomy tubes should not be changed as long as they are functioning properly and there is no infection present. This is to prevent undue trauma.

11. a. teflon
    b. nylon
    c. polyethylene
    d. silicone
    e. polyvinylchloride

12. polyvinylchloride

13. a. inner cannula
    b. outer cannula plug
    c. fenestrated tube
    d. the tracheal button

14. a. Cath-Guide Guedel
    b. Rosser
    c. Safar
    d. Connel Waters

15. a. can autoclave
    b. human tissue will not adhere to it
    c. will not remain wet when in contact with body fluids

16. PVC products need to be completely aerated or dried prior to processing with ETO

17. c

18. a. Remove solid inner cannula.
    b. Deflate cuff.
    c. Place cork in opening of outer cannula.

19. a. lymphatic flow obstruction, edema
    b. venous flow obstruction, edema
    c. stop arterial flow, necrosis

20. Kaamen-Wilkinsen

21. deflate cuff and flatten it, insert tube, remove syringe and allow cuff to resume shape, cuff exerts below 20 mmHg

22. a. stabilize artificial airway
    b. protect the airway

23. 5

24. a. edema
    b. epithelial ischemia and necrosis
    c. sloughing of mucosa
    d. necrotic cartilage

25. suction above cuff, deflate cuff, suction airway, insert 10-cc syringe filled with air, auscultate,

fill with air until no sound, slowly withdraw air until hear small leak

26. high, low

27. a. straight
    b. curved

28. the tip of the straight blade is placed under the epiglottis

29. the tip of the curved blade fits into the vallecula

30. a. sniffing position
    b. used to align the pharyngeal, laryngeal, and oral axis during direct laryngoscopy

31. left

32. a. laryngoscope: aids in visualization with light
    b. straight blade (Miller): place below epiglottis
    c. curved blade: place in vallecula (MacIntosh)
    d. Magill forceps: used in nasotracheal intubation to guide
    e. stylette: used to alter shape of tube
    f. endotracheal tube

33. a. epiglottis
    b. arytenoid cartilages

34. a. auscultate
    b. x-ray
    c. visual chest inspection

35. a. nasotracheal intubation
    b. oral intubation

36. a. laryngospasm
    b. aspiration
    c. hypertension
    d. bradycardia
    e. broken teeth
    f. laceration of mucosa
    g. hemorrhage

37. a. relief of upper airway obstruction
    b. protection of airway
    c. bronchial hygiene
    d. support ventilation

38. laryngospasm: may cause death; aspiration: may cause infection

39. a. humidity
    b. suction
    c. cuff pressures

40. Explain procedure to patient, preoxygenate, suction trachea, oropharynx, and nasopharynx, preoxygenate, ask patient to take in deepest breath possible, at peak inspiration deflate cuff and remove tube, postoxygenate; evaluate patient for signs of obstruction, stridor, and difficulty breathing.

41. a. laryngospasm
    b. glottic edema
    c. subglottic edema

42. a. laryngospasm: severe respiratory distress
    b. glottic edema: marked inspiratory stridor

43. racemic epinephrine

44. cricothyroidotomy

45. a. thyroid cartilage
    b. cricoid cartilage
    c. incision point
    d. circothyroid membrane

46. cricothyroid membrane

47. a. lidocaine to act as an anesthetic
    b. diazepam to sedate
    c. cocaine to provide vasoconstriction

48. laryngospasm

49. a. humidity
    b. muscle relaxant
    c. increase oxgyen percent

50. a. hypoxemia
    b. dysrhythmias
    c. hypotension
    d. atelectasis

51. a. pre and post oxygenate
    b. correct technique
    c. pre and post oxygenate and correct technique
    d. use correct size catheter

52. one half

53. $mm = \dfrac{F - 2}{4}$

54. $F = 4\,(mm + 2)$

55. French

56. mm

57. a. safe non trauma causing material
    b. minimal friction production
    c. 20 – 22 cm long
    d. smooth ends
    e. side holes

58. a. clear airway of secretions
    b. produce a cough
    c. obtain a sputum specimen

59. Indications
   a. secretion build-up
   b. decreased or depressed cough
   c. obstruction

Clinical Signs
   a. coughing and high pressures
   b. build-up of secretions
   c. cough, increased pressures, decreased air movement, unable to pass suction catheter

60. a. 80 to 120 mmHg
   b. 60 to 80 mmHg
   c. 40 to 60 mmHg

61. a, d, e

62. a. catheter
   b. one-way valve
   c. endotracheal tube

63. It allows for suctioning without disconnecting the patient who is being mechanically ventilated.

64. a. vacuum adapter
   b. the catheter connection
   c. the specimen trap

65. Lukens trap, collect a sterile sputum specimen

66. a. Yankauer-type tonsil suction
   b. oropharyngeal suctioning

67. A.M.

68. a. 2
   b. 3
   c. 4

69. a. soft tissue obstruction
   b. laryngeal obstruction

70. noisy inspiration-snoring sound, low-grade tonal quality

71. a. marked inspiratory effort without air movement
   b. sternal, intercostal and epigastric retractions
   c. strong contraction of accessory muscles of ventilation

72. Treatment of a soft tissue obstruction is to relieve the cause of the obstruction.

73. The nasopharyngeal airway is better tolerated by the alert or semiconscious patient.

74. artificial airway: a tube inserted into the trachea that bypasses the upper airway and laryngeal structures as integral parts of the total airway

75. a. relief of airway obstruction
   b. protect the airway
   c. facilitate tracheal suctioning
   d. facilitate prolonged artificial ventilation

76. a. pharyngeal reflex
   b. laryngeal reflex
   c. tracheal reflex
   d. carinal reflex

77. oral endotracheal tube

78. for long-term conscious patient

79. a. easier to suction
   b. easier to stabilize
   c. better toleration by patients
   d. safer to attach to equipment

80. a. nasal necrosis
   b. sinus obstruction
   c. blocks the opening of the eustachian tubes
   d. cuff rupture during insertion
   e. deviation of septum
   f. poor toleration of maintenance feeding

81. tracheostomy tube

82. a. easy to stabilize
   b. easy to suction
   c. less resistance to airflow
   d. easy to attach to equipment
   e. tolerated well
   f. patient can eat freely

83. a. infection
   b. loss of personal dignity
   c. inability to speak
   d. trauma

84. a. hemorrhage
   b. pneumothorax
   c. air embolism
   d. subcutaneous and mediastinal emphysema

85. a. infection
   b. hemorrhage
   c. airway obstruction
   d. dysfunction of swallowing
   e. tracheoesophageal fistula

86. a. humidity
   b. heat

87. Normal mechanisms to provide these qualities are bypassed.

88. a. kink in tube
   b. slip/herniated cuff
   c. plugs in lumen
   d. collapsed tube
   e. bevel impinged on wall of carina

89. a. manipulate the tube
    b. deflate the cuff
    c. attempt to pass a catheter

90. remove the tube

91. a. sore throat
    b. glottic edema
    c. subglottic edema
    d. ulceration of tracheal mucosa
    e. vocal cord ulceration
    f. vocal cord paralysis
    g. laryngotracheal web

    h. stenosis

92. inspiratory stridor

93. a scarring of the trachea caused by the healing process, which results in stricture of the airway

94. a. cuff pressure
    b. time
    c. movement
    d. decreased perfusion
    e. tube toxicity
    f. infection

PRACTICE QUIZ

1. Which of the following airways would be the airway of choice for a semicomatose patient with a partial airway obstruction?
   a. tracheostomy tube
   b. endotracheal tube
   c. nasopharyngeal tube
   d. oropharyngeal tube
   e. nasotracheal tube

2. A patient is intubated with a nasotracheal tube that is size 8 mm. What size suction catheter is the largest that should be used to suction this patient's airway?
   a. 18 French
   b. 16 French
   c. 14 French
   d. 12 French
   e. 10 French

3. All of the following are indications for the use of artificial airways, *except*:
   a. facilitate prolonged artificial ventilation
   b. facilitate tracheal suctioning
   c. airway protection
   d. relief of airway obstruction
   e. oxygenation

4. Which of the following are complications of airway suctioning?
      I. Dysrhythmia
     II. Atelectasis
    III. Hypoxemia
     IV. Bradycardia
      V. Hypotension
   a. I, IV, V
   b. I, II, III
   c. I, II, III, IV
   d. II, IV, V
   e. I, II, III, IV, V

5. A patient arrives in the emergency room with an esophopharyngeal airway in place. The patient is apneic. The correct procedure at this time would be to:
   a. suction and remove the EOA, then intubate

b. intubate the airway and leave the EOA in place
c. intubate the airway and then remove the EOA
d. insert NG tube, remove EOA, and intubate the airway
e. remove EOA and intubate the patient

6. The curved laryngoscope blade is placed:
   a. in the vallecula
   b. under the rima vestibula
   c. under the glottis to expose the epiglottis
   d. under the epiglottis
   e. under the larynx

7. "Z-79" on the side of an endotracheal tube stands for:
   a. a committee that sets standards for purity of tubes
   b. a designation that the tube has a low pressure cuff
   c. a committee that sets standards for tube usage
   d. a committee that sets standards for tubes and cuffs
   e. all of the above

8. The correct amount of suction of vacuum pressure for a child is:
   a. 40 to 60 mmHg
   b. 60 to 80 mmHg
   c. 80 to 100 mmHg
   d. 80 to 120 mmHg
   e. 100 to 120 mmHg

9. Immediately following extubation, the therapist notices that the patient has inspiratory stridor. This is the cardinal sign of which of the following?
   a. glottic edema
   b. bronchospasm
   c. tracheoesophageal fistula
   d. respiratory distress
   e. nothing; this is a normal part of extubation

10. Which of the following should be at the bedside during an endotracheal extubation procedure?
    I. Racemic epinephrine
    II. Suction source with sterile catheter
    III. Laryngoscope and endotracheal intubation equipment
    IV. Manual resuscitator
    V. Oxygen source
    a. II, III, IV, V
    b. I, III, IV
    c. I, II, IV, V
    d. I, II, III, IV
    e. I, II, III, IV, V

11. The _____ is a relatively safe procedure that could be used in establishing an airway with a minimum amount of training.
    a. nasotracheal intubation
    b. orotracheal intubation
    c. esophageal airway
    d. cricothyrotomy
    c. none of the above

12. Magill forceps are generally used in which procedure?
    a. cricothyrotomy

    b. extubation
    c. nasotracheal intubation
    d. tracheostomy
    e. oral intubation

13. When using a tracheostomy tube, what is the function of the obturator?
    a. It is used for breaking up dried secretions.
    b. It is used in decannulation.
    c. It aids the patient in speaking.
    d. It facilitates tube insertion
    e. When the patient is eating, it prevents aspiration.

14. Which of the following can be considered true of the tracheobronchial suctioning procedure?
    I. Suctioning should only take place during insertion of the catheter.
    II. Oxygenation should take place before and after the procedure.
    III. Catheters should be left in 20 to 30 seconds.
    IV. Suction only when there is evidence of secretions.
    V. The ECG should be monitored during the procedure.
    a. I, II, IV
    b. II, IV, V
    c. I, II, IV, V
    d. II, III, V
    e. I, II, III, IV, V

15. Which manufacturer produces an ET tube that has a cuff inflated with air at atmospheric pressure?
    a. Kaamen-Wilkinson
    b. Foregger
    c. Shiley
    d. Lanz
    e. Portex

16. Which of the following are considered "late" complications of tracheostomy?
    I. Hemorrhage
    II. Airway obstruction
    III. T-E fistula
    IV. Infection
    V. Dysfunction of swallowing process
    a. II, III, IV
    b. III, IV
    c. I, II, V
    d. I, II, III, IV
    e. I, II, III, IV, V

17. Which of the following are considered "early" complications of tracheostomy?
    I. Hemorrhage
    II. Pneumothorax
    III. Infection
    IV. Subcutaneous emphysema
    V. Air embolism
    a. I, III, IV
    b. II, III, V
    c. I, II, III
    d. I, II, IV, V
    e. I, II, III, IV, V

18. Which of the following statements are true of the Carlins endotracheal tube?

I. It has 16 holes in the lumen.
II. It has a double lumen.
III. It is used for emergency intubation.
IV. The right lumen extends into the right mainstem.
V. It has a foam cuff.
a. I, III
b. II, V
c. II, IV
d. I, III, IV
e. III, IV

19. When properly placed, the fenestrated tracheostomy tube allows the patient to:
    I. Breathe around the tube and through the fenestration
    II. Demonstrate the ability to handle secretions
    III. Speak
    IV. Demonstrate the ability to protect his airway
    V. Demonstrate the ability to function without an artificial airway
    a. I, IV, V
    b. I, II, III
    c. II, IV, V
    d. I, III, IV
    e. I, II, III, IV, V

20. Which of the following statements concerning laryngeal complications of endotracheal intubation are true?
    I. Treat sore throat with humidity.
    II. Inspiratory stridor is the sign of glottic edema.
    III. Subglottic edema is more common in children than in adults.
    IV. Laryngotracheal web is a common complication.
    V. Subglottic edema is the most serious postextubation complication.
    a. I, II, V
    b. I, II, III
    c. II, IV
    d. I, III, IV
    e. I, II, III, IV, V

ANSWERS TO THE PRACTICE QUIZ

1. d	11. c
2. d	12. c
3. e	13. d
4. e	14. b
5. c	15. a
6. a	16. a
7. d	17. d
8. b	18. c
9. a	19. e
10. e	20. b

Chapter 10

INFECTION CONTROL

Outline

TERMINOLOGY
PHYSICAL METHODS OF STERILIZATION
  AND DISINFECTION
Incineration
Filtration
Dry Heat
Ionizing Radiation
Autoclave
Pasteurization

CHEMICAL METHODS OF STERILIZATION
  AND DISINFECTION
Alcohols
Aldehydes
Ethylene Oxide
Iodines
Phenols
HANDWASHING TECHNIQUES
PRACTICE QUIZ

Learning Objectives

Upon completion of this unit, the individual will:

1. Define the terminology associated with infection control.
2. List the physical and chemical methods of sterilization.
3. List the physical and chemical methods of disinfection.
4. Describe the processes involved with each method of sterilization and disinfection
5. List the limitations of each method of sterilization and disinfection.
6. Discuss how each technique destroys bacteria.
7. List the methods used in monitoring the effectiveness of sterilization.
8. Differentiate between acid and alkaline glutaraldehyde.
9. Explain handwashing techniques and their importance in the hospital environment.
10. Describe the universal isolation procedure as outlined by the Centers for Disease Control.

REFERENCES

Barnes, TA: Respiratory Care Practice. Year Book Medical Publishers, Chicago, 1988.

Burton, G, and Hodgkin, J: Respiratory Care: A Guide to Clinical Practice, ed 2. JB Lippincott, Philadelphia, 1984.

Egan, DF, Sheldon, RL, and Spearman, CB: Egan's Fundamentals of Respiratory Therapy, ed 4. CV Mosby, St Louis, 1982.

Eubanks, D, and Bone, R: Comprehensive Respiratory Care. CV Mosby, St Louis, 1985.

Kacmarek, RM, Mack, CW, and Dimas, S: The Essentials of Respiratory Therapy, ed 2. Year Book Medical Publishers, Chicago, 1985.

STUDY QUESTIONS

1. Define the following terms: (Burton, p 427; Kacmarek, p 347)

   a. antisepsis: _____

   b. asepsis: _____

   c. antimicrobial: _____

   d. bactericidal: _____

   e. bacteriostatic: _____

   f. disinfection: _____

   g. nosocomial: _____

   h. sterilization: _____

2. Match the word on the left with the definition on the right. (Barnes, p 754; Kacmarek, p 347)

   a. transient flora
   b. resident flora
   c. sterility
   d. sanitization
   e. surveillance

   _____ bacterial residue in the openings of the skin, not eliminated by handwashing

   _____ destruction of all microorganisms

   _____ a baseline of information on infection and frequency

   _____ reduction of the population of microorganisms on inanimate objects

   _____ application of measure to promote health

3. List five physical methods of sterilization or disinfection. (Barnes, p 574; Kacmarek, p 347)

   a. _____   d. _____

   b. _____   e. _____

   c. _____

4. Describe the process of incineration as a method of sterilization. (Barnes, p 574; Burton, p 429; Kacmarek, p 347)

   _____

   _____

_____

_____

5. Describe the process and application of filtration techniques in respiratory care. (Barnes, p 574; Kacmarek, p 347)

_____

_____

_____

6. List the conditions that must be met to ensure that dry heat sterilization will occur. (Barnes, p 575; Burton, p 430)

   a. time: _____

   b. temperature: _____

7. Discuss the materials on which dry heat is used most often, and why. (Barnes, p 575; Burton, p 430; Kacmarek, p 347)

_____

_____

8. Ionizing radiation is a sterilization technique most often used by manufacturers. Why don't hospitals use this method of sterilization? (Barnes, p 575; Burton, p 430)

_____

_____

9. Describe the conditions that must be met to achieve sterilization through use of the autoclave. (Barnes, p 575; Burton, p 430; Kacmarek, p 347)

   a. steam pressure _____ temperature _____ time _____

   b. steam pressure _____ temperature _____ time _____

10. How does the autoclaving process destroy microorganisms? (Barnes, p 576; Burton, p 430; Kacmarek, p 347)

_____

11. List disadvantages of the autoclaving process. (Barnes, p 576; Burton, p 430; Kacmarek, p 347)

   a. _____

   b. _____

   c. _____

12. List four types of plastics that may be autoclaved without damage. (Barnes, p 576)

   a. _____

   b. _____

   c. _____

   d. _____

13. How is the autoclave process monitored for sterilization? (Barnes, p 576)

_____

_____

14. List the advantages of disinfection via pasteurization. (Barnes, p 574; Burton, p 430; Kacmarek, p 347)

    a. _____

    b. _____

    c. _____

    d. _____

15. Describe the disinfection process of pasteurization. (Barnes, p 574; Burton, p 430; Kacmarek, p 374)

_____

_____

16. List the chemical methods of disinfection and sterilization. (Barnes, p 576; Burton, p 430; Kacmarek, p 437)

    a. _____   d. _____

    b. _____   e. _____

    c. _____   f. _____

17. List two alcohols most commonly used as disinfectants, and describe that process of disinfection. (Barnes, p 577; Burton, p 430, Kacmarek, p 347

_____

_____

_____

18. List the effect of alcohols on the following: (Barnes, p 577; Burton, p 430; Kacmarek, p 347)

    a. spores: _____

    b. tubercle bacilli: _____

    c. bacteria: _____

    d. viruses: _____

    e. hepatitis: _____

19. Aldehydes sterilize objects through _____ of

_____. (Barnes, p 576; Burton, p 430)

20. Describe the process of sterilization through the use of glutaraldehydes. (Barnes, p 577)

_____

_____

_____

21. Describe the use of alkaline glutaraldehydes. (Barnes, p 577; Burton, p 430; Kacmarek, p 347)

_____

_____

_____

_____

22. Discuss the use of acid glutaraldehydes. (Barnes, p 578; Burton, p 430; Kacmarek, p 347)

_____

_____

_____

23. How does ethylene oxide destroy microorganisms? (Barnes, p 578; Burton, p 430; Kacmarek, p 347)

_____

24. What conditions must be met to achieve sterilization with the use of ethylene oxide process? (Barnes, p 578; Burton, p 430)

   a. relative humidity: _____

   b. temperature: _____

   c. time: _____

25. List some of the disadvantages of ETO sterilization. (Barnes, p 578; Burton, p 430; Kacmarek, p 347)

   a. _____

   b. _____

   c. _____

   d. _____

   e. _____

26. How is the efficiency of the ETO sterilization ensured? (Barnes, p 578; Burton, p 430; Kacmarek, p 347)

_____

27. Briefly desribe the following methods of disinfection: (Barnes, p 578; Burton, p 430)

   a. iodines: _____

   b. phenols: _____

28. Explain the importance of handwashing in the medical environment. (Barnes, p 573)

_____

_____

29. Describe the correct handwashing technique. (Barnes, p 573)

_____

_____

30. Describe the universal isolation procedures, as outlined by the Centers for Disease Control (CDC).

_____

_____

_____

ANSWERS TO STUDY QUESTIONS

1. a. application of a chemical substance to tissue that will inhibit the growth of microorganisms
   b. free from microorganisms, or a technique to prevent sepsis
   c. chemical agents that can destroy microbes.
   d. causing death to bacteria
   e. inhibition of the growth of bacteria
   f. the chemical or physical process of destroying microorganisms and their products
   g. infections acquired during the patient's stay in the hospital
   h. the complete destruction of microorganisms

2. a, c, b, e, d

3. a. incineration
   b. dry heat
   c. pasteurization
   d. autoclave
   e. filtration

4. the preferred method for material or objects that are highly contaminated with virulent pathogens: used when object is of no further use (careful procedures should ensure a temperature high enough to have complete incineration occur so that no pathogens are released into the air)

5. the process of passing liquid or a gas through a material made up of minute pores (the pores trap the microorganism and the device is disposed of at a later time); used in various types of equipment to protect the patient and the environment

6. a. 1 to 2 hours
   b. 160°C to 180°C

7. metal and glass, because it does not dull edges; also on powder and oils, or anything that cannot tolerate moist heat

8. because this process causes small changes in some products and, more likely, it is a very expensive process

9. a. 2 atm, 121°C, 15 min
   b. 3 atm, 134°C, 3 min

10. The organisms are killed by disruption of the cell membrane and/or coagulation of the cell.

11. a. items must be properly packed
    b. deterioration of many plastic and rubber products
    c. dulls edges of sharp instruments

12. a. teflon
    b. polycarbonate
    c. polypropylene
    d. nylon

13. It is monitored in three ways: thermocouples monitor temperature, heat-sensitive tape monitors temperature, and biologic indicator tapes.

14. a. simple and inexpensive
    b. environmentally safe
    c. tolerated well by heat-sensitive equipment
    d. kills vegetable bacteria and tubercle bacillus

15. It involves the application of heat with hot water submersion at 62°C for 30 minutes or 72°C for 15 minutes.

16. a. gas sterilization
    b. aldehydes
    c. alcohols
    d. phenols
    e. iodines
    f. chlorhexidrine
    (Others: hexachlohene, halogens, quaternary ammonium compounds)

17. The two alcohols used are 70% ethyl alcohol and 90% isopropyl alcohol. These disinfect through damage of the cell membrane. They may also coagulate microbial proteins and denature proteins.

18. a. does not destroy
    b. destroys
    c. destroys

d. destroys
e. does not destroy

19. alkylation, enzymes

20. This process causes disruption of the cell membrane and the cytoplasm. It is dependent upon the time and contact. All items must be free of anything that would interfere with contact.

21. It is activated as a buffer is applied. The buffer is 0.03% bicarbonate. The entire solution is a 2% solution. It is potent for 14 days. It destroys bacteria, viruses, and spores in a 10- to 20-hour period. All items must be rinsed before dried, as this material may cause mucous membrane irritation. Users of the system should wear gloves.

22. This material is extremely potent and toxic. Wearing gloves is a must. All items must be rinsed and dried. It remains potent for 28 days. It is bactericidal and virocidal in 20 minutes. It sterilizes in 1 hour if heated to 60°C.

23. ETO destroys microorganisms via alkylating cellular components.

24. a. 50%
    b. 50 to 56°C
    c. 4 hours

25. a. temperature above 60°C causes polymerization of ETO, making it ineffective
    b. leaves a residual toxic to human tissue

c. expensive
d. requires an aeration chamber
e. ETO exposure associated with mutagenicity and carcinogenity

26. use of the biologic indicator tape B subtilus

27. a. germicidal, an effective agent against vegetative organisms, tuberculosis, some viruses, and fungi
    b. germicidal, bactericidal, acts as protoplasmic poison, kills tuberculosis, not sporicidal

28. Handwashing is considered the single most important exercise in preventing nosocomial infections.

29. Remove all jewelry; best to have a foot-control basin; be careful not to touch faucet handles except with paper drying towels, do not touch waste receptacle.

30. These procedures are as follows: All patients are given consistent care. All body substance specimens are treated as if infected and are handled accordingly. Diagnostic labels are not needed. Wash hands and wear gloves when likely to touch body substances, mucous membranes, or nonintact skin. Wear a plastic apron when clothing is likely to be soiled. Wear mask/eye protection when likely to be splashed. Place intact needle/syringe units and sharp items in designated disposal container. Do not bend or break needles.

PRACTICE QUIZ

1. Which of the statements listed below is/are true about nosocomial infections?
   I. The connection with respiratory therapy equipment is well established.
   II. Good handwashing would greatly decrease the risk.
   III. RT patients are at increased risk.
   IV. Transient flora are most often implicated.
   V. Warm liquid in respiratory therapy equipment often harbors infection.
   a. I, II, III, IV, V
   b. I, II, III
   c. I, III, V
   d. II, IV, V
   e. I, II only

2. Filtration devices placed between the ventilator and the circuit should be changed how often?
   a. every 8 hours
   b. every 40 hours
   c. every 160 hours

    d. every 250 hours

    e. every 500 hours

3. Which of the following antimicrobial agents is sporicidal?
    a. acid glutaraldehyde
    b. alkaline glutaraldehyde
    c. ethyl alcohol
    e. isopropyl alcohol
    e. a and b only

4. Which of the following methods of disinfection and sterilization requires a 50% relative humidity, temperatures of 50 to 56°C at 1 atmosphere, for 4 hours of exposure?
    a. autoclave
    b. pasteurization
    c. ETO
    d. dry heat
    e. acid glutaraldehyde

5. Which of the following methods is/are recommended for rubber, metal, and plastic equipment?
    I. Autoclave
    II. Acid glutaraldehyde
    III. Alkaline glutaraldehyde
    IV. Pasteurization
    V. ETO
    a. I, II, III, IV, V
    b. II, III, IV
    c. II, III, V
    d. I, II, III
    e. IV only

6. Choose the correct statements about ETO sterilization.
    I. It can be used on most moisture- or heat-sensitive items.
    II. It requires 121°C for 15 minutes at 2 atmospheres.
    III. It is nontoxic, simple, and fast.
    IV. An aeration chamber is required.
    V. When it combines with H_2O, it forms ethylene glycol.
    a. I, II, III
    b. I, IV, V
    c. I, II, IV
    d. II, III, IV
    e. I, II, III, IV, V

7. True statements about acid glutaraldehyde include which of the following?
    I. It sterilizes in 10 minutes.
    II. It sterilizes in 1 hour.
    III. It is sporicidal in 10 hours.
    IV. It lasts about 28 days.
    V. It lasts about 14 days.
    a. I, III, IV
    b. II, III, V
    c. I, V
    d. I, III
    e. II, IV

8. What method of disinfection requires a hot water immersion at 62°C for 30 minutes or 72°C for 15 minutes?

a. autoclave
b. pasteurization
c. ETO
d. acid glutaraldehyde
e. alkaline glutaraldehyde

9. Which of the processes listed below form(s) a toxic residue?
    I. Acid glutaraldehyde
    II. Alkaline glutaraldehyde
    III. ETO
    IV. Autoclave
    V. Pasteurization
    a. I, II, III
    b. I, II
    c. I, II, IV
    d. IV, V
    e. III only

10. The preferred method of sterilization of equipment that has been contaminated with an extremely virulent pathogen and that is no longer of use is which of the following?
    a. ETO
    b. pasteurization
    c. dry heat
    d. incineration
    e. autoclave

11. The chemical or physical process of destroying pathogenic organisms and their products is termed:
    a. sterilization
    b. disinfection
    c. asepsis
    d. nosocomial
    e. antisepsis

12. Which of the following are physical methods of sterilization?
    I. Incineration
    II. Pasteurization
    III. Autoclave
    IV. ETO
    V. Ionizing radiation
    a. I, II, IV
    b. II, III, IV
    c. I, II, III, V
    d. I, III, V
    e. I, II, III, IV, V

13. Which of the following is/are true about the use of dry heat as a method of sterilization?
    I. It does not dull edges.
    II. It is used on things that do not tolerate moist heat.
    III. It is used on metal and glass.
    IV. It is used on powder and oils
    V. It requires $160°C$ to $180°C$ for 1 to 2 hours.
    a. I, III
    b. III, IV
    c. II, IV, V
    d. I, II, III, V
    e. I, II, III, IV, V

14. Which disinfection products are the most commonly used?
    a. alcohols
    b. aldehydes
    c. phenols
    d. ETO
    e. halogens

15. Which disinfection agent requires bicarbonate to become activated?
    a. alkaline glutaraldehyde
    b. iodine
    c. phenol
    d. ethylene oxide
    e. propylene

16. Which of the following are disadvantages of the ETO sterilization process?
    I. It is expensive.
    II. It deteriorates rubber products.
    III. Ethylene oxide is toxic.
    IV. It requires long-term aeration.
    V. It is not useful for moisture-sensitive products.
    a. I, II, V
    b. I, III, IV
    c. II, IV, V
    d. I, III, IV, V
    e. I, II, III, IV, V

17. What is the purpose of the indicator tape in ETO sterilization?
    a. ensures sterilization has taken place
    b. indicates the need for more aeration time
    c. indicates the need for a higher humidity level
    d. tells the germ level killed
    e. indicates the tape has been exposed to ETO

18. Microbial sterilization with the use of glutaraldehydes occur via what mechanism?
    a. alkylation
    b. disruption of cell membrane
    c. coagulation of proteins
    d. melting of the cell
    e. dehydration

19. An agent that inhibits the growth of bacteria is termed:
    a. bactericidal
    b. bacteriostatic
    c. fungicidal
    d. germicidal
    e. homeostatic

20. Which of the following would most decrease the nosocomial infection rate in the hospital?
    a. change H_2O in humidifiers daily
    b. increase the number of filters used
    c. increase handwashing
    d. require sterile showers before beginning a shift
    e. decrease physician contact with infectious patients

ANSWERS TO THE PRACTICE QUIZ

1. a		11. b	
2. e		12. c	
3. e		13. e	
4. c		14. a	
5. b		15. a	
6. b		16. b	
7. e		17. e	
8. b		18. b	
9. a		19. b	
10. d		20. c	

SPECIAL PROCEDURES

OUTLINE

LEARNING OBJECTIVES

Upon completion of this unit, the individual will:

1. Identify laboratory values most often reported on an SMA-6 and a CBC report.
2. List the normal range for commonly requested laboratory values.
3. Discuss laboratory test to be ordered to investigate common clinical diagnosis.
4. Discuss the clinical picture associated with a fluid imbalance.
5. Discuss the components of the extracellular and intracellular fluid compartments.
6. Define sensible and insensible water loss.
7. List according to the order of contrast density on the x-ray film, bone, air, fat, soft tissue, and fluid.
8. Define and discuss radiopaque and radiolucency.
9. Describe the common chest x-ray examination positions.
10. Describe a systematic chest x-ray review technique.
11. Describe the appearance of atelectasis and pneumothorax on the chest x-ray film.
12. Differentiate between rigid and fiberoptic bronchoscopy.

13. List the indicators for bronchoscopy.
14. List the complications of bronchoscopy.
15. Describe how bronchial bleeds might be controlled via bronchoscopy.
16. Describe indications and complications in bronchoscopy of the mechanically ventilated patient.
17. Identify and label a common adapter for bronchoscopy of the mechanically ventilated patient.
18. Describe the function of chest drainage systems.
19. Describe the correct chest tube position to drain the pleura of air and fluid.
20. Describe the function of the one-bottle chest drainage system.
21. Differentiate between the one- and two-bottle systems.
22. List reasons for fluid movement in the systems.
23. List reasons movement might discontinue in the chest drainage systems.
24. Identify the components of the three-bottle and disposable chest tube drainage systems.
25. Discuss "clamping" and "stripping" procedures.

REFERENCES

Barnes, TA: Respiratory Care Practice. Year Book Medical Publishers, Chicago, 1988.

Burton, G, and Hodgkin, J: Respiratory Care: A Guide to Clinical Practice, ed 2. JB Lippincott, Philadelphia, 1984.

Deshpande, VM, Pilbean, SP, and Dixon, RJ: A Comprehensive Review in Respiratory Care. Appleton and Lange, Norwalk, CT, 1988.

Egan, DF, Sheldon, RL, and Spearman, CV: Egan's Fundamentals of Respiratory Therapy, ed 4. CV Mosby, St Louis, 1982.

Eubanks, DH, and Bone, RC. Comprehensive Respiratory Care. CV Mosby, St Louis, 1985.

Kacmarek, R, Stoller, J: Current Respiratory Care. BC Decker, Philadelphia, 1988.

Shapiro, BA, Harrison, RA, Kacmarek, RM, and Cane, RD: Clinical Application of Respiratory Care, ed 3. Year Book Medical Publishers, Chicago, 1985.

Stroot, V, Lee, CAB, and Barrett, CA: Fluids and Electrolytes, ed 3. FA Davis, Philadelphia, 1984.

Wilkins, RL, Sheldon, RL, and Krider, SJ: Clinical Assessment in Respiratory Care. CV Mosby, St Louis, 1985.

STUDY QUESTIONS

1. What laboratory values are provided on an SMA-6? (Deshpande, p 92; Stroot, p 302)

   _____

2. What laboratory values are most often reported on a complete blood count (CBC) report? (Deshpande, p 92; Stroot, p 301)

   _____

3. Give the normal range for the following test results: (Deshpande, p 92; Stroot, p 301; Wilkins, p 89)

   a. sodium (Na): _____

   b. potassium (K): _____

   c. chloride (CL): _____

   d. total CO_2: _____

   e. glucose: _____

   f. blood urea nitrogen (BUN): _____

g. hemoglobin (Hgb): male _____ female _____

h. hematocrit (Hct): male _____ female _____

i. white blood count (WBC): _____

j. red blood count (RBC): male _____ female _____

k. calcium (Ca): _____

4. Provide the correct laboratory test to be ordered to obtain the desired information. (Deshpande, p 92)

a. renal function _____

b. fluid balance _____

c. acid base balance _____

d. ventilatory status _____

e. liver function _____

f. cardiac conduction _____

g. degree of tissue injury _____

h. nutritional status _____

5. List the signs and symptoms associated with fluid and electrolyte imbalance. (Stroot, p 23)

_____

6. List the anions/cations of the extracellular/intracellular fluids. (Stroot, p 23)

_____

_____

7. Describe the anion gap calculation and use. (Wilkins, p 99)

_____

_____

8. What laboratory test result best determines the presence of fluid imbalances? (Stroot, p 69)

_____

9. Which fluid compartment contains fluid space that makes up 20 percent of the body weight (Stroot, p 13)

_____

10. List and define the two types of fluid losses. (Stroot, p 333)

a. _____

_____

b. _____

_____

11. List the four main objects normally seen on the chest x-ray film, in the order of increasing density. (Egan, p 310)

a. _____

b. _____

c. _____

d. _____

12. X-rays pass through low-density objects and turn the film _____. When x-rays strike a dense object they are partially absorbed and turn the film _____. (Egan, p 310)

13. What is the "standard" position of the chest film, and how is it done? (Egan, p 311; Barnes, p 98; Wilkins, p 164)

_____

_____

14. What are the two most commonly used "routine" chest film positions? (Egan, p 311; Deshpande, p 109; Wilkins, p 165)

a. _____

b. _____

15. What x-ray position is used for the portable chest film? Describe film and x-ray position in relation to the patient. (Egan, p 311; Barnes, p 98; Deshpande, p 109; Wilkins, p 166)

_____

_____

16. For what purpose is the lateral decubitus chest film used? (Wilkins, p 165)

_____

17. Define the following: (Deshpande, p 109; Wilkins, p 172)

a. radiopaque: _____

b. radiolucent: _____

18. Indicate whether the following would be radiolucent or radiopaque on the chest film: (Deshpande, p 109; Wilkins, p 172)

a. pneumothorax: _____

b. atelectasis: _____

c. tumor: _____

d. foreign body: _____

e. bleb: _____

19. Using Figure 11–1, label each of the following according to the correct order for systematic chest inspection on x-ray. (Deshpande, p 108)

_____ pleural surfaces   _____ mediastinum

_____ dome of diaphragm   _____ lung fields

_____ hilum   _____ subdiaphragm

_____ soft tissue   _____ bones

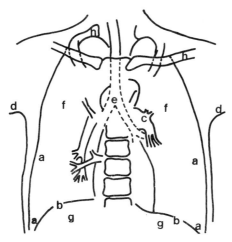

FIGURE 11 – 1. The thorax

20. If the radiograph has been taken with the correct procedure at deep inspiration, the diaphragm will be visible at what rib location? (Egan, p 328; Wilkins, p 171)

_____

21. Indicate whether the following are True or False: (Barnes, p 111; Egan, p 317, 328)

_____ a. Normally the right hilum is slightly higher than the left.

_____ b. The right hemidiaphragm is slightly higher than the left.

_____ c. The pleural space is evident as an air line on x-ray examination.

_____ d. The carina is visible at C-2.

_____ e. Pleural effusions cause blunting of the costrophrenic angles.

22. How will atelectasis change the position of the mediastinum and/or trachea on x-ray examination? (Barnes, p 115; Wilkins, p 174)

_____

23. How might a pneumothorax be exhibited on x-ray examination? (Egan, p 116; Wilkins, p 178)

_____

_____

24. Differentiate between rigid and fiberoptic bronchoscopy. (Egan, p 567; Barnes, p 99; Kacmarek and Stoller, p 101)

_____

_____

_____

_____

_____

_____

25. List four indications for therapeutic bronchoscopy. (Egan, p 567; Kacmarek and Stoller, p 97)

a. _____

b. _____

c. _____

d. _____

26. List two clinical situations in which rigid bronchoscopy is the procedure of choice. (Egan, p 567; Kacmarek and Stoller, p 97)

    a. _____

    b. _____

27. List five complications of bronchoscopy. (Egan, p 568)

    a. _____

    b. _____

    c. _____

    d. _____

    e. _____

28. How might bleeding be controlled through bronchoscopy? (Kacmarek and Stoller, p 98)

_____

_____

29. List four uses of the fiberoptic bronchoscope in the intubated and mechanically ventilated patient. (Kacmarek and Stoller, p 98)

    a. _____

    b. _____

    c. _____

    d. _____

30. The smallest endotracheal tube size of choice for the bronchoscopy procedure in the adult mechanically ventilated patient is _____. (Kacmarek and Stoller, p 98)

31. Give four possible side effects of introduction of the fiberoptic bronchoscope in the mechanically ventilated patient, and list a way to minimize each. (Kacmarek and Stoller, p 98)

    a. _____

    b. _____

    c. _____

    d. _____

32. Identify the device depicted in Figure 11–2. (Kacmarek and Stoller, p 98)

_____

33. Label the components of the device depicted in Figure 11–2. (Kacmarek and Stoller, p 98)

    a. _____

    b. _____

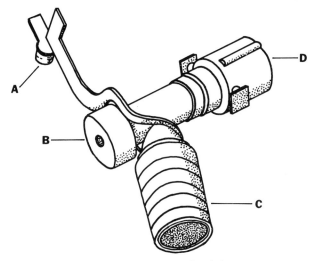

FIGURE 11-2. Adapter

c. _____

d. _____

34. What is the purpose of a chest drainage system? (Deshpande, p 274; Shapiro, p 462)

_____

35. Discuss the correct position for chest tube or needle placement to remove air from the pleural space. (Deshpande, p 275; Burton, p 893)

_____

_____

36. Discuss the correct chest tube placement to drain fluid from the pleural space. (Deshpande, p 275; Burton, p 893)

_____

37. List hazards associated with chest tubes. (Deshpande, p 275)

    a. _____

    b. _____

    c. _____

38. Describe the functioning of the one-bottle chest drainage system illustrated in Figure 11-3. (Deshpande, p 275; Shapiro, p 463)

_____

_____

39. Why does the fluid move up and down the drainage tube in a one-bottle chest tube drainage system in a spontaneously breathing patient? (Deshpande, p 275)

_____

_____

_____

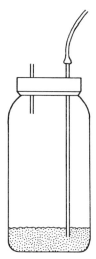

FIGURE 11–3. Single-bottle chest drainage system

40. List four reasons the fluid would discontinue moving up and down the water seal tube in the spontaneously breathing patient. (Deshpande, p 275)

    a. _____

    b. _____

    c. _____

    d. _____

41. Why is the depth of the water seal tube under the fluid in the bottle important in the one-bottle chest drainage system? (Deshpande, p 275)

    _____

    _____

42. How far under the fluid level should the water seal tube be placed to allow drainage to occur? (Deshpande, p 276)

    _____

43. Differentiate between a one- and a two-bottle chest tube drainage system. (Deshpande, p 276; Shapiro, p 464)

    _____

    _____

    _____

44. Describe the function of each of the bottles in Figure 11–4. (Deshpande, p 276; Shapiro, p 465)

    a. _____

    b. _____

    c. _____

45. How is suction pressure set in a three-bottle chest drainage system? (Deshpande, p 277; Shapiro, p 464)

    _____

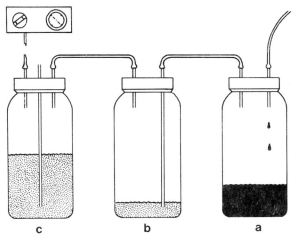

FIGURE 11–4. Triple-bottle chest drainage system

46. What is the range of common suctioning pressures in the chest drainage system? (Deshpande, p 277)

_____

47. What device is illustrated in Figure 11–5? (Deshpande, p 279)

_____

48. Label the parts in Figure 11–5. (Deshpande, p 279; Shapiro, p 465)

   a. A, B, and C function as _____

   b. D and E function as _____

   c. F functions as _____

   d. J is the _____

   e. K is the _____

   f. L is the _____

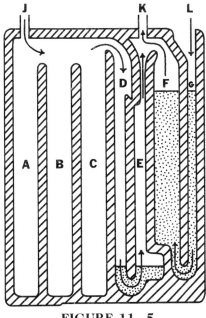

FIGURE 11–5.

49. Discuss chest tube clamping in the following situations: (Deshpande, p 276; Shapiro, p 464)

   a. chest tube becomes disconnected or water seal broken:

   _____

   _____

   b. chest tube disconnected on a pneumonectomy patient:

   _____

   _____

   c. chest tube disconnected on patient with a big air leak:

   _____

   _____

50. Discuss the procedure of "milking" or "stripping" the chest tube. (Deshpande, p 276; Shapiro, p 464)

   _____

   _____

ANSWERS TO STUDY QUESTIONS

1. serum levels of Na, K, Cl, total CO_2, glucose, BUN

2. RBC, WBC, Hct, Hgb

3. a. 135 to 145 mEq/L
   b. 3.5 to 5.0 mEq/l
   c. 95 to 105 mEq/l
   d. 23 to 27 mEq/l
   e. fasting: 65:110 mq/dl
   f. 10 to 20 mg/dl
   g. male: 13.5 to 16.5 g/dl female: 12.0 to 15 g/dl

4. a. BUN, creatinine, electrolytes
   b. H&H, electrolytes, specific gravity of urine, osmolarity
   c. ABGs, electrolytes
   d. ABGs, pulmonary mechanics, PFT
   e. bilirubin
   f. electrolytes, ECG
   g. LDH, CPK, SGOT
   h. glucose, cholesterol, total protein, albumin

5. changes in weight, headache, nausea, sensorium, BP

6. extracellular fluid cation = sodium, anion = chloride
   intracellular fluid cation = potassium

7. Calculate: serum chloride and bicarbonate are subtracted from serum sodium: N = 8-16 mEq/l (calculation identifies etiology of metabolic acidosis)

8. serum sodium

9. the extracellular compartment

10. a. sensible water loss: perceptible body fluid and electrolyte loss (e.g., urine and diaphoresis
    b. insensible water loss: loss of fluids that occurs without the individual's perception (e.g., loss during expiration of gases from the respiratory system)

11. a. bone
    b. soft tissue
    c. fat
    d. air

12. black, white

13. Posterior-anterior (PA): patient's back to x-ray tube, chest against the metal film cassette. X-rays leave the tube, strike the patient's back, and move through the chest to the film.

14. a. PA
    b. lateral

15. AP: x-rays enter the patient at the anterior

chest and move through to the film placed posterior

16. to see free fluid in the chest

17. a. absorbs x-rays, white on radiograph
    b. x-rays pass through, dark on radiograph

18. a. radiolucent
    b. radiopaque
    c. radiolucent
    d. radiopaque
    e. radiolucent

19. a. e
    b. d
    c. b
    d. g
    e. a
    f. c
    q. h
    h. f

20. It will be descended to bottom of the 6th rib anterior or the 10th rib posterior.

21. a. False
    b. True
    c. False
    d. False
    e. True

22. Both structures will shift toward the affected side.

23. increased radiolucency, mediastinumal/tracheal shift away from the affected side, visceral pleural line with area devoid of vascular markings outside the line

24. rigid—less flexible scope, only goes into the major airways and requires an experienced thoracic surgeon; performed under general anesthesia; used for direct visualization, requires a bronch room; more useful for removal of foreign bodies and intrabronchial bleeds
    Fiberoptic—able to reach wide area of respiratory tract; local anesthesia, can be done at bedside; can be done by pulmonologist and internist, has steerable tip with brushes, forceps, and aspiration ability

25. a. to insert double lumen tubes
    b. bronchial toilet
    c. foreign body removal
    d. biopsy
    e. diagnostic procedure
    f. massive hemoptysis

26. a. foreign body removal in the large airway
    b. to control large airway bleeds

27. a. laryngospasm
    b. bronchospasm
    c. vasovagal reaction
    d. hemorrhage
    e. others: fever, hypoxemia, infection

28. epinephrine at $1:20,000$ mg/ml dilution can be instilled, iced saline solution, tamponade of bleeding with a modified fogarty catheter

29. a. tracheobronchial toilet
    b. reexpansion of atelectatic lung
    c. removal of mucous plugs
    d. foreign body removal
    e. confirmation of tube placement

30. preferably no less than 8.5 mm internal diameter

31. a. decreased VT—decrease suction time and procedure time
    b. decreased PaO_2—use 100% O_2
    c. increased $PaCO_2$—decrease bronch time
    d. barotrauma with PEEP in use—decrease use of PEEP during procedure

32. Figure 11–2 represents the ventilator adapter used for fiberoptic bronchoscopy.

33. a. diaphragm plug
    b. diaphragm
    c. ventilator adapter
    d. patient adapter

34. to remove fluid or air from the pleural space

35. the 2nd to 3rd intercostal space, anteriorly, along the midclavicular line because air will rise to the highest thoracic space

36. in the 6th to 8th intercostal space laterally along the midaxillary line

37. a. pneumothorax
    b. infection
    c. hemothorax

38. allows drainage by gravity and normal pleural pressure fluctuations; serves as a collector and a water seal

39. The intrapleural pressure is more negative during inspiration and it draws the fluid up. During expiration the fluid moves out of the tube. Fluid movement of 2 to 6 cm is normal in most spontaneously breathing patients.

40. a. chest tube plugged
    b. chest tube kinked
    c. a leak
    d. pt. is apneic

41. The depth of the water seal tube under the fluid will determine the amount of intrapleural pressure the patient must generate to drain the pleural space.

42. betweeen 2 and 3 cm

43. In the two-bottle system, the first bottle is connected to the patient to collect drainage. The second bottle acts as a waterseal. The one-bottle system functions as both patient drainage and as a waterseal.

44. a. bottle a — collection bottle
    b. bottle b — H_2O seal
    c. bottle c — suction regulatory bottle

45. by the depth the tube in the suction bottle is submerged in the fluid in that bottle

46. The accepted range is −15 to −20 cm H_2O pressure.

47. The commercial chest drainage system, used often as a disposable unit

48. a. collection chambers
    b. water seal
    c. suction control
    d. outlet to the patient
    e. suction outlet
    f. ambient air outlet

49. a. Clamp the tube briefly and place it into glass of H_2O quickly, as it is possible to unclamp.
    b. Clamp to prevent air into pleural space; correct as soon as possible.
    c. Do not clamp — may lead to tension pneumothorax; replace tube as soon as possible.

50. This is the procedure for clearing an obstruction in the flexible chest tubing. It should be done only when necessary to maintain patency.

PRACTICE QUIZ

1. The best determinant of water imbalance is:
   a. potassium
   b. urinary sodium
   c. serum sodium
   d. weight change
   e. hematocrit

2. The two types of fluid losses are which of the following?
   I. Sensible
   II. Intracellular
   III. Extracellular
   IV. Osmosis
   V. Insensible
   a. I, II
   b. II, III
   c. IV, V
   d. I, V
   e. none of the above

3. Which level of potassium is considered to be toxic?
   a. 3.0 to 3.5 mEq/l
   b. 3.5 to 4.0 mEq/l
   c. 3.5 to 5.0 mEq/l
   d. 5.5 to 6.5 mEq/l
   e. none of the above

4. Which of the following should be considered when evaluating the nutritional status of the patient?
   I. Glucose
   II. Cholesterol
   III. Total protein

    IV. Albumin

    V. Bilirubin

a. I, II, III, IV, V

b. I, II, III, IV

c. I, II

d. III, IV

e. II, III, IV

5. Which of the following are not considered a part of the CBC report?

    I. Hematocrit

    II. Serum sodium

    III. Hemoglobin

    IV. Glucose

    V. Platelet count

a. I, III, V

b. II, IV, V

c. II, IV

d. II, III, IV, V

e. I, II

6. List the following in the order of decreasing radiodensity:

    I. Soft tissue

    II. Bones

    III. Air

    IV. Fat

    V. Fluid

a. I, II, III, IV, V

b. II, IV, I, V, III

c. II, I, IV, III, V

d. IV, I, II, III, V

e. III, IV, II, I, V

7. What x-ray film position is used to detect a pleural effusion?

a. PA

b. AP

c. lordic

d. lateral decubitus

e. none of the above

8. What x-ray film position is used for a portable chest film?

a. PA

b. AP

c. lordic

d. lateral decubitus

e. transverse

9. Which of the following are indications for bronchoscopy?

    I. Bronchial hygiene

    II. Foreign body removal

    III. Diagnostic procedure

    IV. Insertion of double lumen endotracheal tube

    V. Biopsy

a. I, II, III, IV, V

b. I, II, III, IV

c. II, III, V

d. III, IV, V

e. IV, V

10. Which of the following are complications of the bronchoscopy procedure?
    a. laryngospasm
    b. bronchospasm
    c. arrhythmia
    d. hypoxemia
    e. all of the above

11. Choose the uses for fiberoptic bronchoscopy in the mechanically ventilated patient.
      I. Tracheobronchial toilet
     II. Re-expansion of the atelectatic lung
    III. Removal of mucous plugs
     IV. Ensure ventilation
      V. Ensure oxygenation
    a. I, II, III, IV, V
    b. I, III, V
    c. I, II, III
    d. II, IV, V
    e. III only

12. Where is the chest tube placed to remove air from the pleural space?
    a. 6th to 8th intercostal
    b. 2nd to 3rd intercostal space, midaxillary
    c. 6th to 8th intercostal space laterally, midaxillary
    d. 2nd to 3rd intercostal space anteriorly, midclavicular
    e. none of the above

13. Choose which of the following is/are complications associated with insertion of the chest tube.
    a. infection
    b. pneumothorax
    c. hemothorax
    d. hemorrhage
    e. a, b, and c

14. Indicate which of the following is/are functionally equivalent:
    a. three-bottle chest drainage system and pleura-vac
    b. one-bottle system and the two-bottle system
    c. two-bottle system and the pleura-vac
    d. none are equivalent
    e. a and b

15. When the one-bottle chest tube system is used to drain fluid from the pleural space and is not connected to a suction device, how does it drain?
    a. by osmosis
    b. by gravity
    c. by pressure release
    d. by resistance
    e. it doesn't work

16. What is the acceptable range of suction pressure in the chest drainage system?
    a. -2 to -8 cm H_2O pressure
    b. -10 to -15 cm H_2O pressure
    c. -15 to -20 cm H_2O pressure
    d. -20 to -25 cm H_2O pressure
    e. -25 to -30 cm H_2O pressure

17. When a large clot obstructs the flexible chest tubing, what procedure is used to clear the lumen and maintain patency?
    a. clamping
    b. stripping
    c. tubing lavage
    d. tubing replacement
    e. none of the above

18. How is suction set in the three-bottle chest drainage system?
    a. by setting the suction regulator
    b. by placing the bottles lower than the patient
    c. by the depth the underwater seal is submerged in the third bottle
    d. by the amount of bubbling in the second bottle
    e. none of the above

19. What symptoms may be associated with chest tube kinking?
    a. increased RR
    b. increased HR
    c. diaphoresis
    d. substernal retractions
    e. all of the above

20. What is the correct procedure to be followed when the chest tube is inadvertently removed from the site of insertion?
    a. Turn off suction.
    b. Push the tube back in.
    c. Cover the opening with a Vaseline gauze pad.
    d. Apply hydrogen peroxide.
    e. Apply pressure with hand-held Vaseline gauze pad.

ANSWERS TO THE PRACTICE QUIZ

1. c	11. c
2. d	12. d
3. d	13. e
4. b	14. e
5. c	15. b
6. b	16. d
7. d	17. b
8. b	18. c
9. a	19. e
10. e	20. e

UNIT 2

ADVANCED PROCEDURES

Chapter 12

RESPIRATORY PHYSIOLOGY

Outline

Learning Objectives

Upon completion of this unit, the individual will:

1. Describe the anatomic changes that must occur to accommodate a lung volume.
2. Define compliance of the lung and express it as an equation.
3. Define elasticity and express it as an equation.
4. Explain the forces that govern the elastic recoil of the chest wall.
5. Calculate the system compliance, given the required data.
6. Describe the forces needed to overcome for inspiration.
7. Define resistance and give the formula used to compute resistance.
8. List three factors that affect airway resistance.

9. Calculate the system resistance, given the required data.
10. Describe the uneven distribution of ventilation.
11. Indicate the normal compliance for the following:
    a. chest wall
    b. lung
    c. total
12. List pathophysiologic conditions that would cause the compliance to increase or decrease.
13. Define surface tension.
14. Explain the factors that are responsible for the work of breathing.
15. Define diffusion.
16. Describe the major circulatory systems that affect the lungs.
17. List the functions of the pulmonary circulation.
18. Explain pulmonary vascular resistance.
19. Discuss the primary lung zones.
20. Describe the relationship of ventilation/perfusion.
21. Explain neurologic control of ventilation.
22. Describe the role of each of the following on the control of ventilation:
    a. medulla oblongata
    b. pons
    c. vagus nerve
    d. peripheral chemoreceptors
    e. central chemoreceptors
    f. cerebral cortex
23. Discuss the respiratory reflexes that control breathing.
24. Discuss the defense mechanism of the lung.
25. List the uses of hyperbaric oxygen therapy.
26. Describe what factors are affected by the normal process of aging.

REFERENCES

Barnes, TA: Respiratory Care Practice. Year Book Medical Publishers, Chicago, 1988.

Burton, G, and Hodgkin, J: Respiratory Care: A Guide to Clinical Practice, ed 2. JB Lippincott, Philadelphia, 1984.

Kacmarek, RM, Mack, CW, and Dimas, S: The Essentials of Respiratory Therapy, ed 2. Year Book Medical Publishers, Chicago, 1985.

Murray, JF: The Normal Lung, ed 2. WB Saunders, Philadelphia, 1986.

Slonim, NB and Hamilton, LH: Respiratory Physiology, ed 5. CV Mosby, St Louis, 1987.

West, JB: Respiratory Physiology, ed 3. Williams & Wilkins, Baltimore, 1985.

STUDY QUESTIONS

1. What three anatomic changes must the thorax make to accommodate lung volume, and how is this accomplished? (Slonim, p 65; Murray, pp 122–133)

   a. _____

   b. _____

   c. _____

2. Describe the forces that oppose ventilation. (Kacmarek, pp 72–75; Slonim, pp 68–71)

   _____

3. Define the following pressures: (Kacmarek, pp 72–75; Murray, pp 84–85)

   a. atmospheric pressure: _____

   b. alveolar pressure: _____

   c. pleural pressure: _____

   d. transpulmonary pressure: _____

4. Define compliance and provide an algebraic formula in your description. (Slonim, p 74; Kacmarek, p 77; West, p 89)

_____

5. List the three types of compliance. (Slonim, p 74; Kacmarek, p 77)

    a. _____

    b. _____

    c. _____

6. In the average "normal" healthy adult male indicate the normal levels for the three types of compliance listed in question 5. (Kacmarek, pp 78–79; Slonim, p 74)

    a. _____

    b. _____

    c. _____

7. Calculate the system compliance using the following clinical data: (Barnes, pp 568–569; Burton, p 1002)   Delivered tidal volume = 600 ml   Plateau pressure = 20 cm H_2O
$$PEEP = 5 \text{ cm } H_2O$$

_____

_____

8. Define surface tension. What effect does surface tension have on the alveoli? How is this phenomenon avoided in the lung? (Kacmarek, p 76; Slonim, pp 74–75; West, pp 89–94)

_____

_____

_____

9. List six pathophysiologic conditions that would cause total lung compliance to decrease (stiffer lungs). (Slonim, p 80; Kacmarek, p 80)

    a. _____

    b. _____

    c. _____

    d. _____

    e. _____

    f. _____

10. List two pathophysiologic conditions that would cause total lung compliance to increase (easier to inflate). (Slonim, p 81; Kacmarek, p 80)

    a. _____

    b. _____

11. Define elastance, and provide an algebraic formula that describes elastance. (Slonim, p 76; Murray, pp 90–91)

_____

_____

12. Define resistance, and provide an algebraic formula that describes resistance. (Slonim, pp 86–87; Barnes, pp 569–570)

_____

_____

13. Pressures generated during breathing must overcome what three types of resistance? (Barnes, p 570; Kacmarek, p 76)

    a. _____

    b. _____

    c. _____

14. At a standard flow rate of 0.5 l/sec, "normal" airway resistance (Kacmarek, p 82) is equal

    to _____.

15. Calculate the following system's resistance, given the following data. (Barnes, p 570)
    Peak airway pressure = 30 cm H_2O Plateau pressure = 20 cm H_2O
    Flow rate = 50 1/min

    _____

    _____

16. Work of breathing is usually expressed in which two ways? Define each. (Kacmarek, pp 293–297; Slonim, p 92; West, p 111)

    a. _____

    b. _____

17. Oxygen consumption in the adult is about _____ depending on basal metabolic levels. (Kacmarek, p 188, Murray, p 203)

18. Define diffusion. (Kacmarek, p 25; Slonim, p 97; West, pp 21–22)

    _____

    _____

19. The rate of diffusion of gases through another gas is affected by what factors? (Kacmarek, p 26; Slonim, pp 99–100)

    a. _____

    b. _____

    c. _____

    d. _____

    e. _____

20. What two gas laws compare the rates of diffusion of carbon dioxide and oxygen so we can determine which diffuses faster? (Kacmarek, pp 26–27; Slonim, pp 99–100)

    _____

21. In order for gas to diffuse through the alveolar-capillary membrane a pressure gradient must exist between the alveolus and the pulmonary capillaries.
    a. What two factors maintain this pressure difference?

b. In the resting condition, how fast (time) does this exchange take in the individual with no lung disease? (Slonim, pp 100–101; Murray, p 166)

a. _____

b. _____

_____

22. What are the two blood circulations associated with the lungs? (Slonim, p 109)

a. _____

b. _____

23. The total blood volume in the pulmonary circulation is approximately _____% of the total circulating blood volume at rest. (Slonim, p 111)

24. What are the major functions of the pulmonary circulation? (Kacmarek, p 121; Slonim, pp 110–111)

a. _____

b. _____

c. _____

25. List/discuss the three primary lung zones. (Kacmarek, p 84; Slonim, p 114; Murray, p 145)

a. _____

b. _____

c. _____

26. Explain pulmonary vascular resistance (PVR). (Murray, p 150; Slonim, pp 116–119; Kacmarek, p 122)

_____

_____

_____

27. What two mechanisms are responsible for the reduction in pulmonary vascular resistance when pulmonary vascular pressures are raised? (West, p 37)

a. _____

b. _____

28. What accounts for the uneven distribution of ventilation in the lungs? (Kacmarek, p 83; Slonim, p 123)

a. _____

b. _____

29. Describe the relationship of ventilation/perfusion ($\dot{V}/\dot{Q}$). What is the overall $\dot{V}/\dot{Q}$ in the lung? (Kacmarek, p 84; Slonim, pp 126–127)

_____

_____

30. There are four possible combinations of ventilation/perfusion. List/explain these combinations (use a drawing to help in your explanation). (Murray, pp 185–200; West, pp 57–59)

    a. _____

    b. _____

    c. _____

    d. _____

31. Clinically there are three useful methods of assessing the ventilation/perfusion inequality in the lung. These are: (West, pp 65–66; Barnes, pp 481–483)

    a. _____

    b. _____

    c. _____

32. List the areas responsible for neurologic control of ventilation. (Kacmarek, p 87; Slonim, chps 13–15, West, pp 113–122)

    a. _____

    b. _____

    c. _____

    d. _____

    e. _____

    f. _____

33. Two distinct areas located in the medulla oblongata are: (Kacmarek, p 87; Slonim, p 174)

    a. _____

    b. _____

34. List/discuss the two respiratory centers located in the pons. (Kacmarek, pp 188–189; Slonim, pp 174–177; West, pp 114–115)

    a. _____

    b. _____

35. What role does the cerebral cortex play in respiratory control? (Kacmarek, p 88; Murray, p 237)

    _____

    _____

36. List/explain, in terms of location, stimulation, and effect of stimulation, the three respiratory reflexes that affect breathing. (West, pp 120–121; Kacmarek, p 90; Slonim, pp 181–183)

    a. _____

    _____

    _____

    b. _____

    _____

    _____

c. _____

_____

_____

37. Where are the peripheral chemoreceptors located? What do these chemoreceptors respond to? (Kacmarek, p 91; Murray, pp 240–245. West, pp 118–119)

_____

_____

38. Central chemoreceptors are located in the _____ and are stimulated by _____. (Kacmarek, p 92; Murray, pp 235–246; West, pp 116–118)

39. As $Paco_2$ increases, ventilation _____, and as $Paco_2$ decreases ventilation _____. (Kacmarek, p 92; West, pp 122–124)

40. How do the nose, larynx, and airways react to inhalation of an irritant? (Murray, chp 13)

_____

_____

_____

41. What mechanism is responsible for the clearance of particulate matter in the tracheobronchial tree? in the alveoli? (Murray, pp 318–322)

_____

_____

42. Why is a mixture of the He-O_2 used when diving to great depths? (Slonim, p 224)

_____

_____

_____

43. What would happen to the $Paco_2$ if you doubled your patient's alveolar ventilation? (Slonim, pp 214–215; West, pp 130–131)

_____

44. What effect does N_2 have on divers at depths of greater than 150 feet? (Slonim, p 224; West, p 137)

_____

45. What would be five clinical uses for increasing the Pao_2 to a very high level with the use of hyperbaric chambers? (Slonim, pp 227–228; West, p 138)

a. _____

b. _____

c. _____

d. _____

e. _____

46. What effect does age have on the following: (Murray, chp 14)

    a. compliance: _____

    b. chest wall: _____

    c. vital capacity: _____

    d. residual volume: _____

    e. forced expiratory flow rates: _____

    f. diffusing capacity: _____

    g. arterial oxygen tension: _____

    h. $(A - a)DO_2$: _____

    i. right to left shunt: _____

    j. carbon monoxide tension: _____

    k. pH: _____

ANSWERS TO STUDY QUESTIONS

1. a. vertical —contraction of diaphragm
   b. lateral—rotation of ribs laterally (2 to 10)
   c. AP—upper ribs elevate sternum

2. Lungs have a tendency to collapse; ribs and thorax have a tendency to expand.

3. a. pressure at opening of mouth
   b. pressure in alveolus, at FRC = atmospheric
   c. pressure in pleural space, at FRC = below atmospheric due to elastic forces
   d. pressure difference betweeen alveolar and pleural

4. the ease with which the lungs-thorax can be distended; $\dfrac{\Delta V}{\Delta P} = \dfrac{L}{cm\ H_2O}$

5. a. lung compliance
   b. thorax compliance
   c. total compliance

6. a. 0.2 l/cm H_2O
   b. 0.2 l/cm H_2O
   c. 0.1 l/cm H_2O

7. 0.04 l/cm H_2O

8. Forces occurring between the interface of a liquid and a gas or of two liquids that tend to cause the liquid to occupy the smallest space; It would cause the alveoli to collapse; avoided by the presence of pulmonary surfactant (type II alveolar cells)

9. a. decrease pulmonary surfactant—hypoxia, acidosis, hyperoxia, atelectasis, hyaline membrane disease
   b. pulmonary edema
   c. ARDS-RDS
   d. pneumothorax
   e. pulmonary consolidation
   f. thoracic deformaties

10. a. alveolar distension
    b. alveolar septal destruction

11. the tendency for a distended lung-thorax system to return to the original shape; $E = \dfrac{\Delta P}{\Delta V}$ $\dfrac{cmH_2O}{L}$

12. dynamic force necessary to overcome resistance (friction) which occurs during air movement. $R = \dfrac{\Delta P}{flow} = cm\ H_2O/l/sec$

13. a. airway resistance
    b. tissue viscous resistance
    c. inertia, change in velocity, change in direction

14. 0.6 to 2.4 cm H_2O/l/sec

15. 0.2 cm H_2O/l/sec

16. a. mechanical work: $w = f \times d$—overcome elastic and nonelastic forces

b. metabolic work: oxygen consumption required for breathing

17. 200 to 350 ml/min

18. passive tendency of molecules to move from a region of higher concentration to one of lower concentration

19. a. concentration gradient
    b. temperature
    c. cross-sectional area
    d. molecular weight
    e. distance gas has to diffuse

20. Graham's and Henry's laws

21. a. alveolar ventilation and pulmonary capillary blood flow
    b. blood traverses the alveolar capillary membrane in about 0.75 sec, but only takes 0.25 to 0.30 sec for oxygen and carbon dioxide to equilibrate

22. a. pulmonary
    b. bronchial

23. 10 percent

24. a. deliver blood from right ventricle to pulmonary capillaries for gas exchange
    b. supply oxygen and nutrients to lung parenchyma and rid the lungs of waste
    c. left ventricular reservoir for cardiac output

25. a. collapse—apices; no perfusion
    b. waterfall—middle; blood flow increases as you go down the lung
    c. distension—bases; blood flow constant

26. determined inflow pressure in pulmonary artery, outflow pressure in pulmonary veins or left ventricle; 60 percent controlled by capillary bed; controlled by alveolar P_{O_2}, hypoxemia, acidosis, and mechanical factor

27. a. distension
    b. recruitment

28. a. variation in compliance and airway resistance
    b. regional variation in transpulmonary pressure

29. Bases are better perfused than apices.
    Apices are better ventilated than perfused
    overall $\dfrac{\dot{V}}{\dot{Q}} = 0.8$

30. a. normal unit—good perfusion, good ventilation
    b. deadspace unit—good ventilation, no perfusion

c. shunt unit—no ventilation, good perfusion
d. silent unit—no perfusion, no ventilation

31. a. calculation of physiologic dead space
    b. calculation of shunt
    c. calculation of $(A-a)D_{O_2}$

32. a. medulla oblongata
    b. pons
    c. cerebral cortex
    d. vagus nerve
    e. peripheral chemoreceptors
    f. central chemoreceptors

33. a. dorsal respiratory group
    b. ventral respiratory group

34. a. pneumotaxic—upper pons; inhibit inspiration
    b. apneustic—lower pons; sustained inspiration, increase rate, increase depth of breathing

35. all conscious respiratory control, ventilatory changes due to pain, anxiety, or other emotions, ventilatory control during speech

36. a. Hering-Bruer reflex—smooth muscle, stimulated by lung inflation and deflation, termination of inspiratory and expiration, bronchodilation, tachycardia
    b. irritant receptors—epithelium trachea, bronchi, larynx, nose, pharynx; irritants, mechanical, anaphylaxis, pneumothorax, congestion; bronchoconstriction, hyperpnea, laryngospasm, cough
    c. juxtapulmonary capillary receptors—walls of alveoli; increase interstitial fluid, chemicals; rapid shallow breathing, expiratory constriction larynx, hypoventilation, and bradycardia

37. located in carotid and aortic bodies, bifurcation of carina and arch of aorta; respond to decrease in blood flow and an increase in temperature

38. ventral side of medulla, changes in H^+ in CSF

39. increase, decrease

40. nose—sneezing
    larynx—cough, laryngeal closure
    airways—cough, hypersecretions, bronchoconstriction

41. tracheobronchial tree—cilia
    alveoli—alveolar macrophages

42. because of O_2 toxicity
    sea level = 0.21×760 mmHg = 159 mmHg
    3 atms = 0.21×2280 mmHg = 478.6 mmHg

43. Pa$_{CO_2}$ would be halved.

44. nitrogen narcosis—nitrogen has euphoric effects at high pressures

45. a. CO poisoning
    b. decompression sickness
    c. gas gangrene
    d. some anemic crises (circulatory shock)
    e. some surgical procedures (organ transplantation, ischemic organs)

46. a. more compliant
    b. less compliant (stiffer)
    c. decreased
    d. increased
    e. decreased
    f. decreased
    g. decreased
    h. widening of gradient
    i. increased
    j. constant throughout one's life
    k. constant throughout one's life

PRACTICE QUIZ

1. Compliance of the human lung is:
    I. Volume change per unit of pressure change
    II. Pressure change per unit of volume change
    III. As lung compliance decreases, the elastic recoil of the lung decreases
    IV. As lung compliance increases, the elastic recoil of the lung decreases
    V. Normal lung compliance is equal to 0.2 l/cm H_2O
    a. I, III, IV
    b. II, IV, V
    c. I, III, V
    d. II, III, V
    e. I, IV, V

2. Which of the following would cause a decrease in compliance?
    a. pneumothorax
    b. chronic bronchitis
    c. emphysema
    d. asthma (late stage)
    e. all of the above

3. If a patient has a tidal volume of 750 ml, and the pressure measured while maintaining the volume is 20 cm H_2O, what is his compliance?
    a. 0.037 l/cm H_2O
    b. 0.043 l/cm H_2O
    c. 0.97 l/cm H_2O
    d. 26.6 l/cm H_2O
    e. 32.8 l/cm H_2O

4. Which of the following factors will cause an increase in airway resistance?
    I. Increased diameter of the airway
    II. No gas flow
    III. Decreased velocity of the gas
    IV. Decreased diameter of the airway
    V. Increased pulmonary compliance
    a. II, III
    b. II, III, IV
    c. IV only
    d. I, II, V
    e. I, II, III, IV, V

5. In relation to systemic circulation, the pulmonary circulation is characterized by:
    I. High pressure
    II. High resistance
    III. Low pressure
    IV. Low resistance
  a. I and II
  b. III and IV
  c. I and IV
  d. II and III
  e. I, II, III

6. If pulmonary artery pressure is increased twofold, the pulmonary vascular resistance would:
  a. increase
  b. decrease
  c. remain the same
  d. increase by half
  e. decrease by half

7. The surface-active material in the lungs (surfactant) is generally believed to be a product of:
  a. white blood cells
  b. type I alveolar cells
  c. mast cells
  d. alveolar macrophages
  e. type II alveolar cells

8. The lung has two different circulatory systems. The system that serves the metabolic needs of the lung itself is known as the:
  a. pulmonary circulation
  b. bronchial circulation
  c. systemic circulation
  d. hepatic circulation
  e. bronchiolar circulation

9. In the elderly, one would expect which of the following lung volumes and capacities to be increased?
    I. FRC
    II. RV
    III. TLC
    IV. TV
  a. I only
  b. I and II
  c. I, II, III
  d. I, III, IV
  e. all of the above

10. CO_2 and O_2 exchange between alveoli and capillaries occurs by what process?
  a. osmosis
  b. hydrolysis
  c. convection
  d. diffusion
  e. defecation

11. Which of the following clinical laboratory data would be the best indicator of adequacy of alveolar ventilation?
  a. Pa_{O_2}
  b. PA_{O_2}

c. P_{H_2O}
d. Pa_{CO_2}
e. pH

12. During a standardized rate of flow of 0.5 l/sec, airway resistance was measured at 0.8 cm H_2O/l/sec. This would be considered:
   a. normal
   b. very low
   c. very high
   d. moderately low
   e. moderately high

13. At rest, a "normal" individual will have an oxygen consumption of approximately:
   a. 2500 ml/min
   b. 25 ml/min
   c. 2.5 ml/min
   d. 250 ml./min
   e. 200 ml/min

14. Small changes in Pa_{CO_2} will stimulate:
   a. central chemoreceptors
   b. pneumotaxic center
   c. apneustic center
   d. medulla
   e. peripheral chemoreceptors

15. Which of the following allows us to have voluntary control of ventilation?
   a. medulla
   b. pons
   c. midbrain
   d. pneumotaxic center
   e. cerebral cortex

16. The primary center for respiratory control is located in the:
   a. lungs
   b. carotid bodies
   c. aortic arch
   d. cerebellum
   e. medulla oblongata

17. The apneustic and pneumotaxic centers are located in the:
   a. medulla
   b. pons
   c. midbrain
   d. hypothalamus
   e. cerebellum

18. Hypoxemia stimulates ventilation via the:
   I. Central chemoreceptors
   II. Medullary center
   III. Peripheral chemoreceptors
   a. I only
   b. III only
   c. II only
   d. I and III
   e. I, II, III

19. The diffusibility of carbon dioxide across the alveolar capillary membrane in relation to oxygen is about:
    a. 10 times faster
    b. 15 times faster
    c. 20 times faster
    d. 25 times faster
    e. 30 times faster

20. Which of the following statements most accurately describes the normal ventilation/perfusion relationship between the bases and apices?
    a. Bases are better ventilated than perfused.
    b. Lung apices are better perfused than ventilated.
    c. Apices are more perfused than the bases.
    d. Apices are better ventilated than perfused.
    e. Both the bases and the apices are equally ventilated and perfused.

ANSWERS TO THE PRACTICE QUIZ

1. e
2. a
3. a
4. c
5. b
6. a
7. e
8. b
9. c
10. d

11. d
12. a
13. d
14. a
15. e
16. e
17. b
18. b
19. c
20. d

Chapter 13

ARTERIAL BLOOD GASES

Outline

LEARNING OBJECTIVES

Upon completion of this unit, the individual will:

1. Define the following terms:
   a. acids
   b. bases
   c. buffers
   d. pH
2. List the major buffering systems in the body.
3. Explain the Henderson-Hasselbalch equation.
4. Describe carbon dioxide transport.
5. Describe oxygen transport.
6. Distinguish between actual and standard bicarbonate.
7. Define base excess
8. List three measurements of oxygenation.
9. Draw/explain the oxyhemoglobin dissociation curve.
10. List/describe the factors that influence the oxyhemoglobin dissociation curve.
11. Describe the Bohr and Haldane effect.
12. List the indications for arterial blood gases.
13. List the complications/hazards of arterial blood gas sampling.
14. Describe the criteria used to access a puncture site.
15. Describe the Allen's test.
16. Describe how a capillary sample is obtained.
17. Explain the use of an umbilical artery catheter in a neonate.
18. Distinguish/discuss the electrodes used to measure the sample.
19. Explain Beer's law.
20. Describe the theories behind transcutaneous carbon dioxide and oxygen monitoring.
21. List the normal arterial blood gas values for adult, pediatric, and neonatal patients.
22. Differentiate between the following:
    a. acidosis versus acidemia
    b. alkalosis versus alkalemia
23. Distinguish between compensation and correction.
24. List the primary causes for the following:
    a. respiratory acidosis
    b. respiratory alkalosis
    c. metabolic acidosis
    d. metabolic alkalosis
25. Explain the effect of carbon dioxide and bicarbonate on pH.
26. Given a set of PaO_2 values, indicate the degree of hypoxemia, in terms of mild, moderate, and severe.
27. Interpret a set of arterial blood gases.
28. Describe the effects of heparin and air bubbles on the arterial blood gas sample.
29. List the types of hypoxia.
30. Calculate the following, given the proper information:
    a. alveolar-air equation
    b. oxygen content
    c. mixed venous content
    d. alveolar/arterial content difference
    e. arterial/venous content difference
    f. shunt
    g. dead space

REFERENCES

Aloan, CA: Respiratory Care of the Newborn. JB Lippincott, Philadelphia, 1987.

Barnes, TA: Respiratory Care Practice. Year Book Medical Publishers, Chicago, 1988.

Bennington, D, et al: Saunders Dictionary and Encyclopedia of Laboratory Medicine and Technology. WB Saunders, Philadelphia, 1984.

Blodgett, D: Manual of Pediatric Respiratory Care Procedures. JB Lippincott, Philadelphia, 1982

Burton, G, and Hodgkin, J: Respiratory Care: A Guide to Clinical Practice, ed 2. JB Lippincott, Philadelphia, 1984.

Kacmarek, RM, Mack, CW and Dimas, S: The Essentials of Respiratory Therapy, ed 2. Year Book Medical Publishers, Chicago, 1985.

Lough, MD, Doershuk, CF, and Stern, RC: Pediatric Respiratory Therapy, ed 3. Year Book Medical Publishers, Chicago, 1985.

Shapiro, BA, Harrison, RA and Walton, JR: Clinical Application of Blood Gases, ed 3. Year Book Medical Publishers, Chicago, 1982.

STUDY QUESTIONS

1. Define the following terms: (Shapiro, p 13; Kacmarek, pp 10–11, 198)

   a. acids: _____

   b. bases: _____

   c. buffers: _____

   d. pH: _____

2. List the four major buffering systems in the body. (Shapiro, p 13)

   a. _____

   b. _____

   c. _____

   d. _____

3. Explain the following equation: (Shapiro, p 16)
   $$pH = pK + \log HCO_3^- / s + PCO_2$$

   _____

   _____

4. What is the role of carbonic anhydrase in the following equation? (Shapiro, p 16; Barnes, p 505)
   $$H_2O + CO_2 \rightleftarrows H_2CO_3 \rightleftarrows H^+ + HCO_3^-$$

   _____

   _____

   _____

   _____

5. The major component of the red blood cell (RBC) is called _____. (Shapiro, p 19; Kacmarek, p 97)

6. Carbon dioxide is transported in the blood dissolved, and in chemical combination with hemoglobin. The portion of carbon dioxide is measured as what value? (Burton, p 274; Kacmarek, p 189)

   _____

7. Describe the chloride shift. (Burton, p 275; Shapiro, p 98)

   _____

   _____

   _____

8. Distinguish between actual and standard bicarbonate. (Burton, p 268; Barnes, p 508; Shapiro, p 98)

   _____

   _____

   _____

9. Define base excess/deficit. (Barnes, p 508; Shapiro, pp 98–99; Kacmarek, p 202)

   _____

10. Three indices of arterial oxygenation are: (Barnes, p 499; Burton, p 259)

    a. _____

    b. _____

    c. _____

11. The relationship between the PaO_2 and the reaction with hemoglobin is graphically described by

    the _____. (Burton, p 261; Barnes, p 501)

12. The shape of the oxyhemoglobin dissociation curve is _____. (Burton, p 261; Barnes, p 501)

13. List the factors that influence the affinity of oxygen to hemoglobin and indicate how the curve will shift (right or left). (Kacmarek, p 187; Barnes, p 501; Burton, p 263)

    a. _____

    b. _____

    c. _____

    d. _____

    e. _____

    f. _____

14. Define P_{50}. (Shapiro, p 170; Barnes, p 502)

    _____

    _____

15. In simple terms describe the Bohr and Haldane effects. (Shapiro, p 27; Barnes, pp 502, 506)

    _____

    _____

16. List as many clinical indications for arterial blood gas analysis as you can. (Barnes, p 497)

    _____

    _____

    _____

    _____

    _____

    _____

    _____

    _____

17. Complications/hazards of arterial blood gas sampling include: (Shapiro, pp 143, 150)

    _____

    _____

18. What criteria are used to access a site for an arterial puncture? (Barnes, p 83; Shapiro, pp 144–145)

_____

19. Describe Figure 13–1. (Burton, p 258; Shapiro, pp 145–147; Barnes, p 84)

_____

20. List the sites most commonly used for arterial puncture. (Barnes, p 83; Shapiro, pp 143–144)

    a. _____

    b. _____

    c. _____

    d. _____

21. A method of assessing the Paco$_2$ and the pH in the newborn can be accomplished by doing a capillary sample. Where is this sample obtained? (Aloan, p 66; Shapiro, p 153)

_____

22. If frequent blood gas sampling is required in the neonate the arterial line is placed in the _____. (Aloan, p 62; Lough, p 224)

23. Identify in Figures 13–2, 13–3, and 13–4 each electrode (name and what each measures). (Shapiro, pp 30–34; Burton, pp 981–983)

    a. _____ Fig. 13–2

    b. _____ Fig. 13–3

    c. _____ Fig. 13–4

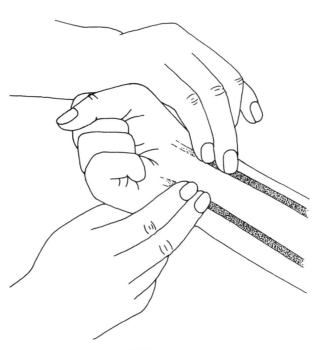

FIGURE 13–1.

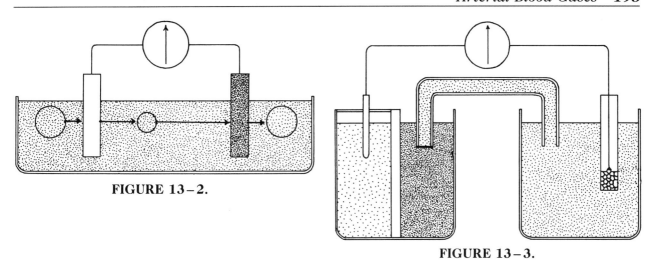

FIGURE 13–2.

FIGURE 13–3.

FIGURE 13–4.

24. Beer's law states that the intensity of light absorbed while passing through a solution will be proportional to the concentration of that molecule within a solution. What device utilizes this principle? (Shapiro, p 38; Barnes, pp 82–83)

_____

25. Other than the noninvasive technique described earlier, what other method is commonly employed to evaluate PaO_2 and $PaCO_2$? (Barnes, p 89; Shapiro, pp 39–40)

_____

26. Describe how the device in question 25 operates. (Barnes, p 89; Shapiro, pp 39–40)

_____

_____

_____

27. Indicate the normal ranges for arterial blood gases in the adult. (Kacmarek, p 203; Shapiro, pp 122–125)

   a. pH: _____

   b. $PaCO_2$: _____

   c. PaO_2: _____

   d. HCO_3: _____

   e. base excess: _____

   f. SaO_2: _____

   g. hemoglobin: _____

28. Indicate the normal ranges for arterial blood gas measurements in the term infant and the child. (Blodgett, pp 221, 228; Bennington, pp 1641–1670)

	Term Infant	Child
a. pH:		
b. $Paco_2$:		
c. Pao_2:		
d. SaO_2:		
e. base excess:		
f. hemoglobin:		

29. Define the following terminology: (Kacmarek, p 209; Shapiro, p 98)

    a. acidemia: _____

    b. acidosis: _____

    c. alkalemia: _____

    d. alkalosis: _____

    e. correction: _____

    f. compensation: _____

30. At a pH baseline value of 7.40 and a $Paco_2$ of 40 mmHg, determine the altered pH value. (Kacmarek, p 208)

    a. $Paco_2$ 60 mm Hg: _____

    b. $Paco_2$ 20 mmHg: _____

    c. $Paco_2$ 80 mmHg: _____

    d. $Paco_2$ 30 mmHg: _____

31. List the primary causes of respiratory acidosis. (Kacmarek, pp 208–209; Shapiro, pp 105–106)

    a. _____

    b. _____

    c. _____

    d. _____

32. What effect does ventilatory failure (hypoventilation) have on $Paco_2$ and pH? (Kacmarek, pp 208–209; Shapiro, pp 105–106)

    _____

33. List the primary causes of respiratory alkalosis. (Kacmarek, p 209; Shapiro, p 107)

    a. _____

    b. _____

    c. _____

    d. _____

34. What effect does alveolar hyperventilation have on $Paco_2$ and pH? (Kacmarek, p 209; Shapiro, p 107)

    _____

35. List the primary causes of metabolic acidosis. (Kacmarek, p 209; Shapiro, pp 276–277)

    a. _____

    b. _____

    c. _____

    d. _____

    e. _____

36. What effect does an increased H^+ ion in the blood have on HCO_3, base excess, and pH? (Kacmarek, p 209; Shapiro, pp 276–277)

    _____

37. List the primary causes of metabolic alkalosis. (Kacmarek, p 210; Burton, pp 277–278)

    a. _____

    b. _____

    c. _____

    d. _____

    e. _____

38. What effect does a decreased H^+ ion in the blood have on HCO_3, base excess, and pH? (Kacmarek, p 210; Burton, pp 277–278)

    _____

39. On a patient less than 60 years old and breathing room air, indicate next to the degree of hypoxemia the range of values of Pao_2. (Kacmarek, p 208; Shapiro, p 137)

    a. mild: _____

    b. moderate: _____

    c. severe: _____

40. How is the $Paco_2$ determined if an individual is over the age of 60 years? (Kacmarek, p 208; Shapiro, p 137)

    _____

    _____

41. The minimal acceptable range for a $Paco_2$ on a given Fio_2 is determined by the formula: _____. (Shapiro, p 127)

42. Using the chart, indicate by using arrows if the value is increased, decreased, or normal (N). (Kacmarek, p 206; Shapiro, p 135)

	pH	$Paco_2$	HCO_3	BE
1. Respiratory acidosis				
a. uncompensated (acute)				
b. partially compensated (acute)				
c. compensated (chronic)				

2. Respiratory alkalosis

    a. uncompensated (acute) _____

    b. partially compensated (acute) _____

    c. compensated (chronic) _____

3. Metabolic acidosis

    a. uncompensated (acute) _____

    b. partially compensated (acute) _____

    c. compensated (chronic) _____

4. Metabolic alkalosis

    a. uncompensated (acute) _____

    b. partially compensated (acute) _____

    c. compensated (chronic) _____

5. Mixed acidosis _____

6. Mixed alkalosis _____

43. Interpret the following arterial blood gas samples:

	pH	$Paco_2$	Pao_2	HCO_3	BE	SaO_2	Interpretation
a.	7.43	41	94	26	+2	95%	_____
b.	7.52	30	45	24	+2	86%	_____
c.	7.15	80	80	26	0	92%	_____
d.	7.20	55	55	20	−8	80%	_____
e.	7.60	40	85	39	+10	94%	_____
f.	7.54	25	52	30	+8	82%	_____
g.	7.25	65	39	35	+15	65%	_____
h.	7.39	38	65	25	0	90%	_____

44. What effect on your sample will too much heparin have on the following values? (increase, decrease, no change) (Kacmarek, p 212)

    a. ph: _____

    b. $Paco_2$: _____

    c. Pao_2: _____

    d. HCO_3: _____

    e. base excess: _____

    f. Oxygen saturation: _____

    g. hemoglobin content: _____

45. What effect on your sample will an air bubble have on the following values? (increase, decrease, no change) (Kacmarek, p 212)

    a. pH: _____

    b. $Paco_2$: _____

    c. Pao_2: _____

    d. HCO_3: _____

    e. base excess: _____

    f. oxygen saturation: _____

    g. hemoglobin content: _____

46. What is the compensatory mechanism for the following: (Kacmarek, p 204)

    a. metabolic acid/base disorders: _____

    b. respiratory acid/base disorders: _____

47. Hypoxia is a state in which the demands of the tissue for oxygen exceed the amount of oxygen supplied. List the four forms of hypoxia. (Burton, p 503; Shapiro, pp 48–50)

    a. _____

    b. _____

    c. _____

    d. _____

48. Write the formulas for the following: (Shapiro, pp 75, 83, 213–225; Kacmarek, pp 185, 218–220, 226)

    a. alveolar air equation: _____

    b. oxygen content: _____

    c. mixed venous content: _____

    d. alveolar/arterial oxygen difference: _____

    e. arterial/venous content difference: _____

    f. Qs/Qt: _____

    g. clinical shunt equation: _____

    h. dead space: _____

ANSWERS TO STUDY QUESTIONS

1. a. donates H^+
   b. removes H^+
   c. prevents extreme changes in pH
   d. measurement of H^+ in solution

2. a. hemoglobin
   b. bicarbonate
   c. phosphate
   d. serum proteins

3. Henderson-Hasselbalch equation, where:
   pK = 6.1
   and HCO_3/H_2CO_3 $\dfrac{\textbf{amount of acid}}{\textbf{base}} = \dfrac{20}{1} = 7.40$;
   the value of $H_2CO_3 = 0.03 \times Paco_2$

4. speeds up the reaction of H_2O and CO_2 to produce carbonic acid

5. hemoglobin

6. Paco$_2$

7. As the reaction $CO_2 + H_2 \rightleftarrows H_2CO_3 \rightleftarrows H^+ + HCO_3$, H^+ is buffered by hemoglobin. Bicarbonate diffuses out of the RBC. To maintain electric neutrality CL^- diffuses into the RBC.

8. actual: value calculated from measurement of Pco$_2$ and pH of arterial blood
   standard: value calculated from measurement of Pco$_2$ and pH of venous blood after Pco$_2$ has been equilibrated to 40 mmHg/g

9. number of mEq/l of total body buffer base above or below 54 mEq/l; with a range of ± 2 mEq/l calculated based on pH, hemoglobin, and bicarbonate

10. a. arterial Po$_2$
    b. percent oxygen saturation
    c. oxygen content

11. oxyhemoglobin dissociation curve

12. sigmoid

13. a. decrease affinity = right shift   increase affinity = left shift
    b. increase P$_{50}$ decrease P$_{50}$
    c. decrease pH   increase pH
    d. increase Pco$_2$ decrease Pco$_2$
    e. increase 2,3 DPG   decrease 2,3 DPG
    f. increase temperature   decrease temperature
                                                carbon monoxide
                                                fetal hemoglobin
                                                methemoglobin

14. Pao$_2$ at which 50 percent of hemoglobin is saturated at 37°C, Pao$_2$ 40 mmHg, pH 7.40, at this point Pao$_2$ = 27 mmHg

15. Bohr—effect of carbon dioxide on oxygen uptake and release
    Haldane—effect of oxygen on carbon dioxide uptake and release

16. I. Arterial oxygenation and oxygen delivery
        a. unexplained tachypnea, dyspnea, restlessness, tachycardia, and anxiety
        b. decreased cardiac output
        c. precardiothoracic or postcardiothoracic surgery
        d. cardiopulmonary arrest
        e. mechanical ventilation
    II. alveolar ventilation
        a. unexplained drowsiness, confusion, tachycardia
        b. bradypnea
        c. cardiopulmonary arrest
        d. mechanical ventilation
   III. acid-base balance
        a. tachypnea or other abnormal breathing patterns
        b. renal failure
        c. drug intoxication
        d. cardiopulmonary arrest
        e. mechanical ventilation

17. damage to nerve, hematoma, infection, thrombosis (embolism), obstruction to blood flow

18. easy access, tissue surrounding site, good collateral circulation

19. modified Allen's test

20. a. radial
    b. brachial
    c. pedal
    d. femoral

21. heal stick

22. umbilical artery

23. a. Clark, Paco$_2$
    b. Sanz, pH
    c. Severinghaus, Paco$_2$

24. oximeter (spectrophotometer)

25. tcPo$_2$ and tcPco$_2$

26. electrode placed on skin and heated to 40 to 50°C promoting oxygen and carbon dioxide transport to the skin; using modified version of Clark and Severinghaus electrode, measures Pao$_2$ and Pco$_2$

27. a. 7.35 to 7.45
    b. 35 to 45 mmHg
    c. 80 to 100 mmHg
    d. 22 to 27 mEq/l
    e. ± 2 mEq/l
    f. ≥ 95 percent
    g. 12 to 16 g percent

28. **Term Infant**
    a. 7.26 to 7.41
    b. 34 to 54 mmHg
    c. 60 to 80 mmHg
    d. 40 to 95 percent
    e. −7 to −1 mEq/l
    f. 14 to 24 g percent

    Child
    a. 7.35 to 7.45
    b. 35 to 45 mmHg
    c. 75 to 100 mmHg
    d. 95 to 98 percent
    e. −4 to +2 mEq/l
    f. 12.5 to 15 g percent

29. a. condition in which blood is too acid
    b. process causing acidemia
    c. condition in which blood is too alkaline
    d. process causing alkalemia
    e. abnormal pH is returned toward normal by altering the component primarily affected
    f. abnormal pH is returned toward normal by altering component not primarily affected

30. a. pH = 7.30
    b. pH = 7.60
    c. pH = 7.20
    d. pH = 7.50

31. a. COPD
    b. oversedation (morphine, anesthesia)
    c. neuromuscular disease
    d. head trauma

32. increase carbon dioxide tension and decrease pH

33. a. hypoxia
    b. CNS stimulation (drugs, trauma)
    c. emotional disorders (anxiety, pain)
    d. pregnancy

34. decrease carbon dioxide and increase pH

35. a. lactic acidosis
    b. ketoacidosis
    c. renal failure
    d. diarrhea
    e. ingestion of drugs (aspirin, alcohol)

36. decrease bicarbonate, decrease base excess, and increase pH

37. a. hypokalemia
    b. hypochloremia
    c. gastric suctioning or vomiting
    d. diuretics
    e. large-dose steroids

38. increase bicarbonate, increase base excess, and decrease pH

39. a. 60 to 79 mmHg
    b. 40 to 59 mmHg
    c. <40 mmHg

40. 1 mmHg subtracted from lower limit of mild and moderate for each year over 60 years

41. $F_{IO_2} \times 5$; clinically $F_{IO_2} \times 3$ is acceptable

42. 1a. decrease, increase, N, N
    b. decrease, increase, increase, increase
    c. N, increase, increase, increase
    2a. increase, decrease, N, N
    b. increase, decrease, decrease, decrease
    c. N, decrease, decrease, decrease
    3a. decrease, N, decrease, decrease
    b. decrease, decrease, decrease, decrease
    c. N, decrease, decrease, decrease
    4a. increase, N, increase, increase
    b. increase, increase, increase, increase
    c. N, increase, increase, increase
    5. decrease, increase, decrease, decrease
    6. increase, decrease, increase, increase

43. a. normal
    b. uncompensated respiratory alkalosis with moderate hypoxemia
    c. uncompensated respiratory acidosis
    d. mixed acidosis with moderate hypoxemia
    e. uncompensated metabolic alkalosis
    f. mixed alkalosis with moderate hypoxemia
    g. partially compensated respiratory acidosis with severe hypoxemia
    h. normal with mild hypoxemia

44. a. decrease
    b. decrease
    c. may change
    d. decrease
    e. decrease
    f. may change
    g. decrease

45. a. increase
    b. decrease
    c. may change
    d. decrease
    e. decrease
    f. may change
    g. no effect

46. respiratory system, metabolic system

47. a. hypoxemic
    b. anemic
    c. circulatory
    d. histotoxic

48. a. $P_{AO_2} = (P_B - P_{H_2O}) \times F_{IO_2} + P_{aCO_2}/0.8$
    b. $C_{aO_2} = (Hgb \times 1.34)S_{aO_2} + (P_{aO_2} \times 0.003)$
    c. $C\bar{v}O_2 = (Hgb \times 1.34)\,S\bar{v}O_2 + (P\bar{v}O_2 \times 0.003)$
    d. $(A - a)DO_2$
    e. $C(a - \bar{v})O_2$
    f. $\dfrac{C_cO_2 - C_aO_2}{C_cO_2 - C\bar{v}O_2}$
    g. $\dfrac{(P_{AO_2} - P_{aO_2})\,0.003}{(P_{AO_2} - P_{aO_2})\,0.003 + 3.5}$
    h. $\dfrac{Vd}{Vt} = P_{aCO_2} - \dfrac{P_{ECO_2}}{P_{aCO_2}}$

PRACTICE QUIZ

1. If a patient's P_{ECO_2} is 18 mmHg and Pa_{CO_2} is 40 mmHg, Vd/Vt will be:
   a. 0.40
   b. 0.45
   c. 0.50
   d. 0.55
   e. 0.60

2. Using your answer in question 1, calculate the physiologic dead space if the tidal volume is 0.5 l.
   a. 175 ml
   b. 225 ml
   c. 275 ml
   d. 350 ml
   e. 400 ml

3. A male with a hemoglobin count of 10 g/100 ml of blood would be considered:
   a. polycythemic
   b. normal
   c. anemic
   d. very healthy
   e. dead

4. At a temperature of 37°C, 100 ml of plasma will contain _____ ml of oxygen per mmHg.
   a. 0.03
   b. 1.34
   c. 0.003
   d. 0.000003
   e. 1.39

5. Using the following data, determine the $\dot{Q}s/\dot{Q}t$:
   $$CO = 4.0 l/min, CaO_2 = 17.0 \ vol\%, CcO_2 = 18.5 \ vol\%, C\bar{v}O_2 = 13.0 \ vol\%$$
   a. 6 percent
   b. 10 percent
   c. 18 percent
   d. 27 percent
   e. 33 percent

6. Oxygen that is carried in the dissolved form is expressed as:
      I. Sa_{O_2}
      II. $P\bar{v}_{O_2}$
      III. $P_{A}O_2$
      IV. Pa_{O_2}
   a. II, IV
   b. I, III
   c. I, II, IV
   d. III only
   e. IV only

7. By analysis, it was found that the DPG level was high and the curve shifted to the right. Later the patient was found to have acute hypoxemia. This would have the effect of:
      I. Increasing the shift to the right
      II. Neutralizing the effect of the elevated DPG
      III. Increasing P_{50}
      IV. Decreasing P_{50}

a. I only
b. II only
c. I, III
d. II, IV
e. I, II, III

8. The blood gas values of $\dfrac{12 \text{ mEq/l}}{1.2 \text{ mEq/l}}$ would be consistent with:
   a. respiratory acidosis
   b. metabolic acidosis
   c. respiratory alkalosis
   d. metabolic alkalosis
   e. mixed alkalosis

9. Pure hypoventilation can be caused by which of the following:
       I. Depressed CNS
      II. Myasthenia gravis
     III. Anesthesia
     IV. Crushed chest
   a. I and II
   b. I, III, IV
   c. I, II, III
   d. II, III, IV
   e. all of the above

10. Breathing 100 percent oxygen will eliminate the hypoxemia caused by all of the following *except*:
    a. hypoventilation
    b. right to left shunt
    c. ventilation/perfusion mismatch
    d. diffusion defect
    e. altitude

11. Which of the following shifts the oxyhemoglobin dissociation curve to the left?
    a. hyperthermia
    b. increase 2,3 DPG
    c. hypocarbia
    d. hypercarbia
    e. acidosis

12. Given Pa_{O_2} 90 mmHg, oxygen saturation 95 percent, Hgb 12 g/100 ml. Calculate total oxygen content.
    a. 12.8 vol%
    b. 14.7 vol%
    c. 16.6 vol%
    d. 18.5 vol%
    e. 20.4 vol%

13. What is the physiologic compensatory response to metabolic acidosis?
    a. accumulation of bicarbonate
    b. shift in the CO_2 dissociation curve
    c. excretion of ammonium chloride
    d. hyperventilation
    e. excretion of excess bicarbonate

14. Given: pH 7.10, Pa_{CO_2} 50 mmHg, Pa_{O_2} 75 mmHg, HCO_3 10 mEq/l. This is an example of:
    a. mixed alkalosis

b. mixed acidosis
c. metabolic acidosis with respiratory compensation
d. respiratory acidosis with metabolic compensation
e. metabolic alkalosis with respiratory compensation

15. Which of the following carbon dioxide transport mechanisms carries the majority of the CO_2 from the tissues to the lungs?
a. reversibly bound to hemoglobin
b. Pa_{CO_2}
c. H_2CO_3
d. bicarbonate
e. carbamino compounds

16. What would be considered normal Pa_{O_2} for a 70-year-old patient?
a. 55 mmHg
b. 60 mmHg
c. 65 mmHg
d. 70 mmHg
e. 80 mmHg

17. Interpret the following blood gas, pH 7.41, Pa_{CO_2} 30 mmHg, Pa_{O_2} 100 mmHg, HCO_3 16 mEq/l:
a. acute respiratory acidosis
b. acute metabolic acidosis
c. partially compensated respiratory alkalosis
d. fully compensated respiratory alkalosis
e. mixed acidosis

18. Which of the following would cause hypoxic hypoxia?
a. decrease in PI_{O_2}
b. decreased cardiac output
c. sickle cell anemia
d. cyanide poisoning
e. carbon monoxide poisoning

19. A substance capable of donating a H^+ is:
a. a base
b. an ion
c. a ketone
d. an ester
e. an acid

20. What is the relationship between Pa_{O_2} and percent saturation of hemoglobin?
a. linear
b. accelerating linear
c. square
d. sigmoid
e. descending square wave

ANSWERS TO PRACTICE QUIZ

1. d
2. c
3. c
4. c
5. d
6. a
7. c
8. b
9. e
10. b

11. c
12. a
13. d
14. b
15. d
16. d
17. d
18. a
19. e
20. d

Chapter 14

PULMONARY FUNCTIONS

OUTLINE

INTRODUCTION
Indications
Evaluation
Factors
TESTING
Lung Volume Tests
Volumes
Capacities
Calculations

Diseases/Conditions
Obstructive
Restrictive
Ventilation Tests
Pulmonary Mechanics Tests
Gas Distribution Tests
Diffusing Tests
Bronchial Provocation Tests
Exercise Testing
PRACTICE QUIZ

LEARNING OBJECTIVES

Upon completion of this unit, the individual will:

1. Define the four lung volumes
2. Define the four lung capacities.
3. Draw/label a diagram of normal lung volumes and capacities.
4. List at least three reasons for doing pulmonary function studies.
5. Define, and explain the technique for measuring, each of the following:
   a. FVC
   b. FEV_T (1 sec and 3 sec)
   c. $\dfrac{FEV_T}{FVC}$
   d. $FEF_{200-1200}$
   e. $FEF_{25-75\%}$
   f. MVV
   g. PEFR
6. Define FRC, and describe three ways it is measured.
7. List the pulmonary and nonpulmonary conditions that would reduce the vital capacity in an individual.
8. List the pulmonary and nonpulmonary conditions that would be considered obstructive and restrictive.
9. Given the appropriate information, calculate the following:

a. V_t
b. frequency
c. minute ventilation
d. $\dfrac{V_D}{V_t}$
e. V_D
f. minute dead space
g. alveolar ventilation
10. Define a flow volume loop.
11. Differentiate a normal and from an abnormal flow volume loop.
12. Describe the significance of performing helium-air flow volume curves (volume of isoflow).
13. Discuss/define each of the following gas distribution tests:
  a. single-breath nitrogen (SBN_2)
  b. closing volume (CV)
c. closing capacity (CC)
14. Identify the following equipment used in pulmonary function testing:
  a. spirometers, water-seal
  b. pneumotachometer
  c. plethysmographs
  d. x-y recorder
15. Explain the application of prebronchodilator and postbronchodilator studies.
16. Describe how diffusing capacity is determined.
17. Define the following:
  a. BTPS
  b. ATPS
  c. STPD
18. Describe the use of bronchial provocation tests.
19. Explain exercise testing in terms of equipment, monitoring, and purpose.

References

Barnes, TA: Respiratory Care Practice. Year Book Medical Publishers, Chicago, 1988.

Burton, G, and Hodgkin, J: Respiratory Care: A Guide to Clinical Practice, ed 2. JB Lippincott, Philadelphia, 1984.

Kacmarek, RM, Mack, CW, and Dimas, S: The Essentials of Respiratory Therapy, ed 2. Year Book Medical Publishers, Chicago, 1985

McPherson, SP: Respiratory Therapy Equipment, ed 3. CV Mosby, St Louis, 1985.

Miller, WF, Scacci, R, and Gast, LR: Laboratory Evaluation of Pulmonary Function. JB Lippincott, Philadelphia, 1987

Ruppel, G: Manual of Pulmonary Function Testing, ed 2. CV Mosby, St Louis, 1982

STUDY QUESTIONS

1. List five clinical indications for performing pulmonary function studies. (Barnes, p 100)

  a. _____

  b. _____

  c. _____

  d. _____

  e. _____

2. Factors that influence normal standardization are: (Miller, pp 86–94)

  a. _____

  b. _____

  c. _____

  d. _____

  e. _____

3. The values on which pulmonary function tests are based for predicted values are: (Ruppel, pp 164–171; Miller, pp 86–94)

   a. _____

   b. _____

   c. _____

   d. _____

4. Label the volumes and capacities based on a typical spirogram in Figure 14–1. (Ruppel, p 2; Miller, p 106)

   a. _____

   b. _____

   c. _____

   d. _____

   e. _____

   f. _____

   g. _____

   h. _____

5. Define the following volumes and capacities: (Kacmarek, p 272; Ruppel, pp 1–3, 13, 17)

   a. total lung capacity: _____

   b. vital capacity: _____

   c. inspiratory capacity: _____

   d. functional residual capacity: _____

   _____

   e. tidal volume: _____

   f. inspiratory reserve volume: _____

   _____

   g. expiratory reserve volume: _____

   _____

   h. residual volume: _____

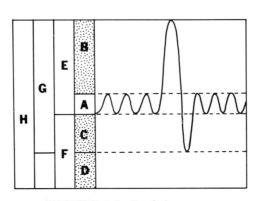

FIGURE 14–1. Spirogram.

6. Using the figure in question 4, answer the following in terms of volumes and capacities: (Ruppel, p 2; Kacmarek, p 274)

    a. Vt + _____ = IC

    b. VC − _____ = ERV

    c. ERV + RV = _____

    d. RV + _____ + _____ + IRV = TLC

    e. ERV + _____ + Vt = _____

    f. FRC − _____ = RV

    g. TLC − _____ = RV

    h. IC + FRC = _____

7. What would a decrease in vital capacity related to lung disease indicate? (Ruppel, p 1; Miller, p 187)

_____

8. What is the device pictured in Figure 14–2? (Barnes, p 35; Ruppel, pp 122–124)

_____

9. Define the following: (Ruppel, p 180; Miller, p 396)

a. BTPS: _____

b. ATPS: _____

_____

c. STPD: _____

10. The technique known as the open-circuit method for determining the FRC is _____. (Ruppel, pp 3–5; Miller, pp 129–138; Barnes, pp 59–61)

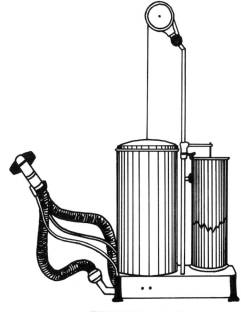

FIGURE 14–2.

11. Using the following formula and data, calculate FRC. (Ruppel, p 187; Barnes, pp 63–64; Kacmarek, p 274)

$$FRC = \frac{\%N_2 \text{ final } (V_E \times V_d) - (T + N_2 \text{ correct})}{\% N_2 \text{ alveolar}}$$

$\%N_2$ final = 7%
volume expired = 30 liters
$\%N_2$ alveolar = 80%
test time (T) = 7 minutes
blood/tissue N_2 washout factor = 0.04 l/min
spirometer/breathing circuit V_d = 0.5 liters
spirometer temperature = 22°C
correction factor = 1.091 (ATPS to BTPS)

_____

_____

_____

_____

12. The technique known as the closed-circuit method for determining FRC is _____ . (Ruppel, p 5; Barnes, pp 55–59; Miller, pp 138–147)

13. Using the following formula and data, calculate FRC. (Ruppel, p 188; Kacmarek, p 276)

$$\left[\frac{-\%He \text{ initial} - \%He \text{ final})}{\%He \text{ final} \times \text{ initial volume}} \right] - He \text{ absorption correction}$$

$$\frac{He \text{ added (ml)}}{\%He \text{ initial}} = \text{ initial volume}$$

He added = 0.30 liters
% He initial = 9%
% He final = 6%
He absorption correction = 0.1 liter
spirometer temperature = 22°C
correction factor = 1.091 (ATPS to BTPS)

_____

_____

_____

_____

14. What is the device in Figure 14–3? (Barnes, p 64; Ruppel, p 142)

_____

15. The gas law that pertains to the device pictured in question 14 is _____ . (Miller, p 110; Rupple, p 8)

16. The device pictured in question 14 is used to measure _____ . (Ruppel, p 9; Barnes, p 64)

17. What other method can be used to determine TLC? (Ruppel, pp 10–11; Miller, pp 148–158)

_____

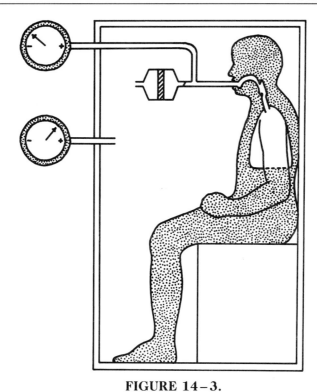

FIGURE 14–3.

18. Distinguish between obstructive and restrictive disease. (Miller, p 107; Burton, pp 236–237)

 a. obstructive: _____

 b. restrictive: _____

19. List disease(s) or syndrome(s) that may show an obstructive pattern on a pulmonary function spirogram. (Burton, p 236; Miller, p 107)

 a. _____

 b. _____

 c. _____

 d. _____

20. List disease(s) or syndrome(s) that may show a restrictive pattern on a pulmonary function spirogram. (Burton, p 236; Miller, p 107)

 a. _____

 b. _____

 c. _____

 d. _____

 e. _____

21. What is the significance of the RV/TLC ratio? (Ruppel, pp 14–15; Miller, pp 108–110)

 _____

 _____

 _____

22. Exhaled volumes are collected over a 5 minute interval. During this time 75 breaths are recorded. The total volume collected from the exhaled volume is 35 liters, Calculate: (Ruppel, p 25; Miller, pp 385–386)

    a. tidal volume: _____

    b. frequency: _____

    c. minute ventilation: _____

23. Given tidal volume = 0.6 liters, frequency = 10 BPM, Pao_2 = 80 mmHg, $Paco_2$ = 45 mmHg, and P_Eco_2 = 30 mmHg, calculate the following: (Ruppel, p 26; Kacmarek, p 226; Barnes, p 481)

    a. $\dfrac{V_D}{V_t}$: _____

    _____

    b. V_D: _____

    _____

    c. minute dead space: _____

    _____

24. Given tidal volume = 0.8 liters, fequency = 12, V_D/V_t = 0.4, calculate alveolar ventilation. (Ruppel, p 26; Miller, p 366)

    _____

    _____

25. Define forced vital capacity. (Miller, p 237; Ruppel, p 27)

    _____

    _____

26. Define FEV_t. (Ruppel, p 27; Miller, pp 267–268)

    _____

    _____

27. In percent, how much volume can be normally exhaled after (a) 1 second, (b) 2 seconds, and (c) 3 seconds of a forced expiratory volume maneuver? (Ruppel, p 31; Kacmarek, pp 281–282; Barnes, p 479)

    a. _____

    b. _____

    c. _____

28. How will the FEV_t be affected by an obstructive disease? Restrictive disease? (Ruppel, p 31; Barnes, pp 479–480)

    _____

29. Identify/describe the spirogram in Figure 14–4. (Ruppel, p 31; Barnes, p 480)

    _____

    _____

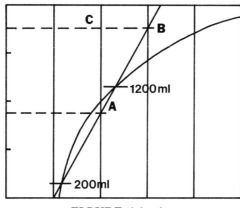

FIGURE 14-4.

30. What is the significance of the test in question 29? (Miller, pp 240-243; Ruppel, p 31; Barnes, p 480)

_____

_____

31. What is the significance of the $FEF_{25-75\%}$? (Ruppel, p 32; Miller, pp 240-243)

_____

_____

32. Indicate from Figure 14-5 which pattern is indicative of obstructive disease and which pattern is indicative of restrictive disease. (Ruppel, p 33; Miller, p 106)

    a. _____

    b. _____

33. What device is used to measure peak expiratory flow rates? (Ruppel, p 34; Barnes, p 36)

_____

34. What recording device is used to plot flow-volume loops? (Ruppel, pp 35, 144; Miller, p 33)

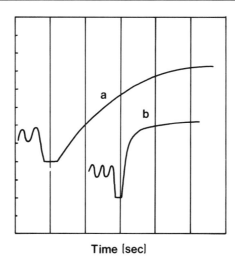

Time (sec)

FIGURE 14-5. Forced vital capacity.

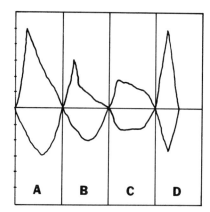

FIGURE 14–6. Flow volume loops.

35. Normal and abnormal flow-volume loops in Figure 14–6. Indicate which flow-volume loop is restrictive, small airway obstruction, normal, and fixed obstruction. (Ruppel, p 76)

   a. _____

   b. _____

   c. _____

   d. _____

36. When performing a volume of isoflow what gas(s) are utilized? (Ruppel, pp 37–39; Miller, pp 277–280)

   _____

37. The point at which the curves meet, when performing a volume of isoflow, is referred to as _____. (Ruppel, p 39; Miller, pp 277–280)

38. An increase in the V. viso is indicative of _____. (Ruppel, pp 37–39; Miller, pp 277–280)

39. Define maximum voluntary ventilation, and explain what this test measures. (Ruppel, pp 39–41; Miller, pp 261–262)

   _____

   _____

40. What is the purpose of performing prebronchodilator and postbronchodilator studies? (Ruppel, p 106; Miller, pp 262–263)

   _____

41. What gas is analyzed when performing closing volumes and closing capacities? (Ruppel, pp 50–52; Miller, pp 323–330)

   _____

42. From Figure 14–7, describe what is occurring in each phase of the single-breath nitrogen test. (Ruppel, p 51; Miller, pp 326–327)

   a. phase I: _____

   b. phase II: _____

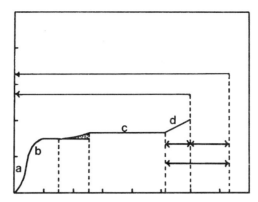

FIGURE 14–7. Single breath nitrogen test.

  c. phase III: _____

  d. phase IV: _____

43. Delta $N_{2750-1250}$ and the slope of phase III are indications of _____
_____. (Ruppel, p 51; Miller, pp 326–327)

44. Define/explain closing volume and closing capacity. (Ruppel, p 52; Miller, p 328)

_____

_____

45. What element is used to perform a lung scan and what does it measure? (Ruppel, pp 56–57; Miller, pp 325–326, 330, 333)

_____

46. What gas is used to determine diffusing capacity, and in what percent? (Ruppel, p 61; Miller, p 409)

_____

47. The average volume of a resting subject by single breath diffusing capacity is _____
_____ ml CO/min/mmHg. (Ruppel, p 68; Kacmarek, p 285)

48. List five states or conditions that would cause diffusing capacity to be decreased. (Ruppel, p 69; Miller, p 437)

  a. _____

  b. _____

  c. _____

  d. _____

  e. _____

49. What is inhalation of methacholine for bronchial challenge tests used to assess? (Kacmarek, pp 285–286; Miller, p 281)

_____

50. Clinically, bronchial challenge testing is used to determine: (Kacmarek, pp 285–286; Miller, p 280)

    a. _____

    b. _____

    c. _____

51. What two methods are commonly employed to vary the workload in exercise testing? (Ruppel, p 83; Miller, p 453)

    a. _____

    b. _____

52. Monitoring the cardiovascular system is important for safe practice during exercise testing. What values are monitored? (Ruppel, p 97; Miller, pp 450–451)

    a. _____

    b. _____

    c. _____

53. What information can be obtained during exercise testing, which may not be obtainable with static pulmonary function testing? (Ruppel, p 81; Miller, p 450)

    _____

    _____

54. How many manuevers should be performed on a subject to get the "best" possible results in pulmonary function testing? (Ruppel, p 119)

    _____

ANSWERS TO STUDY QUESTIONS

1. a. identify and classify certain types of lung diseases
   b. evaluate effectiveness of treatment
   c. documenting progress of disease
   d. compensation for disability
   e. assessing risk factors prior to surgery

2. a. height
   b. age
   c. weight
   d. race/ethnic origin
   e. altitude

3. a. age
   b. sex
   c. height
   d. weight

4. a. tidal volume
   b. inspiratory reserve volume
   c. expiratory reserve volume
   d. residual volume
   e. inspiratory capacity
   f. functional residual capacity
   g. vital capacity
   h. total lung capacity

5. a. maximum volume of gas in the lungs after maximal inspiration
   b. maximum volume that can be expired after maximal inspiration
   c. maximum volume that can be inspired from a resting expiration
   d. amount of gas remaining in lung from resting expiration
   e. resting inspiratory and expiratory volume

f. maximum volume that can be inspired from a normal resting inspiration

g. maximum volume that can be expired from a resting expiration

h. volume of gas remaining in lung after maximal expiration

6. a. IRV
   b. IC
   c. FRC
   d. ERV, TV
   e. IRV, VC
   f. ERV
   g. VC
   h. TLC

7. a loss of distensible lung tissue

8. water-seal spirometer

9. a. body temperature, saturated, body pressure (37°C, 47 mmHg, mmHg)
   b. ambient temperature, saturated, atmospheric pressure (0°C, mmHg, mmHg)
   c. standard temperature, pressure, dry gas (0°C, 760 mmHg, 0 mmHg)

10. nitrogen washout

11. FRC = 2.31 (ATPS), 2.31 × 1.091 = 2.51

12. helium dilution

13. 3.33 liters = initial volume, FRC = 1.56 liters (ATPS)
    1.56 liters × 1.091 = 1.70 (BTPS)

14. body plethysmograph

15. Boyle's law

16. total thoracic gas volume

17. radiologic estimation with the use of a PA and lateral x-ray examination

18. a. any disease that causes an obstruction to airflow through the airways
    b. any disease that limits the expansion of the lungs

19. a. emphysema
    b. chronic bronchitis
    c. bronchial asthma
    d. cystic fibrosis

20. a. neuromuscular diseases
    b. thoracic deformity
    c. infiltrative disease
    d. obesity
    e. respiratory depressants

21. normal value = 20 to 35%; values greater than

35% indicative of obstructive disease; values less than 20% indicative of restrictive disease

22. a. 0.467 liters
    b. 15 BPM
    c. 7 liters

23. a. $PaCO_2 - \dfrac{P_ECO_2}{PaCO_2} = \dfrac{V_D}{V_t}$ ratio $\dfrac{45 - 30}{45} = 0.33$
    b. $V_t = \dfrac{V_D}{V_t} = V_D$
       0.6 × 0.33 = 0.198 liters
    c. V_D × frequency = minute dead space
       0.198 liters × 10 = 1.98 liters

24. V_D = 0.8 liters × 0.4 = 0.32 liters
    VA = (0.8 liters − 0.32 liters) × 12 = 5.76 liters

25. volume of gas that can be forcibly and rapidly expired after a maximum inspiration

26. volume of gas that can be exhaled in a given period of time: 0.5 sec, 1 sec, 2 sec, 3 sec, and so forth

27. a. 1 sec = 75 to 85%
    b. 2 sec = 85 to 94%
    c. 3 sec = 95 to 97%

28. decreased in obstructive; normal or supranormal in restrictive

29. $FEF_{200-1200}$ is the average flow rate for a liter of gas expired after the first 200–1200 ml.

30. a good index of air flow characteristics of large airways; indicative of mechanical problems

31. average flow rate in the middle part of the curve; indicative of the status of the medium airways

32. a. obstructive
    b. restrictive

33. pneumotachometer

34. x-y recorder

35. a. normal
    b. small airway
    c. fixed obstruction
    d. restrictive

36. air and He-oxygen

37. V viso

38. small airway disease

39. largest volume that can be breathed per minute, measures status of respiratory muscles

40. to determine reversibility of lung function; values greater than 15 to 20% considered significant

41. nitrogen

42. a. 100% oxygen
    b. dead space gas (concentration of oxygen and nitrogen change abruptly)
    c. exhalation of alveolar gas
    d. abrupt increase in nitrogen form basal airways and lung apices

43. evenness of ventilation distribution

44. closing volume—point at which small airway starts to close
    closing capacity MCV + RV; lung volume at which airway closure begins

45. ^{133}Xe, regional distribution of ventilation

46. carbon monoxide, 0.1 to 0.3%

47. 25 ml CO/min/mmHg

48. a. sarcoidosis
    b. asbestosis
    c. oxygen toxicity
    d. pulmonary edema
    e. emphysema
    f. lung resection
    g. anemia

49. responsiveness of bronchial airways and lung parenchyma to inhaled aerosols and fumes

50. a. substantial diagnosis of asthma
    b. indicate severity and determine treatment
    c. document inducing effect of occupational asthma and subsequent treatment

51. a. treadmill
    b. bicycle ergometer

52. a. ECG
    b. heart rate
    c. blood pressure

53. efficiency of cardiopulmonary system during periods of increased metabolic demands

54. three

PRACTICE QUIZ

1. Pulmonary function tests can determine all of the following, except:
   a. mechanical ability
   b. gross mechanical abnormalities
   c. efficiency of gas exchange
   d. mechanical efficiency
   e. etiology

2. The predicted values are based on which of the following?
   - I. Height
   - II. Weight
   - III. Sex
   - IV. Age
   a. I, II, III, IV
   b. I, III, IV
   c. II, III, IV
   d. I, II, IV
   e. I and IV

3. Studies on a patient reveal the following: IRV 1.6 liters, TV 500 ml, and ERV 1.0 liters. On the basis of this data, the patient's TLC would be:
   a. 2100 ml minus RV
   b. 2600 ml plus RV
   c. 3100 ml
   d. 3100 ml minus RV
   e. 3100 ml plus RV

4. The 7-minute nitrogen washout test is used to measure which of the following?
   a. closing volume
   b. cardiac output
   c. functional residual capacity
   d. $\dfrac{V_D}{V_T}$ ratio
   e. vital capacity

5. What is the purpose of the soda lime that is found in the spirometers?
   a. absorption of water
   b. release of oxygen preventing oxygen starvation
   c. absorption of carbon dioxide
   d. retains heat
   e. purifies oxygen

6. When one determines thoracic gas volume via a body plethysmograph, what basic gas law is employed to determine the FRC and total lung volume?
   a. Poiseuille's law
   b. LaPlace's law
   c. Charles' law
   d. Boyle's law
   e. Bernouilli's law

7. Which of the following could be considered a restrictive disease or condition?
   I. Pneumothorax
   II. Obesity
   III. Emphysema
   IV. Chronic bronchitis
   V. Rib fractures
   a. I and II
   b. II, III, V
   c. I and III
   d. I, II, V
   e. III and IV

8. What would be the expected alveolar ventilation for a 68 kilogram patient who has a tidal volume of 500 ml and a respiratory rate of 20 BPM?
   a. 6 liters
   b. 7 liters
   c. 8 liters
   d. 9 liters
   e. 10 liters

9. Calculate the amount of physiologic dead space for a patient with the following laboratory values: pH 7.28, Pa_{CO_2} 70 mmHg, Pa_{O_2} 45 mmHg, Sa_{O_2} 82%, HCO_3 29 mEq/l, $P_E{CO_2}$ 35 mmHg, V_t 460 ml, and a respiratory rate of 32 BPM.
   a. 115 ml
   b. 153 ml
   c. 230 ml
   d. 300 ml
   e. 320 ml

10. A forced expiratory tracing that exhibits decreased flow indicates:

a. airway obstruction
b. pulmonary congestion
c. dyspnea
d. diminished maximum voluntary ventilation
e. diminished alveolar ventilation

11. Which of the following should a respiratory care practitioner recommend for measuring the degree of reversibility of a patient's airway obstruction?
    a. body plethysmography
    b. helium dilution lung volumes
    c. carbon monoxide diffusing capacity
    d. spirometry, prebronchodilation, and postbronchodilator
    e. single-breath closing volume

12. FRC and what other lung volume usually increase together in the presence of an obstructive disease?
    a. ERV
    b. RV
    c. TLC
    d. IRV
    e. TV

13. Phase IV is increased on the graph of a single-breath nitrogen test; this would imply:
    a. early closure of the small airway
    b. normal lung function
    c. large airway obstruction
    d. nonuniform emptying of the lungs
    e. none of the above

14. A normal adult should expire what percentage of his or her forced vital capacity in 1 second?
    a. 40 to 50%
    b. 50 to 60%
    c. 60 to 70%
    d. 75 to 85%
    e. 85 to 95%

15. According to standards, flow rates and volumes should be reported at:
    a. BTPS
    b. ATPS
    c. STPD
    d. ATPD
    e. BTPD

16. Which of the following is the most likely diagnosis on the basis of the pulmonary function results shown here?

    $FVC = 80\%$ of predicted
    $FEF_{25-75\%} = 40\%$ of predicted
    $D_{LCO} = 95\%$ of predicted
    $\dfrac{FEV_1}{FVC} = 55\%$ of predicted

    a. chronic bronchitis
    b. silicosis
    c. emphysema
    d. kyphoscoliosis
    e. myasthenia gravis

17. A device that uses heated platinum wires to determine exhaled volume:
    - I. Is a vortex device
    - II. Is a Fleisch pneumotach
    - III. Is a Boehringer spirometer
    - IV. Displays inaccurate readings when wet
    - V. Is expensive
  a. I and II
  b. I, II, IV
  c. III, IV, V
  d. IV and V
  e. II and IV

18. The advantage of the flow volume curve is that it:
  a. reflects instantaneous flow at certain lung volumes
  b. provides for more accurate peak flow readings
  c. can be performed simply and inexpensively in the office setting
  d. is not an effort-dependent measure
  e. all of the above

19. An 8-year-old child should be _____ during all pulmonary function tests:
  a. rested frequently
  b. standing up
  c. reclining on a stretcher
  d. sitting in a chair
  e. in a position that would flex his or her neck

20. A patient's vital capacity can be calculated by using which of the following equations?
    - I. TLC − RV
    - II. IC + FRC
    - III. IRV + TV + ERV
    - IV. FRC + TV
    - V. IC + FRC
  a. I and II
  b. II and IV
  c. III and V
  d. I, II, IV
  e. I, III, V

ANSWERS TO THE PRACTICE QUIZ

1. e	11. d
2. b	12. b
3. e	13. a
4. c	14. d
5. c	15. a
6. d	16. a
7. d	17. e
8. b	18. a
9. c	19. b
10. a	20. e

Chapter 15

ELECTROCARDIOGRAPH

OUTLINE

ELECTROCONDUCTION SYSTEM OF
  THE HEART
Sinoatrial Node
Atrioventricular Node
Common Bundle Branch
Right and Left Bundle Branch
Purkinje Fibers
ECG
Electrical Cardiac Cycles
    Polarization
    Depolarization
    Repolarization
    Resting

Schematic Representation of ECG
Machine
Paper
Electrodes
Wave Productions
INTERPRETATION
Systematic Approach
Rhythm
Rate
Wave Forms
COMMON DYSRHYTHMIAS
PRACTICE QUIZ

LEARNING OBJECTIVES

Upon completion of this unit, the individual will:

1. List and describe two types of cardiac cells
2. List and describe the three states of nature in the cardiac cell.
3. List the components of the cardiac conduction system.
4. Discuss pacing of the heart
5. Describe the function of the electrodes.
6. Discuss Eithoven's triangle

7. Discuss and differentiate between the 12 standard leads.
8. Describe the electrocardiograph paper.
9. Describe the three techniques to calculate cardiac rate.
10. Discuss and describe the normal ECG pattern.
11. List five steps to analyze a rhythm strip.
12. Interpret sample rhythm strips.

REFERENCES

Brown, K, and Jacobson, S: Mastering Dysrhythmias. A Problem Solving Guide. FA Davis, Philadelphia, 1988.

Deshpande, VM, Pilbeam, SP, and Dixon, RJ: A Comprehensive Review in Respiratory Care. Appleton and Lange, Norwalk, CT, 1988.

Eubanks, D, and Bone, R: Comprehensive Respiratory Care. CV Mosby, St Louis, 1985.

Kacmarek, RM, Mack, CW, Dimas, S: The Esssentials of Respiratory Therapy, ed 2. Year Book Medical Publishers, Chicago, 1985.

Walraven, G: Basic Arrhythmias, ed 2. Appleton and Lange, East Norwalk, CT 1985.

STUDY QUESTIONS

1. List and describe the function of the two types of cardiac cells. (Walraven, p 2; Kacmarek, p 259)

   a. _____

   b. _____

2. Define the following terms: (Deshpande, p 132; Walraven, p 4)

   a. polarized: _____

   b. depolarized: _____

   c. repolarization: _____

3. What is automaticity and what is its function in the myocardium? (Brown, p 3; Deshpande, p 132; Eubanks, p 545)

   _____

   _____

   _____

4. List the components of the cardiac conduction system in the correct functional order. (Brown, p 3; Deshpande, p 132; Eubanks, p 545; Kacmarek, p 257)

   _____

   _____

   _____

5. What is an escape mechanism? (Eubanks, p 545; Walraven, p 8)

   _____

   _____

   _____

6. The following sites are known to pace the heart as needed. Give the inherent rate for each. (Brown, p 3; Walraven, p 8)

   a. sinus node: _____

   b. AV node: _____

c. ventricles: _____

7. Although lower sites in the escape mechanism are _____ reliable than the higher sites, the _____ inherent rate will pace the heart. (Walraven, p 8)

8. All impulses that arise from sites other than the SA node are termed _____ _____ pacemakers. (Brown, p 3; Walraven, p 10)

9. Label Figure 15–1. (Deshpande, p 132, Eubanks, p 545)

   1. _____
   2. _____
   3. _____
   4. _____
   5. _____
   6. _____
   7. _____

10. The autonomic nervous system influences the heart through sympathetic and parasympathetic stimulation. List the effects each has on the heart: (I) increase (D) decrease. (Eubanks, p 545; Walraven, p 7)
    a. sympathetic stimulation:

       _____ heart rate

       _____ AV conduction

       _____ irritability
    b. parasympathetic stimulation:

       _____ heart rate

       _____ AV conduction

       _____ irritability

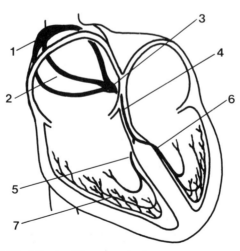

FIGURE 15–1. The electrical conduction system.

11. The parasympathetic branch influences only the ————————————. (Eubanks, p 546; Walraven, p 15)

12. The sympathetic branch influences are the ———————————— and the ————————————. (Eubanks, p 546; Walraven, p 15)

13. What is an electrode? (Deshpande, p 133; Eubanks, p 546; Walraven, p 37)

    _____

    _____

14. List three ways to improve contact of the electrode with the skin. (Deshpande, p 133; Eubanks, p 547; Walraven, p 37)

    a. _____

    b. _____

    c. _____

15. The flow of electricity toward a positive electrode will produce a(n) ———————————— pattern on the graph paper. If electrical flow is toward the negative electrode a(n) ———————————— pattern will be produced. (Deshpande, p 133; Walraven, p 22)

16. Label Figure 15–2. Identify sites for leads I, II, III, AVL, AVR, AVF. (Deshpande, p 134; Eubanks, p 546; Walraven, p 22)

17. There are 12 standard positions for electrode placement. These 12 positions or leads are divided into three groups. Describe the leads here. (Deshpande, p 134; Eubanks, p 546)

    a. _____

    b. _____

    c. _____

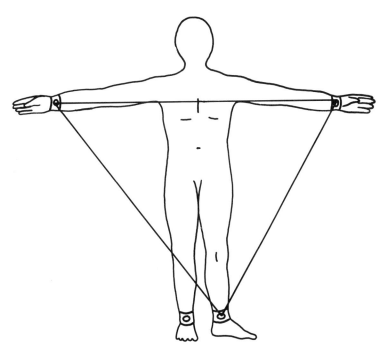

FIGURE 15–2. The limb leads.

18. Differentiate among the leads listed in question 17. (Brown, p 6; Eubanks, p 546; Walraven, p 22)

_____

_____

_____

_____

_____

_____

_____

_____

19. Identify correct placement of precordial leads on Figure 15–3. (Deshpande, p 134; Eubanks, p 546).

20. Which limb lead produces a negative pattern? (Brown, p 6; Eubanks, p 548; Walraven, p 23)

_____

21. Differentiate betweeen limb lead II and modified limb lead II. (Brown, p 6; Eubanks, p 548; Walraven, p 23)

_____

_____

_____

_____

_____

22. The horizontal lines on the electrocardiograph paper measure _____ and the vertical lines are used to measure _____. (Brown, p 8; Deshpande, p 136; Walraven, p 24)

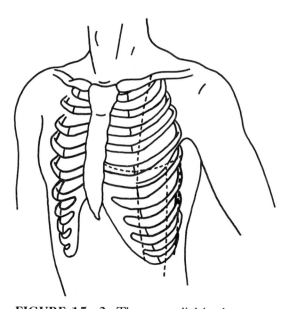

FIGURE 15–3. The precordial leads.

23. The standard strip is _____ seconds long. The smallest squares represent _____ second and the squares between the darkened lines represent _____ second. (Eubanks, p 548)

24. Describe the three most common techniques used to calculate rate. (Brown, p 243; Deshpande, p 136; Walraven, p 58)

   a. _____

   b. _____

   c. _____

25. Calculate the rate on Figures 15–4, 15–5, and 15–6. (Brown, p 243)

   a. Fig. 15–4: _____

   b. Fig. 15–5: _____

   c. Fig. 15–6: _____

26. A single cardiac cycle is seen in Figure 15–7. Label the cycle. (Brown, p 4; Deshpande, p 135; Eubanks, p 548; Walraven, p 29)

   _____

   _____

FIGURE 15–4. Practice strip 1. (From Brown, KR and Jacobson, S: Mastering Dysrhythmias: A Problem-Solving Guide. FA Davis, Philadelphia, 1988, p. 57, with permission.)

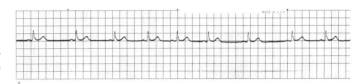

FIGURE 15–5. Practice strip 2. (From Brown, KR and Jacobson, S: Mastering Dysrhythmias: A Problem-Solving Guide. FA Davis, Philadelphia, 1988, p. 238, with permission.)

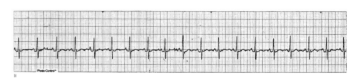

FIGURE 15–6. Practice strip 3. (From Brown, KR and Jacobson, S: Mastering Dysrhythmias: A Problem-Solving Guide. FA Davis, Philadelphia, 1988, p. 240, with permission.)

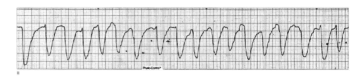

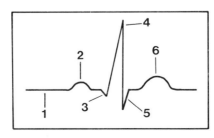

FIGURE 15–7. Practice strip 4.

27. What electrical process(es) do the following represent? (Brown, p 5)

    a. P wave: _____

    b. QRS wave: _____

    c. T wave: _____

28. Give the normal range for the following: (Brown, p 5)

    a. P R interval: _____

    b. QRS complex: _____

29. What is the isoelectric line? (Brown, p 5; Walraven, p 27)

    _____

    _____

30. Define artifact and list the causes for it to appear on the ECG tracing. (Eubanks, p 549; Walraven, p 38)

    _____

    _____

    _____

    _____

31. List five steps used to analyze a rhythm strip. (Walraven, p 64)

    a. _____

    b. _____

    c. _____

    d. _____

    e. _____

32. Describe the analysis of each of the above items in question 31. (Walraven, p 64)

    a. _____

    b. _____

    c. _____

    d. _____

    e. _____

33. Define the following terms: (Eubanks, p 551; Walraven, p 36)

    a. absolute refractory period: _____

    b. relative refractory period: _____

    c. irritability: _____

    d. tachycardia: _____

    e. bradycardia: _____

    f. fibrillation: _____

    g. flutter: _____

34. Identify the dysrhythmia in Figure 15–8. _____ (Walraven, p 112)

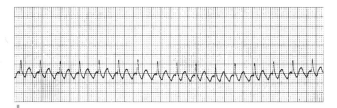

FIGURE 15–8. Practice strip 5. (From Brown, KR and Jacobson, S: Mastering Dysrhythmias: A Problem-Solving Guide. FA Davis, Philadelphia, 1988, p. 50, with permission.)

35. Identify the dysrhythmia in Figure 15–9. _____ (Walraven, p 219)

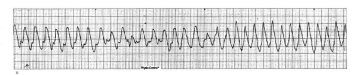

FIGURE 15–9. Practice strip 6. (From Brown, KR and Jacobson, S: Mastering Dysrhythmias: A Problem-Solving Guide. FA Davis, Philadelphia, 1988, p. 133, with permission.)

36. Identify the dysrhythmia in Figure 15–10. _____ (Walraven, p 220)

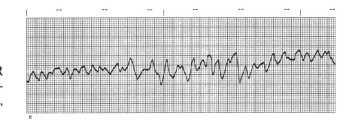

FIGURE 15–10. Practice strip 7. (From Brown, KR and Jacobson, S: Mastering Dysrhythmias: A Problem-Solving Guide. FA Davis, Philadelphia, 1988, p 127, with permission.)

37. Identify the dysrhythmia in Figure 15–11. _____ (Walraven, p 82)

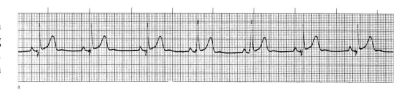

FIGURE 15–11. Practice strip 8. (From Brown, KR and Jacobson, S: Mastering Dysrhythmias: A Problem-Solving Guide. FA Davis, Philadelphia, 1988, p. 260, with permission.)

38. Identify the dysrhythmia in Figure 15–12. _____ (Walraven, p 81)

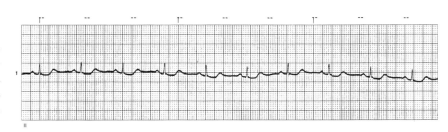

FIGURE 15–12. Practice strip 9. (From Brown, KR and Jacobson, S: Mastering Dysrhythmias: A Problem-Solving Guide. FA Davis, Philadelphia, 1988, p. 56, with permission.)

39. Identify the dysrhythmia in Figure 15–13. _____ (Walraven, p 114)

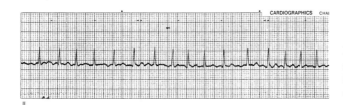

FIGURE 15–13. Practice strip 10. (From Brown, KR and Jacobson, S: Mastering Dysrhythmias: A Problem-Solving Guide. FA Davis, Philadelphia, 1988, p. 48, with permission.)

40. Identify the dysrhythmia in Figure 15–14. _____ (Walraven, p 108)

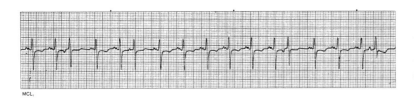

FIGURE 15–14. Practice strip 11. (From Brown, KR and Jacobson, S: Mastering Dysrhythmias: A Problem-Solving Guide. FA Davis, Philadelphia, 1988, p. 71, with permission.)

41. Identify the dysrhythmia in Figure 15–15. _____ (Walraven, p 217)

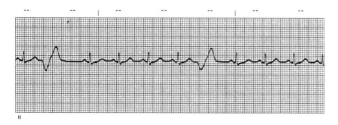

FIGURE 15–15. Practice strip 12. (From Brown, KR and Jacobson, S: Mastering Dysrhythmias: A Problem-Solving Guide. FA Davis, Philadelphia, 1988, p. 115, with permission.)

ANSWERS TO STUDY QUESTIONS

1. a. Mechanical cells function to produce muscle contraction
   b. Electrical cells provide electrical stimulation to the muscle mass.

2. a. the resting state, electrical charges are balanced; positive charges are outside the cell and are equal to the number of negative charges on the inside
   b. sodium (Na) ions move from outside to inside cell; outer surface is negatively charged and at full depolarization potassium moves outside the cell.
   c. this occurs as potassium continues to move out; when potassium ions exceed sodium ions, repolarization begins, electrical charges return to original state.

3. Automaticity is the ability to initiate spontaneous depolarization of the resting cell membrane. This allows the myocardium to pace itself and to establish an escape mechanism.

4. sinoatrial node, intranodal/intronodal pathways, atrioventricular node, atrioventricular bundle/bundle of HIS, right and left bundle branches, Purkinje fibers

5. It is a function of automaticity that allows the lower levels of the electrical conduction system to take over pacing of the heart if there is failure of a higher site to pace.

6. a. 60 to 100 beats per minute
   b. 40 to 60 beats per minute
   c. 20 to 40 beats per minute

7. less, fastest

8. ectopic

9. 1. SA node
   2. intra-atrial pathways
   3. AV node
   4. bundle of HIS
   5. right bundle branch
   6. left bundle branch
   7. Purkinje fibers

10. a. I, I, I
    b. D, D, D

11. atria

12. atria, ventricles

13. An electrode is a device applied to the skin to detect electrical activity and convey it to a machine for display.

14. a. abrading the skin
    b. cleaning or drying medium
    c. contact medium

15. upright, inverted

16. Refer to Figure 15–16.

17. a. standard limb leads: LLI, LLII, LLIII
    b. augmented leads: AVL, AVR, AVF
    c. precordial leads: V1–V6

18. Standard leads are bipolar, measure activity between two electrodes, one positive and one negative, and make up Einthoven's triangle. Augmented leads are designed to increase the amplitude of deflections, are unipolar, and measure the point directly under the lead. Precordial leads are unipolar. Correct placement is imperative. They are called chest leads and are most useful in detecting location of myocardial infarction.

19. See Figure 15–17.

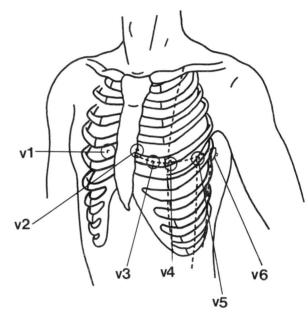

FIGURE 15–17. Precordial leads.

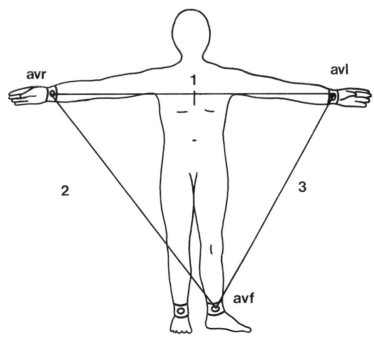

FIGURE 15–16. Limb leads.

20. AVR

21. LLII had been traditionally used because it allows for easy assessment of AV conduction. It has limited detail about ventricular conduction. It is of no use when recognizing bundle branch blocks or detecting supraventricular impulses. Modified limb lead II (MCL1) overcomes the problems associated with LLII, and has gained favor for this reason.

22. voltage, time

23. 6 seconds, 0.04 second, 0.2 second

24. a. count the number of R waves in a 6 sec strip and multiply by 10
    b. count the number of large squares between two consecutive R waves and divide into 300
    c. count the number of small squares between two consecutive R waves and divide into 1500

25. a. 60
    b. 120
    c. 100

26. (1) base line, (2) P wave, (3) Q wave, (4) R wave, (5) S wave, (6) T wave

27. a. atrial depolarization
    b. ventricular depolarization and atrial repolarization buried
    c. ventricular repolarization

28. a. 0.12 to 0.20 sec
    b. less than 0.12 sec

29. the straight line on the ECG, made when no electrical current is flowing

30. Artifact is mechanical or electrical interference causing artificial movement on the ECG. It may be caused by too little contact medium, patient movement, friction, loose electrodes, unclean site, muscle movement or a 60 cycle electrical current.

31. a. regularity and rhythm
    b. rate
    c. P wave
    d. PR interval
    e. QRS complex

32. a. regularity and rhythm: measure R-R intervals and P-P interval, see if irregular and if pattern of irregularity.
    b. rate: measure in three accepted methods.
    c. P wave: should be one preceding each QRS complex, upright, uniform, and regular.
    d. PR interval: constant across the strip, 0.12 to 0.20 sec
    e. QRS complex: less than 0.12 sec

33. a. the heart cannot accept any stimulus at all.
    b. some of the cardiac cells are capable of responding to strong stimulus.
    c. when a site picks speed and takes over pacemaker responsibility
    d. rate over 100 BPM
    e. rate under the 60 BPM
    f. quivering and irregular
    g. tremulous movement, extremely rapid, yet often regular

34. atrial flutter

35. V-tach

36. V-fib

37. sinus brady

38. NRS no dysrhythmia present

39. atrial fibrillation

40. PAC

41. sinus rhythmn with two PVCs

PRACTICE QUIZ

1. The purpose of the AV junction is to:
   a. delay electrical impulses through to the ventricles
   b. initiate normal cardiac impulses
   c. determine atrial firing rate
   d. regulate the normal heart rate
   e. stimulate cardiac irritating mechanisms

2. Initiation of the heart rate normally begins at the:
   a. sinoatrial node

   b. atrioventricular node
   c. bundle of HIS
   d. none of the above

3. Which of the following best describes the location of the SA node?
   a. overriding the right and left atria
   b. in the left atrium near the mitral valve
   c. in the left ventricle at the anterior position
   d. in the right atrium near the superior vena cava
   e. in the right atrium near the tricuspid valve

4. Arrange the following list to indicate the normal sequence of electrical conduction through the heart:
    I. Internodal pathways
    II. Bundle of HIS
    III. Ventricular purkinje system
    IV. Sinus node
    V. Bundle branches
    VI. AV junction
   a. IV, VI, I, V, II, III
   b. IV, I, VI, II, V, III
   c. IV, I, II, VI, V, III
   d. VI, II, I, IV, III, V
   e. I, II, III, IV, V, VI

5. The QRS segment of an ECG represents:
   a. myocardial contractility
   b. atrial repolarization
   c. ventricular depolarization
   d. firing of the AV node
   e. passage of electrical flow through the atria

6. The P wave of the normal ECG represents:
   a. depolarization of the right ventricle
   b. depolarization of the left ventricle
   c. repolarization of the atria
   d. depolarization of the atria
   e. ectopic foci

7. The T wave on the ECG:
    I. Represents depolarization.
    II. Represents repolarization.
    III. Is always seen just prior to the QRS.
    IV. May not be visible.
    V. Represents atrial contraction.
   a. I, II, III, IV, V
   b. I, III, IV, V
   c. I, III, V
   d. II, IV
   e. III, V

8. The T wave of the normal ECG represents:
   a. depolarization of the atria
   b. depolarization of the ventricles
   c. septal depolarization
   d. repolarization of the atria
   e. repolarization of the ventricles

9. The PR interval of the ECG is measured from the:
   a. beginning of the P wave to the start of the QRS
   b. beginning of the P wave to the R wave
   c. beginning of the P wave to the end of the Q wave
   e. beginning of the P wave to the end of the P wave

10. The ECG strip shows a regular series of P waves appearing in a sawtooth pattern between each QRS complex. The ECG pattern is consistent with:
   a. sinus dysrhythmia
   b. atrial fibrillation
   c. trigeminy
   d. sinus tachycardia
   e. atrial flutter

11. The most common cardiac arrhythmia associated with hypoxia of recent onset is:
   a. sinus bradycardia
   b. sinus tachycardia
   c. ventricular tachycardia
   d. sinus rhythm with PVCs
   e. heart block

12. Bradycardia is a heart rate less than:
   a. 60 beats/min
   b. 65 beats/min
   c. 70 beats/min
   d. 75 beats/min
   e. 80 beats/min

13. You review the 12-lead ECG and note the AVR lead is negative. You should:
   a. redo the ECG
   b. call the physician immediately
   c. switch the leads; one is backward
   d. do nothing; this is normal
   e. have maintenance personnel correct cross wires

14. When using a electrocardiographic device, the strip recorder should ensure the paper travels at what speed?
   a. 25 mm/sec
   b. 30 mm/sec
   c. 20 mm/sec
   d. 15 mm/sec
   e. 10 mm/sec

15. If you counted the number of small squares between two R waves, what number should you divide that into to calculate rate?
   a. 10
   b. 100
   c. 200
   d. 300
   e. 1500

16. What is the first wave you should try to locate to analyze a rhythm strip?
   a. P wave
   b. Q wave
   c. R wave

d. S wave

e. T wave

17. The QRS complex is normally measured to be:
    a. less than 0.20 sec
    b. less than 0.15 sec
    c. less than 0.12 sec
    d. between 0.12 and 0.20 sec
    e. none of the above

18. Sometimes, frequently occurring PVCs will be seen in a specific pattern among normal beats. When the PVCs fall into a four complex cycle, with one PVC and three normal beats, it is called:
    a. bigeminy
    b. trigeminy
    c. quadrigeminy
    d. multiple PVCs
    e. a run of PVCs

19. A ventricular escape rhythm is one in which the ventricle takes over pacing the heart in the absence of a higher pacing site. The inherent rate in this case would be:
    a. 20 to 40 beats/min
    b. 40 to 60 beats/min
    c. 60 to 80 beats/min
    d. 80 to 100 beats/min
    e. none of the above

20. Tachycardia is defined as:
    a. rate of more than 60 beats/min
    b. rate of more than 80 beats/min
    c. rate of more than 100 beats/min
    d. rate of more than 90 beats/min
    e. rate of more than 70 beats/min

ANSWERS TO THE PRACTICE QUIZ

1. a	11. b
2. a	12. a
3. d	13. d
4. b	14. a
5. c	15. e
6. d	16. a
7. d	17. c
8. e	18. c
9. a	19. a
10. e	20. c

HEMODYNAMIC MONITORING

OUTLINE

LEARNING OBJECTIVES

Upon completion of this unit, the individual will:

1. Discuss the operational aspects of the following monitoring equipment:
   a. transducers
   b. arterial catheters
   c. central venous catheters
   d. balloon-tipped, flow-directed pulmonary artery catheters
2. Discuss the insertion procedures and complications of the following:
   a. arterial catheters
   b. central venous catheters
   c. balloon-tipped, flow-directed pulmonary artery catheters
3. Identify the abbreviations and normal ranges of the following values:
   a. central venous pressure
   b. right atrial pressure
   c. mean arterial pressure
   d. pulmonary artery pressure
   e. pulmonary capillary wedge pressure
4. Identify the abbreviations, formulas, and normal ranges of the following:

a. cardiac output
b. cardiac index
c. pulmonary vascular resistance
d. systemic vascular resistance

5. List factors that would increase or decrease the following:
   a. central venous pressure
   b. right arterial pressure

c. pulmonary artery pressure
d. pulmonary capillary wedge pressure
e. cardiac output
f. pulmonary vascular resistance
g. systemic vascular resistance

6. Identify pressure tracings from the balloon-tipped, flow-directed pulmonary catheter.

REFERENCES

Barnes, TA: Respiratory Care Practice. Year Book Medical Publishers, Chicago, 1988.

Deshpande, VM, Pilbean, SP, and Dixon, RJ: A Comprehensive Review in Respiratory Care. Appleton and Lange, Norwalk, CT, 1988.

DesJardins, TR: Cardiopulmonary Anatomy and Physiology: Essentials for Respiratory Care. Delmar Inc., Albany, 1988.

Shapiro, BA, Harrison, RA, and Walton, JR: Clinical Application of Blood Gases, ed 3. Year Book Medical Publishers, Chicago, 1985.

Shapiro, BA, Harrison, RA, and Kacmarek, RM: Clinical Application of Respiratory Care, ed 3. Year Book Medical Publishers, Chicago, 1985.

Wilkins, RL, Sheldon, RL, and Krider, SJ: Clinical Assessment in Respiratory Care. CV Mosby, St Louis, 1985.

STUDY QUESTIONS

1. What is the purpose of hemodynamic monitoring equipment? (Barnes, p 486; Deshpande, p 358; Wilkins, p 249)

   _____

   _____

2. Describe the operation of the pressure transducer used in hemodynamic monitoring equipment. (Deshpande, p 358)

   _____

   _____

   _____

   _____

   _____

3. Describe the arterial catheter system. (Barnes, p 486)

   _____

   _____

   _____

4. List purposes of the arterial catheter system. (Deshpande, p 360; Wilkins, p 270)

   a. _____

   b. _____

5. List the sites for arterial cannulation. Indicate which one is most commonly used in the adult and why. (Wilkins, p 270)

a. _____

b. _____

c. _____

d. _____

e. _____

f. _____

g. _____

6. List eight complications associated with the arterial catheter insertion and maintenance. (Barnes, p 487; Shapiro, p 150; Deshpande, p 361)

a. _____ e. _____

b. _____ f. _____

c. _____ g. _____

d. _____ h. _____

7. When maintaining the arterial catheter, what procedures should be followed to decrease the risk of embolization? (Barnes, pp 286, 487; Deshpande, p 361)

_____

_____

_____

8. Give three common functions of the central venous catheter: (Barnes, p 487; Wilkins, p 276)

a. _____

b. _____

c. _____

9. List three points of insertion for the central venous catheter (CVP). (Barnes, p 488; Deshpande, p 361; Wilkins, p 276)

a. _____

b. _____

c. _____

10. List four complications of CVP line insertion. (Barnes, p 488; Deshpande, p 361; Wilkins, p 277)

a. _____

b. _____

c. _____

d. _____

11. Where is the CVP catheter positioned to monitor hemodynamic values? (Barnes, p 487; Shapiro [CARC], p 301; Wilkins, p 276)

_____

12. How is the CVP measurement obtained? (Barnes, p 488; Wilkins, p 277)

_____

_____

_____

_____

13. Does mechanical ventilation affect the CVP reading? If so, how? (Barnes, p 488; Wilkins, p 282)

_____

_____

14. What is the purpose of pulmonary artery pressure (PAP) monitoring? Why is this measurement preferred to CVP monitoring? (Barnes, p 489; Deshpande, p 362; Wilkins, p 283)

_____

_____

_____

_____

_____

_____

15. In the 1960s Swan and Ganz developed the balloon-tipped flow-directed (BTFD) pulmonary artery catheter. Describe the catheter as it is available today. (Wilkins, p 283)

_____

_____

_____

_____

16. Label Figure 16–1. (Barnes, p 489; Deshpande, p 362; Wilkins, p 284)

a. _____

b. _____

c. _____

d. _____

e. _____

f. _____

17. List three common sites of insertion of the BTFD pulmonary artery catheter. (Barnes, p 489; Deshpande, p 362)

a. _____

b. _____

c. _____

18. Which of the insertion routes for the BTFD pulmonary artery catheter is most used, and why? (Deshpande, p 362; Wilkins, p 286)

_____

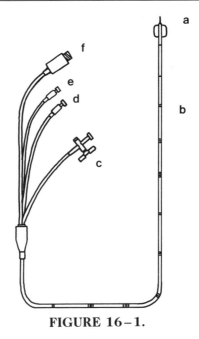

FIGURE 16–1.

19. What three aspects of the BTFD catheter should be checked prior to insertion? (Deshpande, p 362)

    a. _____

    b. _____

    c. _____

20. Describe the insertion process for the BTFD pulmonary artery catheter. (Barnes, p 489; Deshpande, p 363; Wilkins, p 286)

    _____

    _____

    _____

21. Match the illustrations in Figures 16–2 through 16–5 to the pressure tracings in Figures 16–6 through 16–9. (Deshpande, p 364; Wilkins, p 286)

    _____

    _____

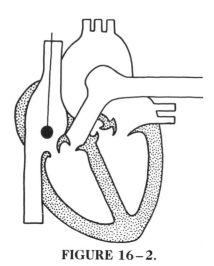

FIGURE 16–2.

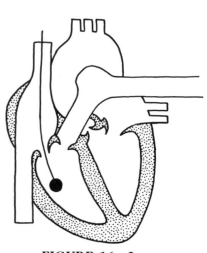

FIGURE 16–3.

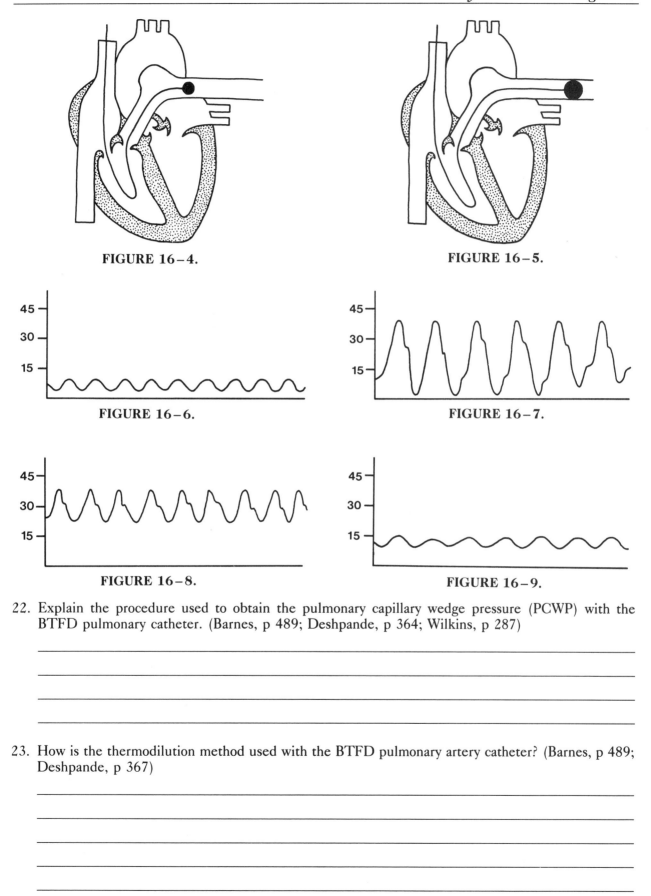

FIGURE 16-4.

FIGURE 16-5.

FIGURE 16-6.

FIGURE 16-7.

FIGURE 16-8.

FIGURE 16-9.

22. Explain the procedure used to obtain the pulmonary capillary wedge pressure (PCWP) with the BTFD pulmonary catheter. (Barnes, p 489; Deshpande, p 364; Wilkins, p 287)

_____

_____

_____

_____

23. How is the thermodilution method used with the BTFD pulmonary artery catheter? (Barnes, p 489; Deshpande, p 367)

_____

_____

_____

_____

_____

_____

24. List four parameters measured with the pulmonary artery catheter. (Barnes, p 489; Deshpande, p 364; Wilkins, p 283)

    a. _____

    b. _____

    c. _____

    d. _____

25. Complete the chart below. (Barnes, p 489; Wilkins, p 286)

Value	Normal Range
Central venous pressure	_____
Right atrial pressure	_____
Pulmonary artery pressure:	
systolic	_____
diastolic	_____
Mean PAP	_____
Pulmonary capillary wedge pressure	_____
Cardiac output	_____

26. Discuss central venous pressure (CVP): where it is measured, what it represents, and how it is determined. (Deshpande, p 361; Shapiro, p 301; Wilkins, p 275)

    _____

    _____

    _____

    _____

    _____

27. List five clinical conditions that would increase CVP. (Deshpande, p 361; Wilkins, p 276)

    a. _____

    b. _____

    c. _____

    d. _____

    e. _____

28. List four factors that might decrease CVP. (Deshpande, p 361; Wilkins, p 276)

    a. _____

    b. _____

    c. _____

    d. _____

29. Discuss right atrial pressure (RAP): how it is measured, and how it is determined. (Deshpande, p 365)

    _____

    _____

_____

_____

30. A rise in RAP is indicative of what types of problems? (Deshpande, p 356)

_____

_____

31. Discuss how pulmonary artery pressure (PAP) is measured and what determines the value. (Deshpande, p 365; Wilkins, p 288)

_____

_____

_____

_____

32. List five conditions that would increase PAP. (Barnes, p 489; Deshpande, p 365; Wilkins, p 288)

   a. _____

   b. _____

   c. _____

   d. _____

   e. _____

33. List three conditions that would decrease PAP. (Deshpande, p 366; Wilkins, p 288)

   a. _____

   b. _____

   c. _____

34. What does PCWP reflect? (Deshpande, p 366; Wilkins, p 288)

_____

_____

_____

35. In the patient with no history of significant pulmonary vascular disease, the PCWP will be _____ pulmonary artery diastolic pressure. (Deshpande, p 366; Wilkins, p 288)
   a. equal to
   b. less than
   c. greater than

36. List five factors that will increase PCWP. (Barnes, p 489; Deshpande, p 366; Wilkins, p 288)

   a. _____

   b. _____

   c. _____

   d. _____

   e. _____

37. Fill in the blanks with the PCWP associated with each x-ray finding in pulmonary congestion. (Deshpande, p 366; Wilkins, p 292)

    a. classic findings of pulmonary edema: _____

    b. no congestion noted: _____

38. Label Figure 16–10 for BTFD pulmonary catheter position. (Deshpande, p 365; Wilkins, p 266)

    a. _____   c. _____

    b. _____   d. _____

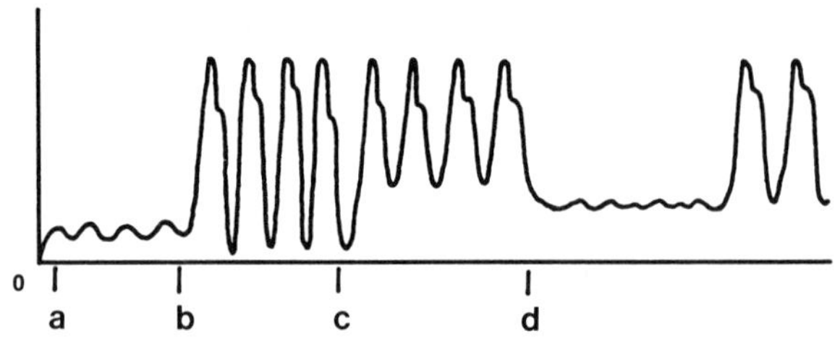

FIGURE 16–10.

39. List two equations used for calculating cardiac output (a, b), and list the normal range (c). (Deshpande, p 366; Barnes, 489)

    a. _____

    b. _____

    c. _____

40. Give the formula for determining pulmonary vascular resistance (PVR) and the normal value range. (Deshpande, p 367; DesJardins, p 153; Wilkins, p 267)

    _____

    _____

    _____

41. What is cardiac index (CI), and why is it used? (Deshpande, p 367; Wilkins, p 251)

    _____

    _____

    _____

42. Give the formula used to determine system vascular resistance (SVR) and the normal range. (Wilkins, p 264)

    _____

    _____

    _____

43. What is the formula for calculating mean arterial pressure, and what is the normal value? (DesJardins, p 149; Wilkins, p 264)

    _____

    _____

    _____

44. List four factors that would increase CO (Deshpande, p 367)

   a. _____

   b. _____

   c. _____

   d. _____

45. List five factors that increase PVR. (Deshpande, p 366; DesJardins, p 153; Wilkins, p 267)

   a. _____

   b. _____

   c. _____

   d. _____

   e. _____

46. List factors that decrease PVR. (Deshpande, p 367; DesJardins, p 154)

   a. pharmacologic agents: _____

   _____

   _____

   _____

   b. humoral substances: _____

   _____

   _____

   _____

ANSWERS TO STUDY QUESTIONS

1. used to detect, treat, and maintain the forces that influence circulation

2. This is a device used to convert a pressure signal to an electrical signal. These units have a fluid column connecting the circulatory system and the transducer diaphragm. The diaphragm is moved by changes in fluid pressure, this movement is recorded as an electrical impulse, amplified, and recorded.

3. A pressure transducer is used, attached to an indwelling arterial cannula, to provide continual pressure readings. It is connected to a oscilloscope for display.

4. a. direct measurement of intra-arterial pressure
   b. avoid frequent needlesticks

5. a. brachial
   b. axillary
   c. femoral
   d. dorsalis pedis
   e. umbilical (artery of choice for newborn)
   f. superficial temporal
   g. radial (artery of choice due to collateral circulation by ulnar artery)

6. a. infection
   b. thrombosis
   c. air embolism
   d. catheter displacement
   e. hemorrhage
   f. impaired circulation
   g. necrosis
   h. arrhythmia

7. flushing line carefully after drawing sample, using heparinized normal saline or Ringer's lactate (2 units/ml; in 1000 units of heparin in 500 ml), drip rate 3 to 5 ml/hr)

8. a. monitor hemodynamic status
   b. fluid administration
   c. medication administration

9. a. jugular
   b. subclavian
   c. right brachial vein

10. a. pneumothorax
    b. pulmonary emboli
    c. arrythmia
    d. air emboli
    e. microelectric shock

11. at the junction of the superior vena cava and the right atrium

12. The patient is placed in a supine position. The zero level of the transducer is placed at the level of the right atrium and the manometer is opened to the patient. Measurement is taken at end exhalation.

13. Yes, positive pressure breathing affects the CVP reading. Mechanical ventilation causes it to fall.

14. PAP monitoring is used to evaluate cardiac output and intravascular volume. It is preferred to CVP because CVP does not provide reliable information on left ventricular filling pressure or left atrial pressure. PAP reflects atrial pressure and adequacy of left ventricular functional in the patient without significant pulmonary vascular dysfunction.

15. The catheter is 110 cm long. It is marked off every 10 centimeters. Two- to five-lumen catheters are available. Most often the 3- or 4-lumen catheter is used. It is made of radiopaque polyvinylchloride, and children's sizes 4 and 5F available.

16. a. balloon
    b. thermistor
    c. balloon lumen stopcock
    d. proximal (CVP) connector
    e. distal (PA) lumen connector
    f. thermodilution cardiac output computer connector

17. a. antecubital
    b. jugular vein
    c. subclavian vein

18. The jugular has the shortest and most direct route.

19. a. balloon-patency and evenness
    b. lumens of catheters for patency
    c. monitoring equipment for correct calibration and operation

20. The catheter is inserted via the jugular or subclavian vein and floated through the superior vena cava, right atrium, right ventricle, pulmonic valve, and into the pulmonary artery.

21. Figure 16–2 and Figure 16–6, Figure 16–3 and Figure 16–8, Figure 16–4 and Figure 16–7, and Figure 16–5 and Figure 16–9.

22. The balloon is partially inflated and floats forward and lodges in a pulmonary capillary. When the balloon is fully inflated, blood flow behind the balloon is obstructed and PCWP is measured. The balloon is immediately deflated and never left inflated.

23. The catheter is positioned in the pulmonary artery. Ten ml of cooled 5% dextrose in H_2O is introduced in the right atrium via proximal CVP port. The thermistor measures the blood temperature in the pulmonary artery. The temperature of the patient, injection solution temperature and volume, and the change in blood temperature are used to calculate cardiac output.

24. a. right atrial pressure
    b. pulmonary artery pressure
    c. pulmonary capillary wedge pressure
    d. cardiac output

25. CVP = 1 to 7 mmHg; RAP = 1 to 7 mmHg; PAP systolic = 15 to 25 mmHg; PAP diastolic = 8 to 15 mmHg; mean PAP = 12 to 15 mmHg; PCWP = 7 to 12 mmHg; cardiac output = 5 to 8 l/min

26. CVP is measured at the junction of the superior vena cava and the right atrium. It measures right atrial pressures and reflects systemic return and right ventricular preload. The CVP is determined by the ability of the heart to pump blood out of the right atrium and venous return to the right heart.

27. a. right heart failure
    b. tricuspid stenosis/regurgitation
    c. pulmonary valve stenosis
    d. pulmonary hypertension
    e. volume overload
    f. pulmonary embolism
    g. cardiac compression
    h. increased intrathoracic pressure

28. a. decrease in circulating blood volume
    b. spontaneous inspiration
    c. vasodilation
    d. air bubbles and or leaks in the pressure line

29. RAP is measured at the proximal port of the catheter. It represents atrial filling and is de-

termined by intravascular volume, tricuspid function, pericardial function, and right ventricular function.

30. tricuspid valve stenosis, tricuspid valve regurgitation, volume overload, pulmonary hypertension, right ventricular failure

31. RAP is monitored via the distal tip of the BTFD pulmonary artery catheter continually. It is determined by right ventriclar function, blood volume, condition of the pulmonary vascular bed, and left heart condition.

32. a. noncardiogenic pulmonary edema
    b. alveolar hypoxia
    c. pulmonary hypertension
    d. alveolar overdistention
    e. cardiogenic pulmonary edema from left heart failure

33. a. dehydration
    b. acute hemorrhage
    c. relative hypovolemia related to shock

34. When the balloon is inflated and correctly positioned, the PCWP reflects left atrial pressure and mean left ventricular diastolic pressure.

35. a. equal to

36. a. left ventricular failure
    b. mitral stenosis
    c. cardiac insufficiency
    d. fluid overload
    e. pulmonary congestion

37. a. above 25 to 30 mmHg
    b. below 18 mmHg

38. a. right atrium
    b. right ventricle
    c. pulmonary artery
    d. pulmonary capillary wedge

39. a. CO = stroke volume × heart rate
    b. CO = oxygen consumption divided by the arterial venous oxygen content difference:

$$CO = \frac{V_{O_2}}{C(a-v)_{O_2}}$$

c. normal range, 5 to 8 l/min

40. $PVR = \dfrac{MAP - PCWP}{CO} \times 80$ (80 is the conversion factor to adjust to dyne × sec × cm); normal range is 2 to 2.5 l/min/m

41. Cardiac index describes the flow output of the heart; it eliminates body size as a variable. The formula is $CI = \dfrac{CO}{BSA}$ where BSA is body surface area

42. $SVR = \dfrac{(MAP - CVP)}{CO}$, the normal range is calculated as 900 to 1400 dynes × sec × cm.

43. $MAP = \dfrac{systolic + 2(diastolic)}{3}$; normal range is 80 to 100 mmHg.

44. a. drugs: dobutamine, epinephrine, dopamine, isoproterenol, digitalis, Inocor
    b. hyperthermia
    c. septic shock
    d. hypervolemia, decreased vascular resistance

45. a. chemical stimuli: alveolar hypoxia, acidemia hypercapnia
    b. medication: epinephrine, norepinephrine, dobutamine, dopamine, phenylephrine
    c. mechanical ventilation
    d. vascular blockage, vascular wall disease, vascular destruction, vascular compression
    e. humoral substances: histamine, angiotensin, serotonin

46. a. oxygen, isoproterenol, aminophylline, calcium-blocking agents
    b. acetylcholine, bradykinin, prostaglandin E, prostacyclin

PRACTICE QUIZ

1. Which of the following is a complication associated with pulmonary artery catheters?
   I. Pulmonary infarction
   II. Local infection at insertion site
   III. Balloon rupture
   IV. Pulmonary artery rupture
   V. Air embolism
   a. I, II, III, IV, V

b. II, III, IV
c. I, III, V
d. III, IV, V
e. II and V

2. Which of the following might cause wave dampening in monitoring via the pulmonary artery catheter?
    I. Air in line
    II. Infection
    III. High altitude
    IV. Blood on transducer
    V. Kinks in the line
    a. I, II, III, IV, V
    b. I, III, IV, V
    c. I, IV, V
    d. II, IV, V
    e. IV, V

3. A 90-year-old woman is admitted to the ICU from a nursing home. BP = 110/60 HR = 110. The patient is confused and lethargic. The neck veins are flattened. PAP = $\frac{22}{5}$, PCWP = 4, CO = 3 l/min. Which of the following is the likely cause of the patient's condition?
    a. cardiac insufficiency
    b. myocardial infraction
    c. fluid overload
    d. hypovolemia
    e. pulmonary embolis

4. The patient is in postoperative trauma, with surgery on the femur. The ER report includes aspiration of a considerable amount of vomitus en route to the hospital. PAP = $\frac{45}{24}$, PCWP = 28, BP = 160/85, CVP = 15, CI = 4. Your diagnosis:
    a. pulmonary embolus
    b. pulmonary edema
    c. hypovolemia
    d. hypervolemia
    e. myocardial infarction

5. Left atrial pressure is best measured by which of the devices listed below?
    a. CVP
    b. pulmonary artery catheter
    c. arterial catheter
    d. blood pressure
    e. none of the above

6. Your patient has a stroke volume of 60 ml/beat, with a heart rate of 80 l/min. What is the cardiac output?
    a. 3.5 l/min
    b. 4.8 l/min
    c. 5.0 l/min
    d. 5.5 l/min
    e. none of the above

7. A patient is admitted to the ICU with an admitting diagnosis of hypovolemic shock. You check her CVP and expect to find it to be:
    a. increased
    b. decreased
    c. normal

   d. fluctuating markedly
   e. none of the above

8. The patient receiving mechanical ventilation in ICU bed 9 is in moderate to severe distress. He is a heroin overdose patient. He is receiving nutritional supplementation and IV fluids. Initial PAP was $\frac{25}{15}$ and PCWP was 10. Three hours later the PAP is $\frac{32}{16}$ and PCWP is 16. These findings are indicative of:
   a. fluid overload
   b. pulmonary edema
   c. right ventricular failure
   d. pulmonary hypertension
   e. ARDS

9. CVP catheter is used to monitor:
   I. Fluid volume
   II. Cardiac output
   III. Circulatory dynamics
   IV. Right heart function
   V. Pulmonary hypertension
   a. I, II, III
   b. II, III, V
   c. I, III, IV
   d. II, III, IV, V
   e. I, II, III, IV, V

10. Mean pulmonary artery pressure is:
   a. 40 mmHg
   b. 35 mmHg
   c. 30 mmHg
   d. 25 mmHg
   e. 15 mmHg

11. As the BTFD catheter is wedged into the pulmonary artery, the wedge pressure approximates:
   a. right ventricular pressure
   b. left ventricular end diastolic pressure
   c. right heart pressure
   d. cardiac output
   e. pulmonary artery pressure

12. What is the normal range for central venous pressure?
   a. 1 to 7 cm H_2O
   b. 10 to 15 cm H_2O
   c. 15 to 20 cm H_2O
   d. 20 to 25 cm H_2O
   e. 25 to 18 cm H_2O

13. Which of the formulas listed here is used to determine mean arterial pressure?

   a. $\dfrac{2(\text{systolic} \times \text{diastolic})}{4}$

   b. $\dfrac{2(\text{diastolic} \times \text{systolic})}{3}$

   c. $\dfrac{\text{diastolic} + \text{systolic}}{2}$

d. $\dfrac{2(\text{diastolic}) + \text{systolic}}{3}$

e. none of the above

14. What is the normal systolic pulmonary artery pressure?
    a. 4 to 7 mmHg
    b. 7 to 12 mmHg
    c. 16 to 25 mmHg
    d. 25 to 30 mmHg
    e. 30 to 40 mmHg

15. Which of the following is considered a complication of arterial catheter usage?
    a. hemorrhage
    b. embolization
    c. infection
    d. necrosis
    e. all of the above

16. Which of the following is true about the BTFD catheters?
    I. It is available in 4 lumen choices only.
    II. It is 110 cm in length.
    III. It is marked off in 20 cm increments.
    IV. It was designed by Swan and Ganz in the 1960s.
    V. Common insertion site is the femoral vein.
    a. I, II, III, IV, V
    b. II, IV, V
    c. II, IV
    d. I, IV
    e. III, V

17. Which of the following is true about the PCWP?
    I. A value of 15 to 18 mmHg is a sign of pulmonary congestion.
    II. A value of 25 to 30 mmHg indicates frank pulmonary edema.
    III. The value should be correlated to chest x-ray report.
    IV. It is measured only intermittently.
    V. It is valuable in fluid management.
    a. I, II, III, IV, V
    b. I, II, III, IV
    c. III, IV
    d. II, III, V
    e. II and III

18. In the calculation of PVR, units of resistance must be multiplied by _____ to convert to dynes $\times$ cm $\times$ sec.
    a. 10
    b. 20
    c. 40
    d. 60
    e. 80

19. The formula for calculation of cardiac index is:
    a. HR $\times$ SV
    b. the Fick equation
    c. $\dfrac{\text{CO}}{\text{BP}} \times 2$

d. $\dfrac{CO}{BSA}$

e. none of the above

20. The following are hazards associated with CVP lines:
    I. Infection
    II. Clot formation
    III. Pneumothorax
    IV. Bleeding
    V. Air emboli
    a. I, II, III, IV, V
    b. I, II, III, IV
    c. II, IV, V
    d. I, II, V
    e. I, II, IV, V

ANSWERS TO PRACTICE QUIZ

1. a
2. c
3. d
4. b
5. b
6. b
7. b
8. a
9. b
10. e

11. b
12. b
13. d
14. c
15. e
16. c
17. b
18. e
19. d
20. a

Chapter 17

PATHOLOGY

OUTLINE

OBSTRUCTIVE DISEASE
COPD
Emphysema
Chronic Bronchitis
Bronchiectasis
Asthma
Status Asthmaticus
RESTRICTIVE DISEASE
Pulmonary Fibrosis
Pulmonary Edema

Pulmonary Embolism
Pneumonia
Adult Respiratory Distress Syndrome
Myasthenia gravis
Guillain-Barré Syndrome
PEDIATRIC PULMONARY DISEASE
Cystic Fibrosis
Croup
Epiglottitis
PRACTICE QUIZ

LEARNING OBJECTIVES

Upon completion of this unit, the individual will:

1. Define the diseases covered in this chapter.
2. Identify the diseases covered as obstructive or restrictive.
3. List the etiology of in each disease.
4. List the clinical presentation of each disease.
5. Identify expected pulmonary function test results for each applicable disease.

6. Identify diagnostic tools needed to confirm diagnosis when applicable for each disease.
7. List expected laboratory results as applicable for each disease.
8. Identify necessary components of management of each disease.

REFERENCES

Deshpande, WM, Philbeam, SP, and Dixon, RJ: A Comprehensive Review in Respiratory Care. Appleton and Lange, Norwalk, CT, 1988.

DesJardins, TR: Clinical Manifestations of Respiratory Disease. Year Book Medical Publishers, Chicago, 1988.

Kacmarek, RM, Mack, CW, and Dimas, S: The Essentials of Respiratory Therapy. Year Book Medical Publishers, Chicago, 1985.

Mitchell, R: Clinical Pulmonary Disease, ed 4. CV Mosby, St Louis, 1988.

STUDY QUESTIONS

1. Define COPD. (Deshpande, p 159; Kacmarek, p 300)

   _____

   _____

   _____

2. List six common etiologic agents associated with COPD. (Deshpande, p 159; Kacmarek, p 300)

   a. _____   d. _____

   b. _____   e. _____

   c. _____   f. _____

3. Using the categories listed below, describe the clinical appearance of COPD. (Deshpande, p 160; Kacmarek, p 300)

   a. general appearance: _____

   _____

   _____

   b. chest assessment: _____

   _____

   _____

   c. ventilatory pattern: _____

   _____

   _____

   d. chest x-ray: _____

   _____

   _____

4. Complete the chart below with the expected PFT study results on the COPD patient. (Deshpande, p 161; Kacmarek, p 302)

   FVC: _____   TLC: _____

   FEV_1: _____   RV: _____

   ERV: _____   RV/TLC: _____

   FRC: _____   MVV: _____

5. Give the direction of movement of the ABG values listed below to follow progression of COPD. (Deshpande, p 161; Kacmarek, p 302)

	Early	End-Stage
pH:		
$Paco_2$:		
Pao_2:		
HCO_3:		

6. What is hypoxic drive? (Deshpande, p 161; Kacmarek, p 303)

_____

_____

_____

7. List six areas of management of COPD. (Deshpande, pp 161–168; Kacmark, p 303)

a. _____ d. _____

b. _____ e. _____

c. _____ f. _____

8. Define emphysema. (Deshpande, p 163; DesJardins, p 134; Kacmarek, p 305)

_____

_____

_____

9. List four etiologic agents associated with emphysema. (Deshpande, p 163; DesJardins, p 134; Kacmarek, p 305)

a. _____

b. _____

c. _____

d. _____

10. List the three types of emphysema. (Deshpande, p 163; DesJardins, p 134; Kacmarek, p 305)

a. _____

b. _____

c. _____

11. Place the type of emphysema in the blank next to the comment that best describes it. (Deshpande, pp 163–165; Kacmarek, p 305)

a. seen most with alpha₁-antitrypsin deficiency: _____

b. prominent bleb formation: _____

c. seen most at alveolar and respiratory bronchiolar level: _____

d. most associated with smoking: _____

e. alveolar septal destruction prominent: _____

    f. changes mainly in upper lobes: _____

    g. also called panacinar: _____

12. Using the categories below, describe the clinical appearance of emphysema. (Deshpande, p 166; DesJardins, p 136; Kacmarek, p 306)

    a. general appearance: _____

    _____

    b. chest assessment: _____

    _____

    c. ventilatory pattern: _____

    _____

    d. chest x-ray: _____

    _____

13. Indicate the direction PFT study results will move in emphysema. (Deshpande, p 165; DesJardins, p 136)

    FVC: _____   TLC: _____

    FEV_1: _____   RV: _____

    FRC: _____   RV/TLC: _____

14. Give the direction ABG values would move in emphysema. (Deshpande, p 165; DesJardins, p 136)

    pH: _____

    $Paco_2$: _____

    Pao_2: _____

    HCO_3: _____

15. Place an "X" next to the response that should be included in management of emphysema. (Deshpande, p 166; DesJardins, p 153; Kacmarek, p 306)

    _____ avoid inhaled irritants

    _____ expectorants

    _____ avoid infection

    _____ proper nutrition

    _____ beta-blocker therapy

    _____ mobilize secretions

    _____ patient/family education

    _____ rehabilitation

    _____ diuretic therapy

16. Define chronic bronchitis. (Deshpande, p 162; Kacmarek, p 306)

    _____

    _____

17. List three etiologic agents in chronic bronchitis. (Deshpande, p 162; Kacmarek, p 307)

a. _____

b. _____

c. _____

18. Describe the clinical appearance of chronic bronchitis. (Deshpande, p 162; DesJardins, p 107; Kacmarek, p 307)

a. cough: _____

_____

b. sputum: _____

_____

c. breath sounds: _____

_____

d. chest x-ray: _____

_____

19. Indicate the direction the following results will move in chronic bronchitis: (Deshpande, p 162; DesJardins, p 108; Kacmarek, p 308)

FVC: _____ FEV_1: _____

FRC: _____ TLC: _____

RV: _____ RV/TLC: _____

20. List four key elements in the management of chronic bronchitis. (Deshpande, p 163; DesJardins, p 127; Kacmarek, 308)

a. _____

b. _____

c. _____

d. _____

21. Define bronchiectasis. (Deshpande, p 166; Kacmarek, p 308)

_____

_____

22. List the three classifications of bronchiectasis. (Deshpande, p 166; Kacmarek, p 308)

a. _____

b. _____

c. _____

23. Use the classifications of bronchiectasis to complete the following: (Deshpande, pp 166–168; Kacmarek, p 308)

a. least severe classification: _____

b. most severe classification: _____

c. replacement of bronchial tissue by fibrous tissue: _____

    d. bronchioie outlines and blunt ends: _____

    e. bronchial walls have bulbous ends: _____

24. List four etiologic components of bronchiectasis. (Deshpande, p 166; Kacmarek, p 308)

    a. _____

    b. _____

    c. _____

    d. _____

25. How is bronchiectasis diagnosed? (Deshpande, p 168; Kacmarek, p 309)

_____

_____

26. List eight manifestations of bronchiectasis. (Deshpande, p 168; Kacmarek, p 309)

    a. _____   e. _____

    b. _____   f. _____

    c. _____   g. _____

    d. _____   h. _____

27. Describe the sputum of bronchiectasis. (Deshpande, p 168; Kacmarek, p 309)

_____

_____

_____

28. List three components of management of bronchiectasis. (Deshpande, p 168; Kacmarek, p 309)

    a. _____

    b. _____

    c. _____

29. The etiologic type of asthma associated with a sensitivity to certain antigens is termed _____. (DesJardins, p 159; Kacmarek, p 310)

30. The etiologic type of asthma that is associated with anxiety, infection, and irrtitant gases is termed _____. (DesJardins, p 159; Kacmarek, p 310)

31. Describe the clinical manifestation of asthma: (Deshpande, 170; DesJardins, p 157; Kacmarek, p 311)

    a. general appearance: _____

    b. chest appearance: _____

    c. breath sounds: _____

    d. chest x-ray: _____

    e. ECG: _____

    f. CBC: _____

32. How is asthma managed? (Deshpande, 170; DesJardins, p 179; Kacmarek, p 313)

_____

_____

33. Differentiate between asthma and status asthmaticus. (Deshpande, 170; DesJardins, p 162; Kacmarek, p 313)

_____

_____

_____

34. Define pulmonary fibrosis. (Deshpande, 174; Kacmarek, p 315)

_____

_____

35. List six etiologic agents of pulmonary fibrosis. (Deshpande, 174; Kacmarek, p 315)

a. _____ d. _____

b. _____ e. _____

c. _____ f. _____

36. Describe the clinical manifestations of pulmonary fibrosis. (Deshpande, p 174)

a. general appearance: _____

_____

b. chest appearance: _____

_____

c. breath sounds: _____

_____

d. chest x-ray: _____

_____

37. Indicate the direction the following values will move in pulmonary fibrosis. (Deshpande, p 174; Kacmarek, p 316)

VC: _____ pH: _____

TLC: _____ $Paco_2$: _____

$FEV_1\%$: _____ Pao_2: _____

38. Describe the management of pulmonary fibrosis. (Deshpande, p 175; Kacmarek, p 317)

_____

_____

39. Define pulmonary edema. (DesJardins, p 210; Kacmarek, p 318)

_____

_____

40. Differentiate between the etiologic factors in cardiogenic and noncardiogenic pulmonary edema. (Deshpande, p 175; DesJardins, p 212; Kacmarek, p 318)

_____

_____

_____

_____

_____

_____

41. Describe the following manifestations of pulmonary edema. (Deshpande, p 176; DesJardins, p 214; Kacmarek, p 318)

    a. breath sounds: _____

    b. chest x-ray: _____

    c. ABG: _____

    d. PCWP: _____

42. Describe the treatment of cardiogenic pulmonary edema. (Deshpande, p 177; DesJardins, p 222; Kacmarek, p 318)

    a. pharmacology: _____

    b. pulmonary: _____

43. Describe the treatment of noncardiogenic pulmonary edema. (Kacmarek, p 321)

_____

44. Define pulmonary embolism: (DesJardins, p 226; Kacmarek, p 324)

_____

_____

_____

45. List five high-risk factors for pulmonary embolism: (DesJardins, p 228; Kacmarek, p 324)

    a. _____

    b. _____

    c. _____

    d. _____

    e. _____

46. Describe the clinical manifestations of pulmonary embolism.(DesJardins, p 228; Kacmarek, p 326)

    a. general appearance: _____

_____

    b. HR/RR/BS: _____

c. ECG: _____

d. chest x-ray: _____

47. What two procedures provide diagnostic information about pulmonary embolism? (DesJardins, p 228; Kacmarek, p 326)

_____

48. Give four components of treatment of pulmonary embolism. (DesJardins, p 244; Kacmarek, p 326)

a. _____

b. _____

c. _____

d. _____

49. Define pneumonia. (Deshpande, p 176; DesJardins, p 187; Kacmarek, p 323)

_____

50. Compare bacterial and viral pneumonia: (Deshpande, p 176; DesJardins, p 188; Kacmarek, p 324)

	Bacterial	**Viral**
onset		
fever		
chills		
hypoxemia		
x-ray		
sputum		
WBC		
pleuritic pain		
cough		
increased HR/RR		

51. List four components of treatment of pneumonia. (Deshpande, p 178; DesJardins, p 205; Kacmarek, p 324)

a. _____

b. _____

c. _____

d. _____

52. List five major pathologic/structural changes associated with adult respiratory distress syndrome (ARDS). (Deshpande, p 187; DesJardins, p 249)

a. _____

b. _____

c. _____

d. _____

e. _____

53. Describe the clinical presentation of ARDS: (Deshpande, p 188; DesJardins, p 249; Kacmarek, p 322)

    a. pulmonary symptomology: _____

    _____

    _____

    b. cardiac symptomology: _____

54. Describe four steps in the management of ARDS: (Deshpande, p 188; DesJardins, p 251; Kacmarek, p 322)

    a. _____

    b. _____

    c. _____

    d. _____

55. Define myasthenia gravis. (Deshpande, p 184; Kacmarek, p 328)

_____

_____

_____

56. Describe the clinical manifestations of myasthenia gravis. (Deshpande, p 184; Kacmarek, p 328)

_____

_____

_____

57. Differentiate between a myasthenic and a cholinergic crisis. (Deshpande, p 184; Kacmarek, p 329)

_____

_____

_____

_____

_____

_____

58. What three parameters should be monitored in the myasthenia gravis patient? (Deshpande, pp 184–185)

    a. _____

    b. _____

    c. _____

59. Define Guillain-Barré syndrome. (Deshpande, p 183)

_____

_____

_____

60. Describe the clinical path of Guillain-Barré syndrome. (Deshpande, p 183)

_____

_____

_____

61. List four diagnostic tests for Guillain-Barré syndrome. (Deshpande, p 183; Kacmarek, p 330)

    a. _____

    b. _____

    c. _____

    d. _____

62. How is Guillain-Barré syndrome treated? (Deshpande, p 183; Kacmarek, p 330)

_____

_____

63. Define cystic fibrosis. (Deshpande, p 389; Kacmarek, p 352)

_____

_____

_____

64. Describe the clinical presentation of cystic fibrosis. (Deshpande, p 389; DesJardins, p 333; Kacmarek, p 352)

    a. gastrointestinal: _____

    _____

    _____

    b. pulmonary: _____

    _____

    _____

    c. chest x-ray: _____

    _____

    _____

65. How is cystic fibrosis diagnosed? (Deshpande, p 389; DesJardins, p 333; Kacmarek, p 352)

_____

_____

_____

66. Give four treatment objectives in managing cystic fibrosis. (Deshpande, p 389; DesJardins, p 353; Kacmarek, p 353)

    a. _____

    b. _____

    c. _____

    d. _____

67. Croup involves inflammation of the _____. (Deshpande, p 388; Kacmarek, p 354)

68. List the four most common etiologic agents in croup. (Deshpande, p 388; Kacmarek, p 354)

    a. _____

    b. _____

    c. _____

    d. _____

69. Describe the clinical presentation in croup. (Deshpande, p 388; Kacmarek, p 354)

    _____

    _____

    _____

70. How is croup diagnosed? (Deshpande, p 388; Kacmarek, p 354)

    _____

    _____

71. List four aspects of management of croup. (Deshpande, p 388)

    a. _____

    b. _____

    c. _____

    d. _____

72. Define epiglottitis. (Deshpande, p 388)

    _____

    _____

73. How is epiglottitis diagnosed? (Deshpande, p 388)

    _____

74. How does the typical epiglottitis case present? (Deshpande, p 388)

    _____

    _____

    _____

    _____

75. What is the most common infectious agent associated with causing epiglottitis? (Deshpande, p 388)

76. How is epiglottitis clinically managed? (Deshpande, p 388)

ANSWERS TO STUDY QUESTIONS

1. chronic obstructive pulmonary disease: a disease characterized by airway obstruction that is exhibited via decreased expiratory flow rates

2. a. smoking
   b. air pollution
   c. allergies
   d. aging
   e. infection
   f. heredity

3. a. anxious, malnourished, complains of lost appetite, use of accessory muscles, muscle atrophy, jugular engorgement cyanosis, digital clubbing
   b. barrel chest, increased AP diameter, hyper-resonant chest, decreased breath sounds, adventitious breath sounds
   c. paradoxical movement of the abdomen, prolonged expiratory time, active exhalation, pursed-lipped breathing
   d. increased AP diameter, hyperinflation, flattened diaphragm, increased retrosternal space

4. FVC decreased, FEV_1 decreased, ERV increased, FRC increased, TLC normal to increased, RV increased, RV/TLC increased, MVV decreased

5. Early: pH normal, $PaCO_2$ decreased, PaO_2 decreased, HCO_3 decreased. Late: pH decreased, $PaCO_2$ increased, PaO_2 decreased, HCO_3 decreased.

6. a clinical case in which the drive to breath is stimulated by a hypoxic mechanism; increased levels of oxygen will decrease the drive to breath

7. a. relieve obstruction
   b. prevent infection
   c. treat hypoxia
   d. maintain cardiac status
   e. decrease exposure to irritant substances
   f. increase exercise tolerance

8. a disease that is characterized by weakening and enlargement of the air spaces distal to the terminal bronchioles and by destruction of the alveolar septal walls

9. a. smoking
   b. air pollution
   c. repeated pulmonary infections
   d. alpha₁-antitrypsin deficiency

10. a. centrilobular
    b. panlobular
    c. bullous

11. a. panlobular
    b. bullous
    c. bulbus
    d. centrilobular
    e. panlobular
    f. centrilobular
    g. panlobular

12. a. cyanosis, digital clubbing, anorexia, muscle atrophy, enlarged neck veins, peripheral edema
    b. barrel-chested, hyperresonant, suprasternal retractions, increased AP diameter, rhonchi, nonproductive cough
    c. increased respiratory rate, pursed-lip breathing, use of accessory muscles,
    d. enlarged heart, flattened hemidiaphragms, hyperinflation, hypertranslucency, increased AP diameter

13. FVC decreased, FEV_1 decreased, FRC increased, TLC increased, RV increased, RV/TLC increased

14. pH normal to decreased, $PaCO_2$ increased, PaO_2 decreased, HCO_3 increased

15. All but beta blockers and diuretic therapy are indicated in management of emphysema.

16. Chronic bronchitis is characterized by a chronic cough with production of large quantities of sputum of unknown cause for 3 months per year for at least 2 consecutive years.

17. a. smoking
    b. air pollution
    c. chronic pulmonary infections

18. a. smoker's cough to morning cough to continual cough
    b. large production with gradual increase, thick gray mucoid until infection present—then purulent
    c. rhonchi to wheeze, use of accessory muscles diminished
    d. early no changes seen, translucent, increased AP, depressed diaphragm, prominent peripheral pulmonary vasculature

19. FVC decreased, FRC increased, RV decreased, FEV_1 decreased, TLC increased, RV/TLC increased

20. a. remove irritant
    b. aerosol and bronchodilator therapy
    c. oxygen therapy
    d. antibiotics

21. an irreversible dilation and distortion of the bronchi and or bronchioles

22. a. cylindrical
    b. cystic (fusiform or varicose)
    c. saccular

23. a. cylindrical
    b. saccular
    c. saccular
    d. cylindrical
    e. cystic

24. a. congenital anomalies
    b. atelectasis
    c. airway obstruction
    d. chronic childhood bronchopulmonary infections

25. The only absolute diagnostic measure is bronchogram. Other tools include x-ray, bronchoscopy, and sputum.

26. a. chronic loose cough
    b. clubbing
    c. cyanosis
    d. recurrent infections
    e. halitosis
    f. hemoptysis
    g. three-layered sputum
    h. increased appetite with poor weight gain and weakness

27. The sputum separates into three distinct layers. The top layer is thin and frothy; the middle layer is turbid and mucoid; and the bottom layer is opaque, mucopurulent, and purulent.

28. a. bronchial hygiene
    b. antibiotic therapy
    c. resection if applicable

29. extrinsic

30. intrinsic

31. a. accessary muscle usage, cyanosis, distress, diaphoresis, barrel chest, anxiety
    b. intercostal, substernal, and subcostal retractions, paradoxical chest movements
    c. inspiratory time and expiratory wheeze, weak cough, increased expiratory time
    d. hyperinflation to normal
    e. sinus tachycardia, PVC, and PAC
    f. increaed eosinophils in extrinsic

32. avoidance of allergens, prophylactic cromolyn sodium, steroids as needed for infection

33. Status asthmaticus is an acute asthma attack that does not respond to optimal treatment. It is treated with sympathomimetics, steroids, subcutaneous epinephrine, and xanthines.

34. a disease characterized by excessive amounts of connective tissue in the lungs.

35. a. tissue necrosis
    b. pneumoconiosis
    c. aspiration
    d. TB
    e. pulmonary infections
    f. pneumonitis

36. a. progressive dyspnea on exertion, clubbing, cyanosis, increased work of breathing
    b. restricted chest wall and diaphragmatic movement, tachypnea, tracheal shift to fibrotic side
    c. nonproductive cough, dry crackles, rales
    d. mediastinal shift toward fibrotic side, irregular diaphragm elevation, fine reticular lines

37. VC decreased, TLC decreased, $FEV_1\%$ normal, pH increased, $PaCO_2$ decreased, PaO_2 decreased; $P(A-a)O_2$ increased

38. No real treatment; mostly supportive mea-

sures, remove any underlying disease, and avoid irritants

39. a disease entity in which there is excessive movement of fluid from the pulmonary vascular system to the alveoli and the extravascular spaces

40. In cardiogenic pulmonary edema, there is movement of fluid across the alveolar-capillary membrane and into the extravascular spaces as a result of increased hydrostatic pressures due to CHF. In noncardiogenic pulmonary edema, the disease develops due to an increased capillary permeability as a result of infection, inflammation, and so on.

41. a. increased RR, cough with expectoration of pink, frothy sputum; rales
    b. increased opacity, enlarged heart, prominent pulmonary vasculature, Kerley B lines
    c. mild alkalosis, hypocapneia, and hypoxemia responsive
    d. increased to 20 to 25 range, indicating frank pulmonary edema

42. a. lasix, morphine, digitalis
    b. oxygen at high percentages, IPPB with ethyl alcohol, PEEP and ventilate as needed

43. oxygen therapy, fluid, diuretics, low-level PEEP

44. Pulmonary embolism is a disease process that occurs when a thrombus or other substance is carried in the blood to occlude a portion of the pulmonary vasculature.

45. a. venous stasis
    b. hypercoagulation
    c. trauma
    d. postoperative or postpartum
    e. obesity
    (others: burns, malignant neoplasm)

46. a. dyspnea, diaphoresis, chest pain, possible hemoptysis, cough, faintness, anxiety
    b. increased HR and RR, decreased breath sounds, wheezes and rales, pleural friction rub
    c. sinus tach, arrhythmias
    d. x-ray nondiagnostic; occasionally signs of decreased volume

47. ventilation/perfusion scan and pulmonary angiography

48. a. IV streptokinase/urokinase
    b. anticoagulation therapy

    c. oxygen therapy
    d. embolectomy

49. acute inflammation of the lungs secondary to infection or insult, RBC, leukocytes, and macrophages pour into the alveoli

50. onset: abrupt (bacterial), gradual (viral)
    fever: high, low-grade
    chills: positive, negative
    hypoxemia: common, uncommon
    x-ray: consolidation, negative
    sputum: purulent, thin mucoid
    WBC: >10,000/cu mm, <10,000/cu mm
    pleuritic pain: positive negative
    cough: positive, positive
    increased HR/RR: positive, negative

51. a. oxygen therapy
    b. antibiotic, fungal therapy as indicated
    c. fluid therapy
    d. mobilize secretions

52. a. interstitial/intra-alveolar edema and hemorrhage
    b. alveolar consolidation
    c. atelectasis
    d. pulmonary surfactant deficiency
    e. beefy lung tissue found on autopsy

53. a. refractory hypoxemia, tachypnea, rales, respiratory distress, SOB, cyanosis, diffuse alveolar infiltrates, cough, intercostal retractions, increased $P(A-a)O_2$, increased WOB
    b. increased HR, CO, BP, and arrhythmias

54. a. ventilation
    b. oxygenation
    c. maintain cardiovascular status
    d. remove cause

55. a disease of the myoneural junction in which transmission of impulses across the motor end plate is disrupted, causing autoimmune disease, weakness, and increased fatigue of the muscles

56. weakness and fatigue on exertion, descending paralysis, facial, ocular muscles involved first, speech problems, respiratory muscles fail; chief complaint = fatiguability

57. They are differentiated by the tensilon test. Myasthenic crisis is an acute exacerbation of myasthenia. A cholinergic crisis is an acute decrease in muscle strength as a result of excessive use of the cholinesterase inhibitors. Tensilon will improve muscle strength in a myasthenic crisis and will worsen it in a cholinergic crisis.

58. a. cardiopulmonary status
    b. VC
    c. NIF

59. an ascending paralyzing disease that affects the peripheral motor and sensory neurons; etiology is unknown – possible virus connection

60. generally flulike illness, with increasing respiratory tract infection, rapid onset, ascending paralysis, deep tendon reflex loss

61. a. increased protein in CSF
    b. leukocytosis
    c. decrease VC
    d. decreased NIF

62. Treatment is supportive, symptomatic; mechanical ventilation as needed; steroids are questionable.

63. a genetic abnormality of the exocrine glands involving malfunction of the pancreas, liver, sweat glands, lungs, and salivary glands; also known as mucoviscidosis and pancreatic enzyme deficiency

64. a. loose, bulky, foul-smelling stools, large appetite with little weight gain, inadequate digestion of fats and proteins, protruding abdomen, malnutrition, and poor body development
    b. increased AP diameter; pursed-lip breathing; progressive, loose, productive cough; cyanosis; frequent infection; SOB; clubbing; diminished breath sounds; use of accessory muscles
    c. translucent, depression of diaphragm, possibly enlarged heart

65. A sweat chloride test result above 60 mEq/l is positive; two positives must be obtained along with documentation of other system involvement.

66. a. mobilization of secretions
    b. mucolytic therapy
    c. oxygen and antibiotic therapy as needed
    d. gastrointestinal management

67. subglottic area including the larynx and trachea

68. a. adenovirus
    b. respiratory syncytial virus
    c. parainfluenza virus
    d. influenza virus

69. usually child between 6 months and 3 years old, dry barking cough following a viral infection, inspiratory stridor, possible slow onset, normal WBC, and more common in fall and winter months

70. Lateral neck radiograph, classic "steeple" appearance seen as narrowing in trachea and larynx

71. a. cool aerosol mist
    b. oxygen therapy if needed
    c. systemic hydration
    d. racemic epinephrine

72. an acute inflammation of the supraglottic area having the potential to completely obstruct the upper airway

73. chest x-ray, lateral neck, most important clinical appearance

74. Child usually betweeen the ages of 2 and 8 years old, complains of sore throat of sudden onset, has labored breathing, hoarseness, and a fever. Child sits up, leans forward, and drools. There is inspiratory stridor; muffled speech and cough; elevated WBC; red swollen epiglottis.

75. Hemophilus influenza type B

76. establish an airway, give antibiotics as indicated; treat fever; intubation by most experienced person in the OR, with tracheostomy kit at hand

PRACTICE QUIZ

1. Which of the following conditions are considered to be obstructive?
    I. Bronchiectasis
    II. Pneumonia
    III. Chronic bronchitis
    IV. Asthma
    V. Guillain-Barré syndrome

   a. I, II, III, IV, V
   b. I, II, IV
   c. I, III, IV
   d. II, IV, V
   e. II and IV

2. Which of the following play a major role in decreasing bronchial gas flow and increasing intrapleural pressures in emphysema?
   a. Poiseuille's law
   b. Boyle's law
   c. Charles' law
   d. Dalton's law
   e. none of the above

3. Which type of emphysema is most closely related to the alpha$_1$-antitrypsin deficiency?
   a. bullous
   b. septalobular
   c. centrilobular
   d. panlobular
   e. all of the above

4. Intrinsic asthma may be triggered by which of the following?
       I. Infection
      II. Vapor
     III. Cat hair
      IV. Pollen
       V. Cold Air
   a. I, II, III, IV, V
   b. I, III, IV, V
   c. II, III, IV
   d. I, II, V
   e. III and IV

5. Early in an acute asthma attack, ABGs would yield which of the following results?
       I. Increased pH
      II. Decreased pH
     III. Increased Pa_{CO_2}
      IV. Decreased Pa_{CO_2}
       V. Normal to decreased HCO_3
   a. I, II, V
   b. I, IV, V
   c. II, III, V
   d. II, IV, V
   e. I and III

6. Increased hydrostatic pressures are correlated with which of the following causes of pulmonary edema?
   a. heroin overdose
   b. uremia
   c. nephritis
   d. pneumonia
   e. fluid overload

7. Which of the following is/are etiologic agent(s) in pulmonary embolism?
       I. Thrombophlebitis
      II. CHF

     III. Polycythemia
     IV. Obesity
     V. Oral contraceptives
  a. I, II, III, IV, V
  b. I, III, IV
  c. II, III, IV
  d. I, II, III
  e. I only

8. What is the most common source of pulmonary emboli?
  a. blood clots
  b. bone marrow
  c. fat
  d. malignant tumors
  e. air

9. How is myasthenia gravis diagnosed?
  a. chest radiograph
  b. administration of parasympathomimetic or cholinesterase inhibitor
  c. WBC
  d. blood culture
  e. C and S sputum

10. Which of the following are true of myasthenia gravis?
     I. There is descending paralysis.
     II. Caused by autoimmune antibody to the motor end plates
     III. Protein count in CSF is increased.
     IV. It is virus-related
     V. Tensilon increases muscle weakness.
  a. I, II, III, IV, V
  b. I, II, V
  c. I, II, III
  d. I, IV, V
  e. I, III, V

11. Which classification of bronchiectasis is the most severe and has the worst prognosis?
  a. saccular
  b. centrilobular
  c. fusiform
  d. cystic
  e. cylindrical

12. Which is the absolute diagnostic tool in bronchiectasis?
  a. chest radiograph
  b. bronchoscopy
  c. bronchogram
  d. sputum exam
  e. blood culture

13. Which PCWP is indicative of frank pulmonary edema?
  a. 5 to 10 mmHg
  b. 10 to 15 mmHg
  c. 15 to 20 mmHg
  d. 20 to 25 mmHg
  e. unknown

14. Which of the following are considered etilogic agents of noncardiac pulmonary edema?
   I. Head trauma
   II. Heroin overdose
   III. High-altitude sickness
   IV. Renal failure
   V. Aspiration syndrome
   a. I, II, III, IV, V
   b. I, III, IV, V
   c. II, IV, V
   d. II, III, IV
   e. II and V

15. Which of the following is/are clinical feature(s) of ARDS?
   a. decreased FRC
   b. diffuse alveolar infiltrates
   c. decreased compliance
   d. refractory hypoxemia
   e. all of the above

16. Which of the following is/are the most common agent(s) associated with epiglottitis?
   I. Adenovirus
   II. Hemophilus influenza
   III. Influenza virus
   IV. RSV
   V. Parainfluenza virus
   a. I, II, III, IV, V
   b. I, III, V
   c. I, II, IV
   d. II and IV
   e. II only

ANSWERS TO PRACTICE QUIZ

1. c		11. b	
2. a		12. d	
3. d		13. d	
4. d		14. b	
5. b		15. a	
6. e		16. c	
7. a		17. d	
8. a		18. a	
9. c		19. e	
10. c		20. e	

$\mathcal{C}$hapter 18

PHARMACOLOGY

OUTLINE

Diuretics
**CENTRAL NERVOUS SYSTEM DEPRES-
SANTS AND STIMULANTS; SKELETAL
MUSCLE RELAXANTS**
CNS Depressants
CNS Stimulants

Skeletal Muscle Relaxants
Nondepolarizing
Depolarizing
CALCULATIONS
PRACTICE QUIZ

LEARNING OBJECTIVES

Upon completion of this unit, the individual will:

1. List and give an example of the major sources of drugs.
2. Explain the two major theories of drug action.
3. Describe various routes of drug administration.
4. Define pharmacokinetics in terms of absorption, distribution, metabolism, and excretion.
5. Define the following terms:
   a. tolerance
   b. cumulation
   c. tachyphylaxis
   d. synergism
   e. antagonism
   f. additive
   g. potentiation
6. List/explain the possible adverse reactions that can occur upon administration of a drug.
7. Describe the pathways for both the parasympathetic and the sympathetic branches of the autonomic nervous system.
8. State the two layers of the mucous blanket.
9. List the composition of mucus, and discuss mucokinesis.
10. Describe the four major concepts of management of respiratory tract secretions according to Zimet.
11. Categorize mucokinetic drugs into six major classes.
12. List the receptors found on an adrenergic receptor and describe the mechanism of action when each is stimulated.
13. List the common side effects associated with sympathomimetic drugs.
14. Identify common trade names of drugs used in respiratory care with their generic counterparts.
15. Explain the primary effects of xanthines and the importance of determining serum levels.
16. Describe how a muscarinic antagonist causes bronchodilation and how these agents are used.
17. Identify/discuss the adrenal medulla and adrenal cortex and the secretions they produce.

18. Differentiate between mineralcorticoids and glucocorticoids, and discuss their uses.
19. Characterize the physical appearance and clinical symptoms of a patient with iatrogenic Cushing's syndrome.
20. Discuss the psychologic and physiologic aspects of steroid dependency.
21. Discuss cromolyn sodium in terms of use, mode of action, and hazards associated with administration.
22. Describe the drugs associated with the treatment of coughs and colds and classify them according to four general categories.
23. State the effects of prostaglandins E and F on the mucosa and smooth muscle in the lung and list the clinical situations that cause their release.
24. Differentiate between bacteriostatic and bactericidal agents.
25. Identify the major pathogens encountered by the respiratory care practitioner.
26. Identify the five modes of action of antimicrobials and clarify the effect of the antimicrobial in each category.
27. Define nosocomial infection and superinfection.
28. Define the following:
   a. inotropic
   b. chronotropic
   c. dromotropic
29. Given a clinical situation, identify the category or specific cardiovascular drug that could be used.
30. Identify the antidysrhythmic and antihypertensive drugs by their mechanism of action.
31. Discuss the use and effects of diuretics and give an example.
32. Discuss the uses of respiratory stimulants and depressants.
33. Differentiate between nondepolarizing and depolarizing neuromuscular blocking agents.
34. Given the appropriate information, calculate solutions dealing with preparation of respiratory medication.

REFERENCES

Barnes, TA: Respiratory Care Practice. Year Book Medical Publishers, Chicago, 1988.

Becker, DE: Pharmacology for the Health Professional. Reston Publishing Company, Virginia, 1985.

Burton, GG, et al: Respiratory Care: A Guide to Clinical Practice, ed 2. JB Lippincott, Philadelphia, 1984.

Kacmarek, RM, Mack, CW, and Dimas, S: The Essentials of Respiratory Therapy, ed 2. Year Book Medical Publishers, Chicago, 1985.

Mathewson, MK: Pharmacotherapeutics. FA Davis, Philadelphia, 1986.

Physicians' Desk Reference, ed 42. Medical Economics, Oradell, New Jersey, 1988.

Rau, JL: Respiratory Therapy Pharmacology, ed 2. Year Book Medical Publishers, Chicago, 1984.

Thomas, CL (ed): Taber's Cyclopedic Medical Dictionary, ed 15. FA Davis, Philadelphia, 1985.

Ziment, I: Respiratory Pharmacology and Therapeutics. WB Saunders, Philadelphia, 1978.

STUDY QUESTIONS

1. Match the abbreviations in column A with their meaning in column B. (Rau, p 31; Ziment, p 37)

Column A	Column B
_____ ac	a. with
_____ cc	b. gram
_____ NPO	c. as needed
_____ BID	d. every 4 hours
_____ prn	e. without
_____ ml	f. twice daily
_____ $\bar{p}$	g. before meals
_____ q	h. immediately
_____ TID	i. nothing by mouth
_____ gm	j. every day
_____ q4h	k. drop
_____ p.o.	l. after meals
_____ qod	m. every 2 hours
_____ $\bar{c}$	n. 3 times daily
_____ stat	o. half
_____ pc	p. every
_____ $\bar{s}$	q. milliliter
_____ gtt	r. every other day
_____ q2h	s. by mouth
_____ qd	t. cubic centimeter
_____ ss	u. after

2. List two sources of drug information. (Barnes, p 545; Rau p 4; Ziment, p 12)

_____

_____

3. List/describe two methods by which a drug produces an effect. Give an example of each. (Becker, pp 8–12; Rau, p 25)

   a. _____

   _____

   b. _____

   _____

4. Pharmokinetics involve four major factors controlling a drug at any given moment. These factors are: (Becker, p 4; Rau, p 17; Kacmarek, pp 529–530)

   a. _____

   b. _____

   c. _____

   d. _____

5. Drugs come from a variety of sources. Give an example of each source listed here. (Rau, p 5)

   a. animal: _____

   b. plant: _____

   c. mineral: _____

   d. chemical: _____

6. List the major routes of drug administration. (Ziment, p 16; Becker, p 5)

   a. _____

   b. _____

   c. _____

   d. _____

7. Match the following drug interactions in column A with their definitions in column B: (Ziment, p 20; Kacmarek, p 527; Rau, p 26)

   Column A
   _____ tolerance
   _____ cumulation
   _____ tachyphylaxis
   _____ synergism
   _____ antagonism
   _____ additive
   _____ potentiation

   Column B
   a. two drugs give an effect equal to the summation of each drug
   b. two drugs, one inactive, that produce results greater than the active drug alone
   c. two drugs elicit response greater than the sum of each drug's effect
   d. a drug whose effect is directly opposite that of another drug
   e. rate of drug removal is slower than the rate of drug's administration
   f. unusual resistance to standard drug dose
   g. development of rapid tolerance to a drug

8. As a result of drug administration side effects occur that are not intended or desired. Not all side effects are detrimental to the individual; however, those side effects that are toxic and/or detrimental

to the individual are called _____ (Ziment, p 20)

9. A severe hypersensitivity reaction resulting in fever, asthma-like symptoms, rash, shock, coma, decreased blood pressure, or death is termed _____. (Ziment, p 20)

10. The peripheral nervous system is composed of: (Becker, pp 21–27; Rau, pp 50–52; Kacmarek, p 147)

   a. _____

   b. _____

11. The two branches of the autonomic nervous system are: (Becker, p 27; Rau, pp 52–53; Kacmarek, p 149)

   a. _____

   b. _____

12. Compare/contrast the parasympathetic branch and the sympathetic branch of the autonomic nervous system. (Becker, p 27; Kacmarek, pp 151–152; Rau, p 52)

   _____

   _____

   _____

   _____

   _____

13. Match the drugs with the same meanings that affect the autonomic nervous system. (Rau, p 53; Kacmarek, pp 151–152)

   _____ sympathomimetic   a. cholinergic

   _____ parasympatholytic   b. adrenergic

   _____ parasympathomimetic   c. anticholinergic

   _____ sympatholytic   d. antiadrenergic

14. The three receptors located on an adrenergic receptor (smooth muscle) are: (Ziment, pp 109–111; Rau, p 66; Becker, pp 43–45)

   a. _____

   b. _____

   c. _____

15. Describe the mechanism of action after stimulation of a beta$_2$ adrenergic receptor. (Ziment, pp 115–117; Rau, p 67)

   _____

   _____

16. What systemic effects result with the activation of a beta$_1$ adrenergic receptor? (Becker, p 43; Kacmarek, p 534)

   _____

17. List three indications for a sympathomimetic drug. (Becker, p 50; Kacmarek, p 534)

    a. _____

    b. _____

    c. _____

18. What systemic effects results with the activation of an alpha adrenergic receptor? (Becker, p 43; Ziment, pp 331–333)

    _____

    _____

19. List six major side effects of sympathomimetics. (Rau, pp 79–82; Zimet, p 152; Kacmarek, p 534)

    a. _____

    b. _____

    c. _____

    d. _____

    e. _____

    f. _____

20. Match the trade name in column A with the generic name in column B. (Barnes, p 545; Kacmarek, pp 536–538; Ziment, pp 158–185)

Column A	Column B
_____ Vaponephrine	a. albuterol (salbutamol)
_____ Adrenalin	b. isoproterenol HCl
_____ Proventil	c. racemic epinephrine
_____ Alupent	d. terbutaline
_____ Isuprel	e. metaproterenol sulfate
_____ Bronkosol	f. phenylephrine
_____ Neo-Synephrine	g. isoetharine
_____ Brethine	h. epinephrine

21. Drugs that block the effects of acetylcholine on the muscarinic receptor site are termed _____. (Rau, p 95; Kacmarek, p 542)

22. Give two examples of drugs referred to in question 21. (Rau, p 95; Kacmarek, p 542; Mathewson, pp 199–201)

    a. _____

    b. _____

23. What would be the clinical use of the drugs in question 21? (Rau, p 100; Mathewson, pp 199–201; Kacmarek, p 542; Becker, p 36)

    _____

    _____

24. The method by which xanthines relax smooth muscle is _____ _____. (Becker, p 188; Ziment, p 190; PDR, pp 1861–1863)

25. Other than bronchodilation, primary effects of xanthines include: (Rau, pp 103–104; PDR, pp 1861–1863; Ziment, pp 195–199)

    a. _____

    b. _____

    c. _____

    d. _____

    e. _____

    f. _____

    g. _____

26. An example of a xanthine is _____. (PDR, p 1861; Barnes, p 545; Ziment, pp 212–213)

27. For the following ranges of theophylline serum levels, indicate the drugs effect(s). (Ziment, p 192; Rau, pp 104–105; PDR, p 1862)

    a. <5 μg/ml: _____

    b. 10 to 20 μg/ml: _____

    c. 20 to 30 μg/ml: _____

    d. 30 to 40 μg/ml: _____

    e. 40 to 50 μg/ml: _____

28. The two major constituents of mucus are: (Ziment, p 42; Becker, pp 191–192)

    a. _____

    b. _____

29. The two major layers of the mucocilliary blanket are: (Ziment, p 41; Kacmarek, p 42)

    a. _____

    b. _____

30. Mucokinesis involves: (Ziment, p 45; Rau, pp 118–121)

    _____

    _____

31. According to Ziment, management of respiratory tract secretions is based on what four concepts? (Ziment, p 48)

    a. _____

    b. _____

    c. _____

    d. _____

32. Classification of mucokinetic drugs involves subdivision into six classes. Next to each class give two examples. (Ziment, p 48; Rau, pp 129–148; Becker, pp 191–192)

    a. dilutent (hydration): _____

    b. surface acting agent: _____

    c. bronchomucotropic agent (expectorant): _____

    d. mucolytic: _____

    e. cilia augmentors: _____

    f. airway dilators: _____

33. Two major uses of steroids are: (Becker, p 158; Ziment, p 219; Rau, p 153)

    a. _____

    b. _____

34. The adrenal gland is an endocrine gland located on top of each kidney. Two distinct glands compose the adrenal gland. The names of these glands are: (Rau, p 155; Ziment, p 219)

    a. _____

    b. _____

35. Which part of the adrenal gland is responsible (a) for secretion of corticosteroids and (b) secretion of epinephrine and norepinephrine? (Rau, p 155; Ziment, p 219; Kacmarek, pp 121; 151; 161)

    a. _____

    b. _____

36. Hormones secreted by the adrenal cortex have two distinct activities to maintain body homeostasis. Next to each hormone describe this activity. (Kacmarek, p 161; Becker, pp 158–160)

    a. glucocorticoid (cortisol): _____

    b. mineralocorticoid (aldosterone): _____

37. List five pulmonary diseases/syndromes that may benefit from the treatment of the anti-inflammatory properties of steroids. (Ziment, p 256; Kacmarek, p 546; Mathewson, p 634)

    a. _____

    b. _____

    c. _____

    d. _____

    e. _____

38. The major side effects associated with steroidal therapy result in a condition similar to that of Cushing's syndrome. List as many side effects that are considered cushingoid effects. (Ziment, p 225; PDR, pp 1858, 2042; Becker, pp 158–160, Mathewson, p 765)

    _____

    _____

    _____

39. Use of glucocorticoids cause both physiologic and psychologic dependency. Explain each form of dependency. (Ziment, pp 227–228)

_____

_____

_____

40. Because of the dependency with prolonged administration of steroid therapy, these drugs must be withdrawn _____. (Becker, p 160; Mathewson, p 774)

41. Match the trade name in column A with the generic name in column B. (Barnes, p 546; Ziment, pp 233, 235–236)

Column A

_____ Solu-Cortef

_____ Decadron

_____ Vanceril

_____ AeroBid

_____ Solu-Medrol

_____ Azmacort

_____ Deltasone

_____ Valisone

Column B

a. methyprednisone

b. beclomethasone

c. triamcinolone

d. hydrocortisone

e. betamethasone

f. flunisolide

g. dexamethasone

h. prednisone

42. The most significant side effect associated with aerosolized corticosteroids is _____. (Rau, p 65; Mathewson, p 634; Ziment, p 251)

43. Cromolyn sodium is used _____. (Rau, p 120; Mathewson, p 634; Kacmarek, pp 531–532)

44. The mode of action of cromolyn sodium is: (Kacmarek, pp 531–532; Ziment, p 276; Becker, p 190)

_____

_____

_____

45. Hazards associated with inhalation of cromolyn sodium are: (Ziment, p 276; Kacmarek, pp 531–532; Becker, p 190)

a. _____

b. _____

c. _____

d. _____

46. There are four classes of drugs used in the treatment of coughs and colds. List these classes and next to each class list it's use. (Rau, p 138; Ziment, pp 287–339)

a. _____

b. _____

c. _____

d. _____

47. Match the representative drug(s) in each category used for the treatment of coughs and colds. (Ziment, pp 287–339; Rau, pp 138–145)

_____ sympathomimetic

_____ antihistamine

_____ expectorant

_____ antitussive

    a. Benadryl
    b. Neo-Synephrine
    c. SSKI
    d. Vistaril
    e. Sudafed
    f. dextromethorphan
    g. Phenergan
    h. guaifenesin
    i. Afrin
    j. Chlor-Trimeton
    k. codeine
    l. Seldane
    m. Bisolvon
    n. hydrocodone

48. Prostaglandins affect the lung by their ability to alter smooth muscle tone. Next to each prostaglandin indicate its effect on bronchial smooth muscle. (Rau, p 277; Ziment, pp 125–128)

a. prostaglandin E: _____

b. prostaglandin F: _____

49. List the clinical situations associated with prostaglandin release. (Rau, pp 278–279; Ziment, pp 125–128)

a. _____

b. _____

c. _____

d. _____

e. _____

50. Differentiate between bacterial and bacteriostatic. (Taber's, pp 171–172; Kacmarek, p 580)

_____

_____

51. Match each major pathogen encountered by the respiratory care practitioner with its classification. (Kacmarek, pp 567–578; Ziment, p 341)

_____ *Pneumocystis carinii*

_____ *Haemophilus influenzae*

_____ respiratory syncytial virus

_____ *Streptococcus*

_____ tuberculosis

_____ *Bacteroides*

_____ *Staphylococcus aureus*

_____ *Klebsiella pneumoniae*

_____ *parainfluenza*

a. gram-positive bacteria

b. gram-negative bacteria

c. anaerobic bacteria

d. mycoplasma and viruses

e. mycobacteria

f. fungi

g. parasite (protozoa)

_____ *Histoplasma capsulatum*

_____ *Toxoplasma gondii*

_____ *Pseudomonas aeruginosa*

_____ *Candida*

_____ *Escherichia coli*

_____ *Proteus*

52. Next to each mode of action list the classes/groups of antibiotics that inhibit or kill microorganisms. (Rau, p 184; Ziment, p 253; Becker, p 164)

  a. inhibition of cell wall synthesis: _____

  b. inhibition of cell membrane function: _____

  c. inhibition of protein synthesis: _____

  _____

  d. inhibition of nucleic acid synthesis: _____

  e. inhibition of intermediary metabolism: _____

53. Define nosocomial infection. (Kacmarek, p 566; Taber's, p 1136)

  _____

54. Evidence suggests that aerosolized antimicrobials may not be the best route of antibiotic administration. There is clinical evidence that inhalation of antibiotic therapy may be associated with potential hazards. List the potential hazards of aerosolized antibiotics. (Ziment, pp 342–343; Rau, p 198)

  a. _____

  b. _____

  c. _____

  d. _____

55. Describe a superinfection. (Becker, p 165; Ziment, p 342; Taber's, p 1657)

  _____

  _____

56. Match the representative drug in column A to the category in which it is found in column B. (Rau, pp 187–195; Ziment, pp 354–383; Becker, pp 166–174)

Column A	Column B
_____ Keflin	a. Penicillin
_____ tetracycline	b. cephalosporin
_____ penicillin V	c. aminoglycoside
_____ streptomycin	d. tetracycline
_____ Gantrisin	e. sulfonamide
_____ Vibramycin	f. chloramphenicol
_____ isoniazid	g. polymyxin

Column A (cont.)

_____ Chloromycetin

_____ Nystatin

_____ gentamicin

_____ ampicillin

_____ Terramycin

_____ Keflex

_____ Gantanol

_____ amoxicillin

_____ bacitracin

_____ kanamycin

_____ amphotericin B

_____ carbenicillin

_____ erythromycin

_____ rifampin

_____ polymyxin B

Column B (cont.)

h. macrolide

i. antifungal

j. antituberculin

57. Pharmacologic agents can change the rate, force, and rhythm of the heart. Next to each, list the effect on the heart. (Becker, p 76; Kacmarek, p 152; Taber's, pp 330, 492, 851)

   a. inotropic: _____

   b. chronotropic: _____

   c. dromotropic: _____

58. Patients who are experiencing congestive heart failure would most likely benefit from what type of cardiovascular drug? (Kacmarek, p 554; Becker, p 76)

   _____

59. Ischemic heart disease is an inadequacy of coronary blood flow to the myocardium. What agent(s) may be used to treat such patients? (Becker, p 80; Barnes, p 547; Mathewson, pp 532–542)

   _____

60. Dysrhythmia is a general term describing an abnormal rate or rhythm in the myocardium. Antidysrhythmic drugs are classified into four major categories based on their primary mechanism of action. List the drug(s) that affect the myocardium by: (Becker, p 82; Kacmarek, pp 555–557; Mathewson, pp 504–526)

   a. blocking inward flow of Na^+ (anesthetic): _____

   b. blocking cardiac beta$_1$ receptors: _____

   c. prolonging duration of action potential lengthening refractory time: _____

   d. blocking inward flow of Ca^+: _____

61. In some instances cardiovascular drugs are used to increase blood pressure. These are called vasoconstricting agents. An example of this type of drug would be _____. (Mathewson, p 1350; Rau, p 260; Barnes, p 547)

62. Listed below are various pharmacologic mechanisms for reducing hypertension. Give an example of an antihypertensive drug(s) next to each mechanism. (Becker, p 85; Mathewson, pp 477–495)

    a. direct relaxation of blood vessels: _____

    b. alpha sympathetic blocker: _____

    c. depression of vasomotor center: _____

    d. autonomic ganglionic blocker: _____

    e. interfere with neurotransmitter release: _____

63. Give two examples of a drug that would be used as an anticoagulant. (Becker, p 85; Rau, pp 261–263; Mathewson, pp 581–591)

    a. _____

    b. _____

64. A drug used to counteract the effect of Coumadin would be _____
    _____. (Becker, p 89; Mathewson, pp 588–590)

65. Any substance that increases urine flow—and specifically those agents whose therapeutic purpose is to cause net loss of H_2O from the body—is called a _____
    _____. (Rau, p 264; Mathewson, pp 676–678)

66. Many diuretics cause the loss of which electrolyte(s)? (Rau, pp 270–272; Mathewson, pp 678–686)

    _____

67. Give an example of a diuretic used in the treatment of pulmonary edema. (Rau, pp 270–272; Kacmarek, pp 319, 547–549)

    _____

68. Clinically the use of barbiturates include: (Rau, p 220; Kacmarek, p 551; Becker, p 105)

    _____

69. A drug used primarily to relieve pain is called an _____.
    (Becker, pp 121–122; Kacmarek, p 549)

70. For the following drugs used for pain relief, indicate which is/are narcotic and which is/are non-narcotic? (Becker, pp 123–129; Kacmarek, pp 549–550; Mathewson, pp 229–254)

    a. aspirin: _____

    b. morphine: _____

    c. Demerol: _____

    d. acetaminophen: _____

    e. Ibuprofen: _____

    f. Stadol: _____

    g. Dilaudid: _____

    h. Fentanyl: _____

71. From the list in question 70, which drug(s) can be used to reduce elevated body temperature (pyrexia)? (Rau, p 236; Mathewson, pp 229–231, 248; Becker, p 123)

    _____

72. Drugs that cause central nervous system stimulation with secondary respiratory center activation are termed _____. (Rau, p 238; Ziment, p 388)

73. A drug that can reverse the effects of a narcotic is termed _____ . (Rau, p 235; Mathewson, p 254; Barnes, p 248)

    An example is _____ .

74. Valium is used for: (Rau, p 224; Mathewson, pp 366–369; Zimet, p 411)

    a. _____

    b. _____

    c. _____

75. Differentiate between a nondepolarizing and a depolarizing neuromuscular blocking agent. Give an example of each. (Rau, pp 203–204; Mathewson, p 271; Becker, pp 37–39)

    _____

    _____

    _____

    _____

76. What is the antidote to succinylcholine? (Rau, p 204; Mathewson, p 271; Becker, pp 37–39)

    _____

77. What is the antidote to Pavulon? (Rau, p 203; Mathewson, p 271; Becker, pp 37–39)

    _____

78. A 1:100 solution means _____ . (Rau, p 43; Kacmarek, pp 4–5)

79. How many milligrams of active ingredient are there in 10 cc of a 1:100 solution of Bronkosol? (Rau, p 44; Kacmarek, pp 4–5)

    _____

    _____

    _____

    _____

    _____

80. How much 30 percent Mucomyst is needed to prepare 3 cc of 10 percent Mucomyst solution? (Rau, p 45; Kacmarek, pp 6–7)

    _____

    _____

    _____

    _____

    _____

ANSWERS TO STUDY QUESTIONS

1. g, t, i, f, c, q, u, p, n, b, d, s, r, a, h, l, e, k, m, j, o

2. United States Pharmacopoeia, Physician's Desk Reference, National formulary, hospital formulary, druggist

3. a. structurally specific — drug will attach to a specific receptor (e.g., nicotine, opium)
   b. structurally nonspecific — drug penetrates cell, accumulates in cell membrane, or reacts biophysically to elicit a response (e.g., anaesthetic drug)

4. a. absorption
   b. distribution
   c. metabolism
   d. excretion

5. a. insulin, thyroid medication, heparin
   b. atropine, morphine, digitalis
   c. copper sulfate, magnesium sulfate, mineral supplements
   d. sodium bicarbonate, synthetic drugs

6. a. oral
   b. parenteral (IV, IM, subcutaneous)
   c. topical
   d. inhalation

7. f, e, g, b, d, a, c

8. adverse reactions

9. anaphylaxis

10. a. somatic nervous system
    b. autonomic nervous system

11. a. parasympathetic
    b. sympathetic

12. parasympathetic — day-to-day functions, digestion, bladder, bowel, mucous secretion, decreased heart rate, bronchoconstriction
    sympathetic — alarm system, "fight or flight," increased heart rate, increased blood pressure, bronchodilation

13. b, c, a, d

14. a. alpha
    b. beta$_1$
    c. beta$_2$

15. receptor — release of adenylcyclase; changes ATP to cyclic 3'5 AMP; causes bronchodilation

16. increased cardiac output, tachycardia, arrhythmias

17. a. bronchoconstriction
    b. edema of mucous membranes
    c. cardiac stimulation

18. mucosal vasoconstriction, uterine contraction, intestinal relaxation, arteriole vasoconstriction

19. a. tachycardia
    b. palpitations
    c. tremors
    d. headache
    e. nausea/vomiting
    f. tachyphylaxis

20. c, h, a, e, b, g, f, d

21. muscarinic antagonist or parasympatholytic

22. a. atropine
    b. Ipratopium (Atrovent)

23. bronchodilator enhancement, preoperatively for drying secretions, reversal of bradycardia, pupil dilation

24. inhibit phosphodiesterase; *note*: mechanism questionable, may also be the result of prostaglandin inhibition or decrease in histamine release

25. a. cerebral stimulation
    b. pulmonary vasodilation
    c. skeletal muscle stimulation
    d. smooth muscle relaxation
    e. coronary vasodilation
    f. cardiac stimulation
    g. diuresis

26. theophylline, aminophylline

27. a. no effect
    b. therapeutic range
    c. nausea
    d. cardiac dysrhythmias
    e. seizures and/or coma and death

28. a. water (95 percent)
    b. mucin (glycoproteins or mucoproteins)

29. a. sol layer (lower)
    b. gel layer (upper)

30. healthy cilia, adequate volume of secretions within normal limits, and adequate cough mechanism

31. a. increase depth of sol layer
    b. alter consistency of gel layer
    c. decrease adhesiveness of gel layer
    d. improve ciliary activity

32. a. H_2O, saline
    b. $NaHCO_3$, ethanol
    c. SSKI, hypertonic saline
    d. Mucomyst, mucolytic enzymes
    e. sympathomimetics, xanthines
    f. sympathomimetics, xanthines

33. a. anti-inflammatory
    b. immunosuppression

34. a. adrenal medulla
    b. adrenal cortex

35. adrenal cortex, adrenal medulla

36. a. glucose metabolism, anti-inflammatory, immunologic suppression
    b. water and electrolyte balance

37. a. asthma
    b. emphysema
    c. adult respiratory distress syndrome
    d. sarcoidosis
    e. allergic alveolitis

38. moonface, buffalo hump, thin extremities, weight gain, hirsutism, fragile skin, bruising, osteoporosis, hypertension, hyperglycemia, sodium retension, water retension, mood changes, and so on

39. psychologic—euphoric effects, decrease everyday aches and pains
    physiologic—suppression of adrenal gland (similar to that of Addison's disease)

40. gradually

41. d, g, b, f, a, c, h, e

42. candidiasis on the gums and in the mouth

43. prophylactically as an antiasthmatic agent

44. to inhibit the degranulation of the mast cell during type I antigen-antibody reaction, thereby preventing the release of histamine and heparin

45. dryness and irritation of the mouth and throat, cough and bronchospasm, nasal congestion

46. a. decongestant
    b. reduce (dry) secretions
    c. increase mucous clearance
    d. suppress cough reflex

47. sympathomimetic: b, e, i; antihistamine: a, d, g, j, l; expectorant: c, h, m; antitussive: f, k, n

48. a. relaxation
    b. contraction

49. a. anaphylaxis
    b. mechanical stimulation
    c. hyperventilation
    d. pulmonary embolism
    e. pulmonary edema

50. bactericidal—kills bacteria during logarithmic phase
    bacteriostatic—inhibits the replication of microorganisms

51. g, b, d, a, e, c, a, b, d, f, g, b, f, b, b

52. a. penicillins, cephalosporins
    b. antifungal, polymixins
    c. aminoglycosides, chloramphenicols, tetracyclines, macrolides
    d. antituberculin
    e. sulfonamides

53. an infection acquired within the hospital

54. a. bronchospasm
    b. systemic side effects
    c. opportunistic bacteria
    d. sensitivity to antibiotic

55. appearance of a new infection with different strains or species during prolonged administration of antimicrobial therapy

56. b, d, a, c, e, d, j, f, i, c, a, d, b, e, a, g, c, i, a, h, j, g

57. a. myocardial contractility
    b. myocardial rate
    c. conduction of electrical impulse

58. digitalis preparation

59. nitrates (e.g., Isordil, Nitro-Bid, Procardia)

60. a. lidocaine, Quinidine, Procainamide (Pronestyl)
    b. propranolol (Inderal)
    c. bretylium
    d. verapamil

61. dopamine (Intropin), levarterenol (Levophed), metaraminol (Aramine)

62. a. hydralazine (Apresoline), nitroprusside (Nipride), minoxidil
    b. phentalamine, prazosin (Minipress)
    c. methydopa (Aldomet), clonidine (Catapres)
    d. mecamylamine (Inversine)
    e. reserpine (Serpasil)

63. a. heparin
    b. coumadin

64. vitamin K

65. a diuretic

66. K^+, Cl^-, and Na^+

67. Lasix, Diuril

68. sedation, sleep, anticonvulsant, anesthesia

69. analgesic

70. a. non-narcotic
    b. narcotic
    c. narcotic
    d. non-narcotic
    e. non-narcotic
    f. narcotic
    g. narcotic
    h. narcotic

71. aspirin and acetaminophen

72. analeptics

73. narcotic antagonist, Narcan

74. a. antianxiety
    b. muscle relaxation
    c. sedation

75. nondepolarizing—competetive antagonist to acetylcholine not allowing the muscle to con-

tract (e.g., Pavulon, Curare)
depolarizing—muscle depolarizes and is then maintained in this refractory state (e.g., succinylcholine)

76. There is none.

77. Tensilon, Prostigmin

78. 1 gram per 100 milliliters

79. $1:100 = 0.1\% = 0.001$
ingredient $= (x)$ gram/amount of solution

$$.001 = \frac{(x)\ gram}{10\ cc}$$

$x = 0.001 \times 10\ cc$
$x = 0.01\ gram$

80. desired amount $=$
$$\frac{amount\ needed \times active\ ingredient}{total\ solution}$$
and
$$0.10 = \frac{x(0.30)}{3\ cc} =$$
$$x = \frac{3cc\ (0.10)}{0.30} =$$
$x = 1\ cc$

PRACTICE QUIZ

1. The neurotransmitter at the myoneural junction is:
   a. cholinesterase
   b. acetylcholine
   c. adentylcyclase
   d. phosphodiesterase
   e. norepinephrine

2. The correct order of these routes of drug administration, beginning with the fastest and ending with the slowest, is:
   I. Intramuscular
   II. Inhalation
   III. Intravenous
   IV. Oral
   V. Topical or "applied to the skin"
   a. III, I, II, IV, V
   b. II, III, I, IV, V
   c. I, III, II, V, IV
   d. III, II, IV, I, V
   e. III, II, I, IV, V

3. Sympathomimetics:
   I. Are specific in action.
   II. Increase the production of cyclic 3'5 AMP.

III. Decrease the production of cyclic 3'5 AMP.

IV. Are nonspecific in action.
  a. I only
  b. II and IV
  c. III and IV
  d. I and II
  e. I and III

4. Which of the physiologic responses is a beta$_1$ effect?
  a. bronchodilation
  b. increased heart rate
  c. central nervous system depressant
  d. decreased myocardial contractility
  e. increase in venous tone

5. Which of the following is an adrenergic drug?
  a. acetylcholine
  b. racemic epinephrine
  c. atropine
  d. water
  e. normal saline

6. Of the following solutions, which will produce aerosol particles that tend to increase in size as it deposits in the airway?
  a. hypotonic saline
  b. hypertonic saline
  c. isotonic saline
  d. metatonic saline
  e. hygrotonic saline

7. Which of the following would *not* be a mechanism for reducing the viscosity of mucous?
  a. hydration
  b. proteolytic enzymes
  c. rupture of disulfide bonds
  d. bronchomucotropic agents
  e. parasympathetic blocking agents

8. The enzyme responsible for converting cyclic 3'5 GMP to the inactive 5' GMP in smooth muscle cells is:
  a. adenylcyclase
  b. phosphodiesterase
  c. acetylcholinesterase
  d. cholinesterase
  e. monoamine oxidase

9. In which of the following patient situations would theophylline administration be contraindicated?
    I. Unstable blood pressure
    II. Glaucoma
    III. Peptic ulcers
    IV. Patient 34 years old with status asthmaticus
    V. Intestinal virus causing nausea and vomiting
  a. I, II, III, IV
  b. II, III, IV, V
  c. I, III, IV, V
  d. I, II, III, V
  e. I, II, III, IV, V

10. Which steroid is best administered by inhalation?
    a. hydrocortisone
    b. beclomethasone
    c. methylprednisone
    d. triamcinolone
    e. prednisone

11. A 1:2000 solution contains how many milligrams per milliter?
    a. 0.1 mg/ml
    b. 0.2 mg/ml
    c. 0.5 mg/ml
    d. 1.0 mg/ml
    e. 5.0 mg/ml

12. Cromolyn sodium:
    I. Is used for the treatment of an acute asthma attack.
    II. Is used for management of asthma prophylactically.
    III. Is used to treat atrioventricular block.
    IV. Interferes with mediator release from mast cells.
    a. I and II
    b. I, II, IV
    c. II and IV
    d. III only
    e. IV only

13. A respiratory care practitioner is assisting the physician in obtaining tissue specimens via bronchoscope, and the patient begins to bleed. The therapist should be prepared to instill which of the following?
    a. lidocaine
    b. penicillin
    c. metaproterenol
    d. epinephrine
    e. dexamethasone

14. Which of the following drugs would be considered an antagonist to isoproterenol?
    a. propranolol
    b. digitalis
    c. narcan
    d. levarterenol
    e. bretylium

15. Potential side effects of furosemide (Lasix) diuretic therapy would include:
    I. Pulmonary edema
    II. Hypokalemia
    III. Metabolic alkalosis
    IV. Increased chlorine reabsorption
    a. III and IV
    b. II and III
    c. I and IV
    d. II, III, IV
    e. I and II

16. A patient receiving continuous mechanical ventilation needs medication for pain. You would suggest:
    a. acetaminophen
    b. phenobarbital
    c. succinylcholine

d. morphine
e. Compazine

17. Which of the following would describe tachyphylaxis?
    a. Larger and larger doses are required to achieve a therapeutic effect.
    b. A response occurs that is opposite to the expected effects of the drug.
    c. A therapeutic effect from the drug cannot be achieved even with larger doses.
    d. The patient is unable to survive without the drug.
    e. The undesirable effect is observed during administration of the drug.

18. A patient has inspiratory stridor caused by edematous vocal cords. Which of the following agents may help relieve his/her obstruction?
    a. a beta$_1$ sympathomimetic
    b. a beta$_2$ sympathomimetic
    c. an alpha sympathomimetic
    d. a parasympathomimetic
    e. a sympatholytic

19. Two hours after isoetharine is administered to a patient with bronchospasm, his symptoms return. Which of the following agents would you recommend to his physician for future use?
    a. metaproterenol sulfate
    b. epinephrine
    c. phenylephrine
    d. racemic epinephrine
    e. isoproterenol HCl

20. A 1:200 solution of isoproterenol is needed for a mininebulizer treatment; 0.5 cc is mixed with 2 cc of normal saline. The final mixture will have what new dilution of isoproterenol?
    a. 1:800
    b. 1:1000
    c. 1:2000
    d. 1:400
    e. 1:900

ANSWERS TO THE PRACTICE QUIZ

1. b		11. c	
2. e		12. c	
3. d		13. d	
4. b		14. a	
5. b		15. b	
6. b		16. d	
7. e		17. a	
8. b		18. c	
9. d		19. a	
10. b		20. b	

MECHANICAL VENTILATION

OUTLINE

MA-1
Bourns Bear 1

Seimens Servo 900B
Seimens Servo 900C

LEARNING OBJECTIVES

Upon completion of this unit, the individual will:

1. Differentiate between negative and positive pressure ventilation.
2. Describe the following cycling mechanisms:
   a. pressure
   b. volume
   c. time
   d. flow
3. Differentiate between the single and double circuit.
4. Describe the various flow characteristics used in mechanical ventilation.
5. Describe the following ventilating modes.
   a. assist
   b. control
   c. assist-control
   d. intermittent mandatory ventilation
   e. synchronized intermittent mandatory ventilation
6. Define the following:
   a. PEEP
   b. CPAP
   c. CPPV
   d. EPAP
7. List indications for mechanical ventilation.
8. List the goals of mechanical ventilation.
9. Describe five steps of ventilator commitment.
10. Describe ventilatory parameters and oxygenation parameters indicative of the need for mechanical ventilation.
11. Discuss the hazards of mechanical ventilation.
12. Describe the goal of PEEP therapy.
13. List the benefits and hazards of PEEP therapy.
13. List the benefits and hazards of PEEP therapy.
14. List the indications of monitoring concerns of PEEP therapy.
15. Define optimal PEEP.
16. Discuss the difference between dynamic and static compliance.
17. Give ventilatory and oxygenation parameters indicative of the need for weaning from mechanical ventilation.
18. Describe three methods of ventilatory weaning.
19. Briefly discuss the Bennett MA-1 and MA-2 ventilators.
20. Briefly discuss the Siemens Servo 900 B and C.
21. Briefly discuss the Bourns Bear 2.

REFERENCES

Barnes, TA: Respiratory Care Practice. Year Book Medical Publishers, Chicago, 1988.

Burton, GG, and Hodgkin, JE: Respiratory Care, ed 2. JB Lippincott, Philadelphia, 1984.

Deshpande, VM, Pilbeam, SP, and Dixon, RJ: A Comprehensive Review in Respiratory Care. Appleton and Lange, Norwalk, CT, 1988.

Egan, DE, Spearman, CB, and Sheldon, RL: Egan's Fundamentals of Respiratory Therapy, ed 4. CV Mosby, St Louis, 1982.

McPherson, SP: Respiratory Therapy Equipment, ed 3. CV Mosby, St Louis, 1985.

Pilbeam, SP: Mechanical Ventilation: Physiological and Clinical Application. CV Mosby, St Louis, 1986.

Shapiro, BA, Harrison, RA, Kacmarek, RM, and Cane, RD: Clinical Application of Respiratory Care, ed 3. Year Book Medical Publishers, Chicago, 1985.

STUDY QUESTIONS

1. Differentiate between a negative pressure ventilator and a positive pressure ventilator. (Burton, p 556; Pilbeam, p 5)

   _____

   _____

   _____

   _____

   _____

   _____

2. What is a cycling mechanism? (Burton, p 563; Shapiro, p 380)

   _____

   _____

3. Define the following: (Burton, p 561; Shapiro, p 380; Pilbeam, p 85)

   a. pressure-cycled: _____

   _____

   b. volume-cycled: _____

   _____

   c. flow-cycled: _____

   _____

   d. time-cycled: _____

   _____

4. Differentiate between a single and a double circuit. (Pilbeam, p 67)

   _____

   _____

   _____

   _____

5. Describe each of the following: (Burton, p 560; Pilbeam, p 78)

   a. square or constant flow: _____

   _____

   b. sine wave: _____

   _____

   c. accelerating flow: _____

   _____

   d. decelerating flow: _____

   _____

6. Describe the following ventilatory modes: (Burton, p 565; Pilbeam, p 27)

    a. control: _____

    _____

    b. assist: _____

    _____

    c. assist-control: _____

    _____

    d. intermittent mandatory ventilation: _____

    _____

    e. synchronized intermittent mandatory ventilation: _____

    _____

7. List five methods used as the power sources for mechanical ventilators. (Pilbeam, p 65)

    a. _____

    b. _____

    c. _____

    d. _____

    e. _____

8. Define the following: (Pilbeam, p 30; Shapiro, p 408)

    a. positive end-expiratory pressure: _____

    _____

    b. continuous positive airway pressure: _____

    _____

    c. continuous positive pressure ventilation: _____

    _____

    d. expiratory positive airway pressure: _____

    _____

9. List four indications for mechanical ventilation. (Burton, p 566; Shapiro, p 367)

    a. _____

    b. _____

    c. _____

    d. _____

10. List four clinical goals of mechanical ventilation. (Barnes, p 217; Deshpande, p 338; Pilbeam, p 46)

    a. _____

    b. _____

    c. _____

    d. _____

11. Give five steps of mechanical ventilation commitment. (Pilbeam, p 118; Shapiro, p 369)

    a. _____

    b. _____

    c. _____

    d. _____

    e. _____

12. List six hazards associated with mechanical ventilation. (Barnes, p 218; Pilbeam, p 127)

    a. _____

    b. _____

    c. _____

    d. _____

    e. _____

    f. _____

13. Complete the following with the normal adult value and the value indicative of the need for mechanical ventilation. (Deshpande, p 338)

	Normal	Critical
VT ml/kg		
VC ml/kg		
RR f/min		
$\dot{V}_E$ l/min		
NIF cm H_2O		

14. List the arterial blood gas results that would indicate a need for ventilatory support in the non-COPD patient. (Deshpande, p 338; Shapiro, p 367)

    pH: _____

    Pa_{CO_2}: _____

    Pa_{O_2}: _____

15. Give the normal range and the value that would indicate a need for mechanical ventilation. (Pilbeam, p 44)

	Normal	Critical
V_D/V_T		
$P(A-a)D_{O_2}$ 100% mmHg		
$\dot{Q}S/\dot{Q}T\%$		
$Pa_{O_2}/PA_{O_2}\%$		

16. Give the calculations that allow for determination of initial ventilator settings. (Deshpande, p 339)

    a. minute ventilation: _____

    b. tidal volume: _____

    c. ideal body weight: _____

d. tubing compliance: _____

e. frequency: _____

17. What is the goal of PEEP? (Pilbeam)

_____

18. List four benefits of PEEP therapy. (Pilbeam, p 229; Shapiro, p 425)

a. _____

b. _____

c. _____

d. _____

19. List four cardiac complications of PEEP therapy. (Pilbeam, p 242; Shapiro, p 433)

a. _____

b. _____

c. _____

d. _____

20. List four renal complications of PEEP therapy. (Deshpande, p 347; Pilbeam, p 245)

a. _____

b. _____

c. _____

d. _____

21. Define optimal or best PEEP. (Pilbeam, p 229; Shapiro, p 429)

_____

_____

22. List four clinical indications for the use of PEEP or CPAP. (Pilbeam, p 222; Deshpande, p 347)

a. _____

b. _____

c. _____

d. _____

23. PEEP should be changed in increments of _____. (Pilbeam, p 231)

24. What should be monitored during PEEP therapy? (Pilbeam, p 233)

a. _____   f. _____

b. _____   g. _____

c. _____   h. _____

d. _____   i. _____

e. _____   j. _____

25. Define the following: (Pilbeam, p 174; Deshpande, p 344)

   a. peak pressure: _____

   _____

   b. plateau pressure: _____

   _____

26. What is static compliance? (Pilbeam, p 175)

   _____

   _____

   _____

   _____

27. What is dynamic compliance? (Pilbeam, p 175)

   _____

   _____

   _____

   _____

28. List the accepted value for beginning weaning from mechanical ventilation. (Deshpande, p 353; Pilbeam, p 286)

   VC: _____

   $\dot{V}_E$: _____

   VT: _____

   NIF: _____

   V_D/V_T: _____

   RR: _____

   CsT: _____

   shunt: _____

   $P(A-a)D_{O_2}$: _____

29. List five other variables that should be monitored prior to attempting to wean. (Deshpande, p 353; Pilbeam, p 286)

   a. _____

   b. _____

   c. _____

   d. _____

   e. _____

30. List three methods of ventilator weaning. (Deshpande, p 353; Shapiro, p 377; Pilbeam, p 285)

   a. _____

   b. _____

   c. _____

31. Describe each of the weaning methods listed in question 30. (Pilbeam, p 285; Shapiro, p 377)

    a. _____
    _____

    b. _____
    _____

    c. _____
    _____

32. Complete the following information about the Bennett MA-1: (Barnes, p 446; Pilbeam, p351)

    a. primarily _____ cycled, _____ cycled
    when preset limit pressure is met

    b. _____ and _____ powered

    c. ventilator rate determined by setting the _____ control

    d. oxygen alarm visual green: _____

    e. oxygen alarm visual red: _____

33. Complete the following information about the Bear 1: (McPherson, p 491; Pilbeam, p 349)

    a. _____ powered and _____ controlled

    b. pressurized _____ source required

    c. compressed air may be supplied _____ or
    _____ to the ventilator

    d. a valve incorporated in the inspiratory line allows _____
    _____

34. Complete the following information about the Siemens Servo ventilator 900B: (McPherson, p 469; Pilbeam, p 357)

    a. _____ powered and _____ controlled

    b. can be _____ or _____ cycled on A/C

    c. Which three controls are of great importance in the functioning?

    _____

    _____

    _____

    d. To set a rate of IMV 8 per minute the following settings can be used:

    rate setting = _____   IMV switch = divide by _____

    _____   _____

    _____   _____

35. Complete the following information about the Siemens Servo ventilator 900C. (McPherson, p 481)

    a. spontaneous ventilation can also be partially aided mechanically during a mode called _____
    _____

b. _____ circuit and _____ flow generator

c. tidal volume result of a preset _____

and _____

d. inspiratory time percent preset as a _____

of _____

ANSWERS TO STUDY QUESTIONS

1. The negative pressure ventilation involves extrathoracic pressures being applied to the patient. The difference between the partial pressure of the atmosphere and the lungs causes movement into the chest. It is noninvasive, durable, and easy to use. The positive pressure ventilation provides a positive intrapulmonary pressure to the lung. The pressure is above atmospheric.

2. It is the mechanism in the mechanical ventilator unit that terminates inspiration.

3. a. pressure-cycled: inspiration is terminated when a preset pressure is reached.
   b. volume-cycled: inspiration is terminated when a preset volume has been delivered.
   c. flow-cycled: inspiration is terminated when a gas flow decreases to a critical level
   d. time-cycled: inspiration is terminated when a preset inspiratory time is concluded

4. In the single circuit it is the gas volume that powers the ventilator and goes to the patient; only one pressurized gas volume is used. In the double circuit, one gas is used to power the ventilator and to operate another mechanism that delivers a second gas source to the patient.

5. a. square or constant flow: flow is constant throughout the inspiratory phase, no changes for patient's lung character
   b. sine wave: flow gradually builds to a peak flow at midinspiration and tapers down
   c. accelerating flow: progressive increase of flow until a set limit is reached
   d. decelerating flow: flow peaks at start of inspiration and tapers down until end inspiration

6. a. control: ventilation is completely controlled for depth and frequency, not sensitive to patient effort.
   b. assist: a pressure volume is delivered in response only to a negative pressure initiated by the patient
   c. assist-control: frequency and depth are set at a minimum; patient may go above rate but has no ability to influence volume or minimum rate
   d. IMV: controlled rate combined with spontaneous breathing
   e. SIMV: assist-control type mode that allows for spontaneous ventilation between breaths and allows synchronous breath with control breath

7. a. electric
   b. fluidic
   c. pneumatic
   d. electronic microprocessor
   e. pneumatic and electric

8. a. pressure on the airway above ambient at the end of exhalation
   b. PEEP is applied during inspiration and exhalation in a spontaneously breathing patient.
   c. the patient is receiving full ventilatory support and PEEP
   d. PEEP applied to spontaneously breathing patient where inspiration airway pressures need to go below atmospheric for inspiration to occur

9. a. apnea
   b. acute respiratory failure
   c. impending respiratory failure
   d. oxygenation
   e. muscle failure or impending fatigue

10. a. ventilation
    b. decrease myocardial work
    c. decrease the work of breathing
    d. improve gas distribution

11. a. establish airway and manually ventilate
    b. ensure cardiovascular stabilization

c. establish appropriate monitors and baseline values

b. establish ventilatory pattern

e. connect patient to ventilator

12. a. barotrauma
    b. adverse effects to circulation
    c. ADH syndrome
    d. infection
    e. hyperventilation
    f. increased intracranial pressure

13. V_T = 5 to 8 (normal), <5 (critical)
    VC = 65 to 75, 15
    RR = 12 to 20, >35
    $\dot{V}_E$ = 5 to 6, <10
    NIF = −75 to −100, −20 to −25

14. pH = <7.25 to 7.29
    Pa_{CO_2} = >55 mmHg
    Pa_{O_2} = <70 mmHg

15. V_D/V_T = 30 to 40, >60
    $P(A-a)D_{O_2}$ 100% = 25 to 65, >450
    QS/QT = 5%, 20% to 30%
    Pa_{O_2}/Pa_{O_2} = 75, <15

16. a. $\dot{V}_E$ = (males)   4 × BSA;   (females)
       3.5 × BSA
    b. V_T = 10 to 15 ml/kg of ideal body weight + tubing compliance volume loss
    c. IBW = (males) 106 + 6 (ht in inches − 60); females = 105 + 5 (ht in inches − 60)
    d. tubing compliance volume loss = peak pressure × 3 ml/cm H_2O
    e. frequency = $\dot{V}_E/V_T$

17. to improve oxygenation to the tissues

18. a. increase FRC
    b. increase compliance
    c. increase Pa_{O_2}
    d. decrease intrapulmonary shunt

19. a. decrease cardiac output (C.O.)
    b. decrease venous return
    c. arrhythmias
    d. altered cardiovascular function

20. a. decreased circulating ADH levels
    b. reduced renal perfusion
    c. redistributed renal perfusion
    d. decreased urine output

21. the PEEP level that produces the maximum oxygenation and lung compliance with the minimum of side effects

22. a. ARDS
    b. IRDS
    c. cardiogenic pulmonary edema
    d. bilateral diffuse pneumonia

23. 3 to 5 cm H_2O

24. a. blood pressure
    b. breath sounds
    c. patient appearance
    d. peak and plateau pressures
    e. RR
    f. V_T
    g. minute ventilation
    h. hemodynamics
    i. compliance
    j. Ca_{O_2}.
    k. QS / QT
    l. ABG
    m. $C(A-v)D_{O_2}$
    n. $P(A-a)D_{O_2}$
    o. cardiac output

25. a. peak pressure: the highest pressure reached on the inspiratory phase
    b. plateau pressure: pressure obtained during inflation hold maneuver when there is no gas movement

26. Compliance is a change in volume per unit of pressure change. Static compliance is made up of chest wall and lung compliance.

$$N = \frac{70 \text{ ml}}{\text{cm } H_2O} \qquad Cs = \frac{Vt}{\text{Plat P} - \text{PEEP}}$$

27. a compliance measurement that correlates well with changes in recoil of thoracic cage and airway resistance

$$N = \frac{50 \text{ to } 100 \text{ ml}}{\text{cm } H_2O}$$

28. $\dot{V}_C$ = <15 ml/kg
    $\dot{V}_E$ = <10 l/min
    V_T = 3 × BW in kg
    NIF = >−20
    V_D/V_T = <60%
    RR = <25/min
    CsT = >0.25 shunt + <15%
    $P(A-a)D_{O_2}$ = <300 to 350 on 100%

29. a. level of consciousness if possible
    b. drive to breathe
    c. cardiac stability
    d. airway secretions
    e. nutritional status

30. a. traditional assist-control
    b. IMV/SIMV methods
    c. discontinuance

31. a. traditional: T piece used 3 to 5 minutes of every 30 min and increased as tolerated
    b. IMV/SIMV methods: IMV rate gradually reduced, monitored with gases and cardiovascular status
    e. discontinuance: patient taken off and placed on T piece to go on trial basis

32. a. volume, pressure
    b. pneumatically, and electrically
    c. cycle rate
    d. supply pressured and in use
    e. loss of pressure source

33. a. pneumatically, electronically
    b. oxygen

c. internally, externally
d. patient the ability to breathe spontaneously through the ventilator.

34. a. pneumatically, electronically
    b. patient, time
    c. minute volume, inspiratory time percent, rate
    d. rate setting to 16 and divide by 2; then 40 and 5; then 80 and 10

35. a. pressure support
    b. single, square
    c. minute volume, frequency
    d. percent, total cycle time

PRACTICE QUIZ

1. An advantage to the tank-type negative pressure ventilator is that:
   a. cardiovascular system is not adversely affected
   b. nursing care is easily administered
   c. an artificial airway is not required
   d. reduced chance of barotrauma
   e. the patient is very accessible

2. When determining how a ventilator is cycled, one must consider:
   a. what begins inspiration
   b. what terminates inspiration
   c. what ends exhalation
   d. alarm systems
   e. power sources

3. Which of the following is/are indications for mechanical ventilation?
       I. Apnea
      II. Acute respiratory alkalosis
     III. Impending respiratory failure
      IV. Acute respiratory failure
       V. Oxygenation
   a. I, II, III, IV, V
   b. I, III, IV, V
   c. I, II, III, IV
   d. II, IV
   e. I only

4. Continuous mechanical ventilation may result in which of the following?
   a. increased mean intrathoracic pressure
   b. decreased mean intrathoracic pressure
   c. decreased pleural pressure
   d. enhanced venous return
   e. increased cardiac output

5. Complications of ventilator care include:
       I. Infection

    II. Stress ulcers
    III. Subcutaneous emphysema
    IV. Barotrauma
    V. Renal dysfunction
  a. I, II, III, IV, V
  b. I, III, IV
  c. II, III, IV
  d. I, IV, V
  e. III and V

6. CPAP:
    I. Increases FRC
    II. Impeded venous return
    III. Decreases cardiac output
    IV. Is used only in controlled ventilation
    V. Improves oxygenation
  a. I, II, III, IV, V
  b. I, II, III
  c. I, IV, V
  d. I, II, III, V
  e. I, II, IV

7. A patient who is being mechanically ventilated has a decrease in urine output, although his renal function, electrolyte balance, and hydration are normal. With respect to the ventilator, which of the following is responsible?
  a. pressure
  b. flow
  c. oxygen concentration
  d. tidal volume
  e. frequency

8. On a volume-cycled ventilator, an increase in airway resistance will:
  a. increase the rate
  b. increase the volume
  c. alter the humidity
  d. shut off the pressure alarm
  e. increase peak airway pressure

9. The oxygen alarm light on the MA-1 will change from green to red when:
  a. there is a drop in FIO_2 delivered
  b. the line connected to compressed air disconnects
  c. there is a drop in oxygen source pressure
  d. the analyzer is disconnected
  e. none of the above

10. On the Bear II ventilator, if only the compressor is functional, what FIO_2 would you be delivering?
  a. 1.0
  b. 0.6
  c. 0.4
  d. 0.3
  e. 0.21

11. On the Bear I ventilator, whenever the patient initiates a breath while in the SIMV mode, which of the following inspiratory source indicator lights up?
  a. assist
  b. sigh

    c. apnea
    d. nonsequence
    e. spontaneous

12. Which of the following conditions would be a minimum requirement to begin weaning from mechanical ventilation?
    a. NIF greater than 20 cm H_2O and VC of 3 ml/kg
    b. NIF greater than 40 cm H_2O and VC of 3 ml/kg
    c. NIF greater than 30 cm H_2O and VC of 7 ml/kg
    d. NIF greater than 20 cm H_2O and VC of 15 ml/kg
    e. NIF greater than 15 cm H_2O and VC of 15 ml/kg

13. Which of the following formulas is used to monitor the static compliance?
    a. $\dfrac{\text{tidal volume}}{\text{plateau pressure} - \text{end expiratory pressure}}$
    b. $\dfrac{\text{tidal volume}}{\text{peak pressure}}$
    c. $\dfrac{\text{peak pressure}}{\text{plateau pressure}}$
    d. $\dfrac{\text{peak pressure}}{\text{tidal volume}}$
    e. none of the above

14. Tests of a patient's capabilities that indicate readiness for weaning include which of the following?
    I. $P(A-a)DO_2$ less than 300 torr at FIO_2 of 1.0
    II. VC greater than 15 ml/kg
    III. NIF greater than −15
    IV. VD/VT greater than 30 percent
    V. Shunt less than 45%
    a. I, II, III, IV, V
    b. I, III, IV
    c. I and II
    d. III and IV
    e. II only

15. The ventilator mode that allows the patient to breathe spontaneously and also receive augmented intermittent positive pressure ventilation that is not in phase with the patient's own breathing is?
    a. control
    b. assist
    c. assist-control
    d. IMV
    e. SIMV

16. Which of the following measurements would be most helpful to evaluate the effects of PEEP on cardiovascular system?
    a. cardiac output
    b. blood pressure
    c. PaO_2
    d. $P(A-a)DO_2$
    e. a and b

17. When considering ventilator discontinuance, the first parameter to be reviewed is:
    a. reversal of pathophysiology that necessitated it
    b. PaO_2
    c. oxygen percent in use

  d. PEEP levels in use
  e. sensorium

18. Choose the goals of mechanical ventilation.
  a. oxygenation
  b. infection level decrease
  c. increase cardiac function
  d. increased distribution of ventilation
  e. a and d

19. Choose the most common complications of PEEP therapy.
  I. decrease cardiac output (CO)
  II. decrease renal perfusion
  III. decrease venous return
  IV. reduced cardiovascular function
  V. decrease in circulating ADH
  a. I, II, III, IV, V
  b. I, III, IV
  c. I, III, IV
  d. II, IV, V
  e. I only

20. The simplest noninvasive monitor of the effects of PEEP is:
  a. CO
  b. RR
  c. BP
  d. HR
  e. FVC

ANSWERS TO THE PRACTICE QUIZ

1. d		11. e	
2. b		12. d	
3. b		13. a	
4. a		14. c	
5. a		15. d	
6. d		16. e	
7. a		17. a	
8. e		18. e	
9. c		19. a	
10. e		20. c	

Chapter 20

NEONATES AND PEDIATRICS

Outline

LEARNING OBJECTIVES

Upon completion of this unit, the individual will:

1. Indicate approximately when the fetal lung starts to develop.
2. Describe the four stages of fetal lung development.
d. Describe the function of the placenta.
4. Explain the importance of the L/S ratio in lung development.
5. Describe fetal circulation.
6. List the stimuli necessary to initiate respiration.
7. Describe the mechanisms responsible for changes in fetal circulation.
8. Explain APGAR scoring.
9. Explain the Silverman-Anderson scoring system.
10. List the approximate tidal volumes and respiratory rates for a newborn and a child.
11. Explain assessment methods for the fetus.
12. Explain the importance of thermoregulation in the neonate.
13. List the five common signs and symptoms associated with respiratory distress syndrome in a newborn.
14. List the methods used to monitor an infant's cardiopulmonary status.
15. Differentiate between periodic breathing and apnea.
16. Explain the following congenital heart defects.
    a. patent ductus arteriosus
    b. transposition of the great vessels
    c. ventricular septal defects
    d. coarctation of the aorta
    e. tetralogy of Fallot
    f. total anomalous pulmonary venous return
17. Describe the following diseases, or syndromes:
    a. respiratory distress syndrome
    b. bronchopulmonary dysplasia
    c. retrolental fibroplasia
    d. meconium aspiration
    e. cystic fibrosis
    f. AIDS
    g. congenital diaphragmatic hernia
    h. respiratory syncytial virus
    i. epiglottitis
    j. bronchiolitis
    k. croup
    l. SIDS
18. Describe the following therapies:
    a. oxygen therapy
    b. aerosol therapy
    c. isolettes
    d. CPAP
    e. high-frequency ventilation
    f. endotracheal tubes
    g. transillumination
    h. arterial blood gas analysis
    i. extracorporeal membrane oxygenator

REFERENCES

Aloan, CA: Respiratory Care of the Newborn. JB Lippincott, Philadelphia, 1987

Blodgett, D: Manual of Pediatric Respiratory Care Procedures. JB Lippincott, Philadelphia, 1982

Burton, G, and Hodgkin, J: Respiratory Care: A Guide to Clinical Practice, ed 2. JB Lippincott, Philadelphia, 1984.

Kacmarek, RM, Mack, CW, and Dimas, S: The Essentials of Respiratory Therapy, ed 2. Year Book Medical Publishers, Chicago, 1985.

Karones, SB: High-Risk Newborn Infants, ed 3. CV Mosby, St Louis, 1981.

Koff, PB, Eitzman, DV, and Neu, J: Neonatal and Pediatric Respiratory Care. CV Mosby, St Louis, 1988.

Lough, MD, Doershuk, CF, and Stern, RC: Pediatric Respiratory Therapy, ed 3. Year Book Medical Publishers, Chicago, 1985.

Merenstein, GB, and Gardner, SL: Handbook of Neonatal Intensive Care. CV Mosby, St Louis, 1985.

Philip, AGS: Neonatology: A Practical Approach, ed 3. WB Saunders, Philadelphia, 1987.

STUDY QUESTIONS

1. Lung development begins at approximately _____. (Kacmarek, p 166; Lough, p 4)

2. Match the phase of fetal lung development. (Lough, p 5; Koff, pp 4–5)

   _____ canalicular

   _____ pseudoglandular

   _____ alveolar

   _____ embryonic

   a. lung bud (0 to 5 weeks)

   b. capillary network; Type I and II cells; (16 to 26 weeks)

   c. dicotomous branching; (6 to 16 weeks)

   d. saccular and alveolar formation; (27 to 40 weeks)

3. The ratio of lecithin to sphingomyelin to support extrauterine life is _____.

   (Lough, pp 16–17; Kacmarek, pp 166–167)

4. During intrauterine life, gas exchange, nutrient exchange, and waste elimination are accomplished by the _____. (Kacmarek, p 167; Karones, pp 1–4)

5. Lung fluid is approximately equal to the _____. (Karones, p 200; Kacmarek, p 167)

6. Fetal circulation differs from the adult circulation in three major ways. What are they, and what is their purpose? (Kacmarek, p 169; Lough, pp 20–21)

   a. _____

   b. _____

   c. _____

7. List the stimuli necessary to initiate and maintain respiration. (Kacmarek, p 170; Lough, p 18; Karones, pp 196–200)

   a. _____

   b. _____

   c. _____

   d. _____

   e. _____

   f. _____

   g. _____

8. What are the mechanisms responsible for changes in fetal circulation after birth, and how are these changes accomplished? (Kacmarek, p 169; Lough, p 21; Karones, pp 202–205)

   _____

   _____

   _____

9. What system is used to evaluate the neonate in the delivery room? When is this system used? (Karones, pp 68–72; Merenstein, pp 35–42)

   _____

10. The evaluation system in question 9 is based on what criteria? (Koff, p 31; Karones, pp 68–72; Merenstein, pp 35–42)

11. What scoring system is used to assess the respiratory system? What criteria are used? (Kacmarek, p 172; Koff, p 31)

12. List the approximate respiratory rates for the following ages: (Kacmarek, p 173; Blodgett, p 226)

    a. neonate: _____

    b. 1 year old: _____

    c. 5 years old: _____

    d. 10 years old: _____

13. What is the average tidal volume of an infant? of a child? (Kacmarek, p 175; Koff, p 291)

14. What are the methods by which the fetus can be assessed in utero? (Koff, pp 28–30; Philip, pp 3–7)

15. Discuss the importance of thermoregulation in the neonate and how this concept applies to respiratory care. (Aloan, pp 98–106; Merenstein, pp 85–96)

16. List the five common signs that relate to an infant with respiratory distress in varing degrees. (Aloan, p 56; Merenstein, pp 306–308)

    a. _____

    b. _____

    c. _____

    d. _____

    e. _____

17. List the methods utilized to monitor an infant for cardiopulmonary status. (Aloan, pp 62–67, 84–94; Koff, pp 260–280; Philip, pp 381–383)

    a. _____   e. _____

    b. _____   f. _____

    c. _____   g. _____

    d. _____   h. _____

18. Differentiate between periodic breathing and apnea. (Aloan, pp 120–121; Merenstein, pp 336–339)

_____

_____

_____

19. Discuss the etiology, clinical presentation, radiographic pattern, treatment(s), and complications of treatment for infant respiratory distress syndrome. (Philip, pp 113–119; Merenstein, pp 330–332)

_____

_____

_____

_____

_____

_____

_____

_____

_____

_____

_____

_____

_____

_____

20. What is a common cardiovascular defect associated with both prematurity and respiratory distress syndrome? How is this defect treated? (Koff, pp 148, 155; Karones, pp 234–237)

_____

_____

_____

21. List the defects that describe tetralogy of Fallot. (Koff, pp 144–145; Merenstein, pp 364–365)

a. _____

b. _____

c. _____

d. _____

22. Explain the following cardiovascular heart defects: (Merenstein, pp 353–372; Koff, pp 144–156)

a. complete transposition of the great vessels: _____

_____

b. coarctation of the aorta: _____

_____

c. ventricular septal defect: _____

d. anomalous pulmonary venous return: _____

23. Discuss the theory behind bronchopulmonary dysplasia. (Merenstein, pp 327–329; Koff, pp 73–76)

24. Describe meconium aspiration syndrome in terms of etiology, clinical presentation, treatment, and prevention. (Aloan, pp 145–151; Merenstein, pp 333–334)

25. Discuss the etiology, pathophysiology, and diagnosis of cystic fibrosis. (Koff, pp 86–87; Lough, pp 99–102)

26. How does AIDS relate to neonatal and pediatric respiratory infections? (Koff, pp 85–86)

27. Describe the clinical presentation, radiographic pattern, and treatment for congenital diaphragmatic hernia. (Aloan, pp 197–199; Merenstein, pp 377–378; Philip, pp 95–98)

28. The most common lower respiratory tract viral pathogen causing bronchiolitis is _____ _____, and it can be treated with _____. (Koff, p 83; Lough, pp 94–95)

29. Define epiglottitis. How is this diagnosed? What is the treatment? (Koff, p 100–102; Lough, pp 84–85)

_____
_____
_____
_____
_____
_____

30. Another name for croup is _____. (Lough, p 86; Koff, pp 102–103)

31. The mainstay of therapy for croup is _____. (Lough, p 86; Koff, pp 102–103)

32. Define/discuss SIDS. (Koff, p 159)

_____
_____
_____

33. When administering aerosol therapy on an infant, what monitoring procedure is utilized to prevent fluid overload? (Koff, p 202)

_____

34. How is oxygen delivered in small infants and neonates? (Koff, p 202; Lough, p 130)

_____

35. Isolettes are used in the neonate to control: (Lough, pp 127–128; Koff, p 205)

   a. _____
   b. _____
   c. _____

36. What toxic effect (eyes) can occur by excessive use of oxygen in a preterm infant? (Merenstein, pp 329–330; Koff, p 200; Aloan, pp 214–215)

_____

37. List the situations in which continuous positive airway pressure may be indicated in infants and children. (Koff, p 226; Merenstein, pp 310–311; Lough, pp 56–58)

   a. _____
   b. _____
   c. _____

d. _____

e. _____

f. _____

38. List the five methods used to deliver CPAP. (Koff, p 238; Aloan, pp 222–229)

a. _____

b. _____

c. _____

d. _____

e. _____

39. Why is it not necessary for an endotracheal tube to have a cuff for a child under 8 years of age? (Koff, p 247; Aloan, pp 295–297)

_____

_____

40. Define high-frequency ventilation. (Lough, p 186; Koff, pp 333–334; Aloan, pp 268–269)

_____

_____

41. Indicate the normal range for arterial blood gas analysis for newborn and pediatric patients. (Koff, p 261; Aloan, p 67)

	Newborn	**Pediatric**
pH	_____	_____
$Paco_2$	_____	_____
Pao_2	_____	_____
HCO_3	_____	_____

42. Besides the use of chest radiology for emergency diagnostic testing, what other method can be employed to determine a pneumomediastinum or pneumothorax in an infant? (Philip, p 393; Blodgett, pp 193–194)

_____

43. When conventional ventilation is not adequate, such as in infants with pulmonary hypertension syndromes due to meconium aspiration syndrome or diaphragmatic hernias, extracorporeal membrane oxygenation can be used. Describe this alternative method of ventilation in treating these infants. (Koff, pp 337–339)

_____

_____

_____

_____

ANSWERS TO STUDY QUESTIONS

1. 26 to 28 days, or 4 weeks

2. b, c, d, a

3. 2/1

4. placenta

5. FRC

6. a. foramen ovale: connects the right atrium to the left atrium, which bypasses lungs
   b. ductus arteriosus: connects the pulmonary artery to the aorta, which bypasses lungs
   c. ductus venosis: bypasses immature liver to inferior vena cava

7. a. temperature change
   b. bright lights
   c. hypoxemia
   d. acidemia
   e. hypercapnia
   f. intrathoracic pressure
   g. clamping of cord

8. clamping of cord: increase systemic vascular resistance
   ventilation: increase arterial oxygenation, which decreases pulmonary vascular resistance and constricts ductus arteriosus

9. APGAR, 1 and 5 minutes of life

10. heart rate, respiratory rate, muscle tone, reflex irritability, color

11. Silverman-Anderson index based on five areas: upper chest movement, lower chest movement, xiphoid retractions, dilation of nares, expiratory grunt; Score 0 to 2 in each category; lower score is better

12. a. 30 to 50 min
    b. 24 to 30 min
    c. 20 to 25 min
    d. 16 to 20 min

13. 6 to 8 ml/kg, 10 to 12 ml/kg

14. ultrasound, amniocentesis, fetal heart rate monitor

15. A baby not maintained in a neutral thermal environment poses problems with energy that affect oxygen consumption; in order to maintain their body temperature these infants must metabolize brown fat, which requires the oxygen. Much of respiratory therapy influences heat gain or loss (humidity and aerosol therapy, CPAP, mechanical ventilation, and so on)

16. a. tachypnea
    b. cyanosis
    c. nasal flaring
    d. expiratory grunt
    e. retractions

17. a. apnea monitor
    b. transcutaneous monitor–oxygen and carbon dioxide
    c. capillary samples
    d. umbilical arterial line
    e. peripheral arterial puncture
    f. cardiac monitor
    g. pulse oximetry
    h. capnography

18. periodic breathing: appears in premature infants; apnea for 5 to 10 sec; tachypnea; heart rate, color, and temperature do not change
    apnea: no breathing for longer than 20 sec; bradycardia, and cyanosis

19. *etiology*: prematurity, decreased surfactant or insufficient amounts
    presentation: immediately or shortly thereafter nasal flaring, intercostal and substernal retractions, tachypnea, tachycardia, grunting
    Infants get worse, resulting in atelectasis, hypoxia, V/Q mismatch, increased WOB, hypercarbia, hypoxemia, acidosis, increased pulmonary vascular resistance, right to left shunting, and the formation of hyaline membrane
    x-ray: diffuse bilateral reticulogranular pattern (ground-glass appearance), air bronchograms
    Rx: maintain oxygen, pH with O_2 therapy; may have to use CPAP or mechanical ventilation; constant monitoring, adequate hydration, and neutral thermal environment
    complications: pnemothorax, pneumomediastinum, oxygen toxicity, bronchopulmonary dysplasia

20. patent ductus arteriosus
    treatment: prostaglandin inhibitor (indomethacin), if treatment does not resolve surgical ligation

21. a. ventricular septal defect
    b. over-riding aorta
    c. pulmonary aorta
    d. right ventricular hypertrophy

22. a. aorta originates from right ventrical and pulmonary artery originates from left ventrical
    b. constriction of aorta in region of the ductus arteriosus

c. left to right shunting causing blood to be shunted from left ventrical to right ventrical; associated with many congenital heart defects

d. failure of pulmonary veins to enter the left atrium

23. influenced by the amount and time of use with oxygen therapy and positive pressure

24. *etiology*: term infant who had experienced asphyxia at some point in pregnancy, causing the fetus to pass meconium into the amniotic fluid
presentation: tachypnea, retractions, nasal flaring, cyanosis, low APGAR scores, gradually gets worse
x-ray: decreased aeration, hyperlucency, pneumothorax, irregular densities
therapy and prevention; suctioning after head is delivered, intubation postdelivery, postural drainage, O_2 therapy, resolves in approximately 72 hours

25. caused by a recessive gene and diagnosed by a sweat chloride test; dysfunction of exocrine glands; altercation of viscosity of mucus
respiratory therapy includes antibiotics, CPT, bronchodilator therapy, nutrition, and oxygen therapy

26. pneumocystic carinii, failure to thrive, recurrent bacterial infections, x-ray of interstitial pulmonary infiltrates, cytomegalovirus

27. *etiology*: failure of diaphragm to close properly, causing the intestines to herniate into the left side of the thorax
presentation: respiratory distress, barrel chest, scaphoid abdomen, decreased breath sounds on affected side of chest
x-ray: bowel in chest; shift of the mediastinum to the unaffected side
Rx: surgery; slowly reinflate the collapsed lung

28. respiratory syncytial virus, ribovirin

29. *etiology*: bacterial infection (usually *Haemophilus influenzae*) of the tissues above the glottis, including the epiglottis
diagnosis: febrile, difficulty swallowing, drooling, and lateral neck x-ray
therapy: establish artificial airway (intubation in surgery), antibiotic racemic epinephrine nebulizer therapy

30. laryngotracheobronchitis

31. cool, humidified air (large particles)

32. leading cause of death in infants between 1 and 12 months, peak time is between 1 and 3 months, winter season, illness (viral) associated with SIDS a week before death

33. daily weight

34. oxyhood

35. a. temp
b. humidity
c. filter gas

36. retrolental fibroplasia or retinopathy of prematurity (ROP)

37. a. RDS
b. pneumonia
c. aspiration syndromes
d. apnea
e. bronchiolitis
f. Reye's syndrome

38. a. head chamber
b. face mask
c. ET tube
d. nasopharyngeal tube
e. nasal prongs

39. anatomic difference and the narrowest portion of the child's airway is the cricoid cartilage

40. a. frequency above 150/min used to generate lower volumes, which in turn generate lower airway and intrathoracic pressure; decreasing barotrauma.

41. newborn: pH: 7.34 to 7.42; $PaCO_2$: 32 to 41; PaO_2: 62 to 92; HCO_3 19 to 23
pediatric: pH: 7.35 to 7.45; $PaCO_2$: 35 to 45; PaO_2 80 to 100; HCO_3: 22 to 26

42. transilluminator

43. chronic heart-lung bypass: cannulating a large artery (carotid) and a large vein (interior jugular); blood pumped through membrane oxygenator where ventilation occurs; lungs are ventilated with low pressures and IMV to prevent atelectasis

---

PRACTICE QUIZ

1. Which of the following is/are true about the developing airway?
    I. Formation starts about the 26th to 28th day of life.
    II. The left mainstem bronchus develops at a greater angle than the right mainstem bronchus.

III. There are 30 levels of branching.

IV. Branching of the bronchi continues until the age of 8 years.
- a. I, IV
- b. I, II, III
- c. I only
- d. I, II, III, IV
- e. II, III, IV

2. Surfactant:

I. Appears about the 22nd to 24th week of life

II. Causes alveolar collapse if a deficiency exists.

III. Originates from maternal serum

IV. Maintains stability of the alveoli by lowering the surface tension

V. Is composed of dipalmitoyl lecithin
- a. I, II, III, IV
- b. I, II, III, V
- c. I, II, IV, V
- d. II, III, IV, V
- e. I, III, IV, V

3. Signs and symptoms of meconium aspiration syndrome might include:

I. Low APGAR scores

II. Hypoxemia

III. Bradypnea

IV. Nasal flaring

V. Hyperinflation of the lung on x-ray
- a. I, II, III, IV
- b. I, II, III, V
- c. I, II, IV, V
- d. II, III, IV, V
- e. I, III, IV, V

4. Management of a neonate with meconium aspiration syndrome include:

I. Ventilation with bag and mask immediately after birth

II. Postural drainage

III. Antibiotics

IV. Heated aerosol with oxygen

V. Suction trachea before delivery
- a. I, II, III, IV
- b. I, II, III, V
- c. I, III, IV, V
- d. II, III, IV, V
- e. I, II, III, IV, V

5. Stimulation for the neonates first breath is caused by:

I. Stimulation of the carotid and aortic baroreceptors

II. Decrease in the neonates skin temperature

III. Hypercarbia

IV. Hypoxia

V. Stimulation of the sympathetic nervous system
- a. I, II, III, IV
- b. II, III, IV, V
- c. I, III, IV, V
- d. I, IV, V
- e. I, II, III, IV, V

6. Which of the following is/are not indications for CPAP?
   I. Obstructive sleep apnea
   II. Hyaline membrane disease
   III. Aspiration pneumonitis
   IV. SIDS
   a. I and II
   b. II and IV
   c. I, II, IV
   d. I, II, III
   e. IV only

7. An infant delivered by cesarean section at 26 weeks of gestation has nasal flaring, retractions, and expiratory grunting. A ground-glass appearance is seen on chest radiograph. On the basis of this information, the infant's difficulty probably is the result of:
   a. prenatal hypoxia
   b. hyaline membrane disease
   c. a congenital heart defect
   d. diaphragmatic hernia
   e. pulmonary edema

8. A newborn exhaling against a partially closed glottis creates a phenomenon known as:
   a. retractions
   b. tachypnea
   c. nasal flaring
   d. grunting
   e. inspiratory stridor

9. A 30-week gestation, 4500 g female infant born with a heart rate of 80/min, respiratory rate of 60/min, weak cry, some flexion of the extremities, and a grimace response to nasal suction. Her APGAR score is:
   a. 3
   b. 4
   c. 5
   d. 6
   e. 7

10. Complications of treatment of an infant on mechanical ventilation for respiratory distress syndrome may be:
    I. Pneumothorax
    II. Retrolental fibroplasia
    III. Pneumopericardium
    IV. Bronchopulmonary dysplasia
    V. Infection
    a. I, II, IV, V
    b. II and IV
    c. I, II, III, IV
    d. I, II, III, IV, V
    e. II, III, IV, V

CASE

A mother brings her 2-year-old son into the emergency room in severe respiratory distress. She tells you that his appetite has been poor and that he has been drooling. His distress was sudden and had inspiratory stridor, hoarseness, and fever. The child sits with his head tilted forward. Questions 11 and 12 pertain to this case.

11. The child most likely is suffering from:
    a. aspiration pneumonia
    b. epiglottis
    c. Reye's syndrome
    d. AIDS
    e. asthma

12. The most appropriate immediate respiratory therapy would be:
    a. perform direct laryngoscopy
    b. perform a tracheostomy
    c. administer a high concentration of oxygen
    d. administer ultrasonic nebulizer
    e. give IPPB therapy with Bronkosol

13. Patients with severe croup clinically present most often with:
    a. bilateral rhonchi
    b. diminished breath sounds
    c. expiratory wheezes
    d. inspiratory stridor
    e. normal breath sounds

14. What is the normal tidal volume for a pediatric patient weighing more than 10 kg?
    a. 3 to 4 ml/kg
    b. 5 to 6 ml/kg
    c. 6 to 7 ml/kg
    d. 8 to 10 ml/kg
    e. 10 to 12 ml/kg

15. Respiratory distress syndrome is characterized by:
    a. hyperinflation of lung
    b. mucus plugs
    c. atelectasis
    d. hemoptysis
    e. increased surfactant production

16. Definitive diagnosis of a child with cystic fibrosis is:
    a. sweat chloride test
    b. chest x-ray
    c. CBC
    d. spinal fluid sample
    e. sputum sample

17. In transcutaneous monitoring of an infant, all of the following will alter the accuracy of the reading, *except*:
    a. hypotension
    b. increase in body temperature
    c. decreased tissue perfusion
    d. increased skin thickness
    e. blister formation

18. In fetal circulation, which of the following vessels carries the highest level of oxygen?
    a. descending aorta
    b. pulmonary artery
    c. superior vena cava
    d. umbilical artery
    e. umbilical vein

19. Which of the following assessment(s) do/does not test for fetal maturity?
    I. L/S ratio
    II. Fetal heart rate monitor
    III. Ultrasound
    IV. Fetal blood sample
    a. I and II
    b. III and IV
    c. III only
    d. IV only
    e. II and IV

20. A full-term male infant was delivered vaginally after a 4-hour labor. His APGAR scores were 6 and 8, respectively. Approximately 8 hours after delivery the infant developed difficulty breathing. Upon physical examination the infant was cyanotic with a pulse of 60/min, BP of 40/0, and a respiratory rate of 10 bpm and gasping. Temperature was 95°F rectally, patient had a scaphoid abdomen, and assessment of breath sounds revealed no sound on the left side of the chest. ABGs revealed pH 7.06, $Paco_2$ 75 mmHg, Pao_2 30 mmHg, HCO_3 28 mEq/l, and O_2 saturation 65 percent. Radiography revealed heart and mediastinal structures markedly shifted to the right. The probable diagnosis is:
    a. T-E fistula
    b. esophageal atresia
    c. cytomegalovirus
    d. diaphragmatic hernia
    e. AIDS

ANSWERS TO PRACTICE QUIZ

1. c	11. b
2. c	12. c
3. c	13. d
4. d	14. e
5. e	15. c
6. e	16. a
7. b	17. b
8. d	18. e
9. a	19. e
10. d	20. d

Chapter 21

PULMONARY REHABILITATION AND HOME CARE

OUTLINE

INTRODUCTION
Major Goal
Assessment
Evaluation of Pulmonary Dysfunction
Patient History
Education
TECHNIQUES
Postural Drainage
Breathing Techniques
    Pursed-lip breathing
    Diaphragmatic breathing

Exercise
    Walking
    Stair-climbing
Cough
Nutrition
Therapeutic Modalities
Cleaning of Equipment
Medication
Respiratory Practitioner Role
PRACTICE QUIZ

LEARNING OBJECTIVES

Upon completion of this unit, the individual will:

1. State the major goal of a pulmonary rehabilitation program.
2. List the diagnostic methods used to determine pulmonary dysfunction.
3. List the factors that make up a patient history.
4. Explain the importance of educating the patients and their families.

5. List/describe the educational topics that should be part of the educational process.
6. Describe the technique of pulmonary drainage.
7. Explain/demonstrate pursed-lip breathing, diaphragmatic breathing, walking, stair-climbing, and coughing techniques.

8. List the goals of breathing excercises.
9. Explain the importance of nutrition in a pulmonary rehabilitation program.
10. List/explain the use of respiratory therapy equipment in the home care setting.
11. Describe the method used for cleaning respiratory therapy equipment at home.
12. Describe the use of a drug, given its classification.
13. Explain the role of the respiratory care practitioner in a pulmonary rehabilitation program.

REFERENCES

Burton, G, and Hodgkin, J: Respiratory Care: A Guide to Clinical Practice, ed 2. JB Lippincott, Philadelphia, 1984.

Eubanks, DH, and Bone, RC: Comprehensive Respiratory Care. CV Mosby, St Louis, 1985.

Frownfelter, DL: Chest Physical Therapy and Pulmonary Rehabilitation, ed 2. Year Book Medical Publishers, Chicago, 1987.

Kacmarek, RM, Mack, CW, and Dimas, S: The Essentials of Respiratory Therapy, ed 2. Year Book Medical Publishers, Chicago, 1985.

O'Ryan, JA, and Burns, DG: Pulmonary Rehabilitation: From Hospital to Home. Year Book Medical Publishers, Chicago, 1984.

Shapiro, BA, Harrison, RA, Kacmarek, RM, and Cane, RD. Clinical Application of Respiratory Care, ed 3. Year Book Medical Publishers, Chicago, 1985.

STUDY QUESTIONS

1. The overall goal of a pulmonary rehabilitation program is: (Frownfelter, pp 295–296; Eubanks, p 731)

   _____

2. Patients requiring pulmonary rehabilitation include: (Frownfelter, p 300; Eubanks, p 734)

   _____
   _____
   _____
   _____
   _____
   _____
   _____
   _____

3. What types of assessments must be made prior to admission into a pulmonary rehabilitation program? (Frownfelter, p 300)

   a. _____

   b. _____

   c. _____

4. What diagnostic methods are useful in determining pulmonary dysfunction? (O'Ryan, pp 32–44)

   _____

5. A good patient history should include: (Frownfelter, pp 153–161; O'Ryan, pp 47–49)

   a. _____   f. _____

   b. _____   g. _____

   c. _____   h. _____

   d. _____   i. _____

   e. _____   j. _____

6. Other than the pulmonary system, which of the major body systems should be evaluated? (O'Ryan, pp 49–50; Frownfelter, pp 301–303)

   a. _____   d. _____

   b. _____   e. _____

   c. _____

7. After a thorough evaluation of the patient, a program should be set up regarding: (Eubanks, pp 736–756)

   _____

   _____

   _____

8. Goals should be established between the patient and the rehabilitation term. However, these goals should be _____. (Frownfelter, pp 303–304; Eubanks, p 732)

9. Education is an important aspect of a pulmonary rehabilitation program. The respiratory care practitioner must educate both the _____ and his or her _____. (Frownfelter, p 306; Eubanks, pp 760–761)

10. List the educational topics that should be part of the educational process: (O'Ryan, pp 73–180; Eubanks, p 760; Frownfelter, pp 306–310)

    a. _____

    b. _____

    c. _____

    d. _____

    e. _____

    f. _____

    g. _____

    h. _____

    i. _____

11. Describe the technique of postural drainage for bronchial hygiene therapy. (Frownfelter, pp 271–282; Eubanks, p 26)

_____

_____

_____

_____

12. Postural drainage therapy should not last longer than _____ minutes. (Frownfelter, p 282; Eubanks, pp 460–470)

13. At what time of the day or evening should postural drainage be administered? (Frownfelter, p 282; Eubanks, pp 460–470)

_____

14. Regarding education on postural drainage techniques and aids should not be limited to the patient but extended to the _____ as well. (Frownfelter, p 282)

15. Patients should be aware of changes in their sputum to include: (Frownfelter, p 283; Eubanks, p 735)

   a. _____

   b. _____

   c. _____

16. What is the breathing technique pictured in Figure 21–1? (O'Ryan, p 67; Eubanks, p 224)

_____

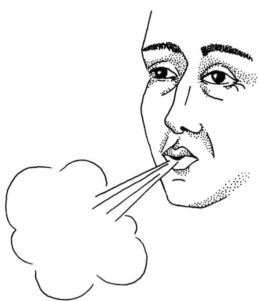

FIGURE 21–1.

17. What is the technique pictured in Figure 21–2? (O'Ryan, p 67; Eubanks, pp 752–755)

_____

18. List the goals of breathing exercises. (Frownfelter, pp 234–235; Eubanks, pp 746–752; O'Ryan, pp 64–81)

   a. _____

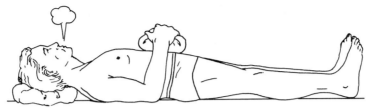

FIGURE 21–2.

b. _____

c. _____

d. _____

e. _____

f. _____

g. _____

19. Explain the technique for walking exercises pictured in Figure 21–3. (O'Ryan, pp 73–74; Frown-felter, p 242)

_____

_____

_____

_____

_____

_____

_____

_____

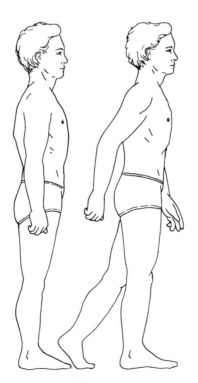

FIGURE 21–3.

20. Explain the technique for stair-climbing. (O'Ryan, pp 76–77; Eubanks, pp 749–752)

_____
_____
_____
_____
_____
_____

21. Describe the cough mechanism found in the sequence of pictures in Figures 21–4 through 21–7. (Frownfelter, p 261; Burton, pp 667–670)

    a. Fig. 21–4: _____
    b. Fig. 21–5: _____
    c. Fig. 21–6: _____
    d. Fig. 21–7: _____

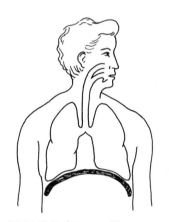

FIGURE 21–4. The cough

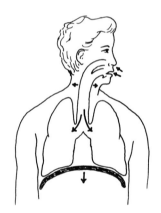

FIGURE 21–5. The cough

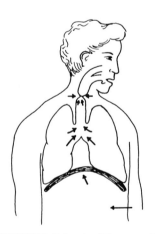

FIGURE 21–6. The cough

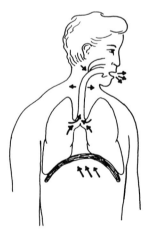

FIGURE 21–7. The cough

22. Pulmonary rehabilitation patients have a tendency to trap air. These patients will generally cough better with lower volumes and a less stressful technique. Discuss this technique known as pump or huff coughing. (Burton, p 671; Frownfelter, p 267)

23. Why are patients with chronic pulmonary disease frequently anorexic and underweight? (O'Ryan, pp 135–140; Frownfelter, pp 302, 307)

24. What information should be attained to assess the patient's nutritional needs? (Frownfelter, p 302; O'Ryan, pp 136–141)

25. How does good nutritional status relate to a patient who is on a pulmonary rehabilitation program? (Frownfelter, p 302; O'Ryan, pp 141–144)

26. Oxygen therapy is indicated in the home care setting if the PaO_2 is _____ mmHg on room air. (Frownfelter, p 314; O'Ryan, p 119)

27. Patients with chronic hypoxemia will benefit from oxygen therapy if the liter flow is run between _____, because a higher flowrate might diminish their hypoxic drive. (Frownfelter, p 314; O'Ryan, p 120)

28. What oxygen delivery systems can be utilized in the home care setting? (O'Ryan, pp 121–123; Eubanks, p 759)

    a. _____
    b. _____
    c. _____

29. Give the types of respiratory therapy services that can be used to aid a patient on a home care program. (Burton, p 683)

30. The cleaning of respiratory therapy equipment is extremely important. Explain the proper procedure for cleaning respiratory equipment in the home care setting. (Eubanks, p 760)

31. Match column A with column B. (Frownfelter, pp 308–310; Burton, pp 682–683)

Column A	**Column B**
_____ bronchodilator	a. reduce inflammation
_____ mucokinetic	b. reduce edema
_____ corticosteroids	c. prevent/treatment of infection
_____ antibiotic	d. reduce bronchospasm
_____ cardiovascular	e. strengthen contraction of heart
_____ diuretic	f. aid in expectoration

32. The roles of the respiratory care practitioner in the rehabilitation/home care program include: (Eubanks, p 759; O'Ryan, p 200)

_____

_____

_____

_____

_____

33. Visits to a patient receiving home care should be scheduled and evaluation procedure should be performed. What areas should be evaluated when a home care patient is visited? (Eubanks, p 758; O'Ryan, pp 230–232)

_____

_____

_____

_____

_____

_____

_____

ANSWERS TO STUDY QUESTIONS

1. to improve the quality of life and decrease cost to patient

2. a. neuromuscular diseases: e.g., myasthenia gravis, Guillain-Barré, amyotrophic lateral sclerosis
   b. chest wall deformities: e.g., kyphoscoliosis
   c. disorders of ventilatory drive, which may stimulate or depress drive: e.g., central nervous system disorders, Pickwickian syndrome
   d. pneumonocioses: occupational lung diseases
   e. chronic lung diseases: e.g., emphysema, chronic bronchitis, asthma, cystic fibrosis

3. a. personal medical history
   b. familial medical history
   c. motivational level

4. history, complete physical, laboratory data (e.g., CBC, hemoglobin), chest radiograph, pulmonary function test, exercise testing

5. a. presenting complaints
   b. symptoms
   c. smoking history
   d. family history
   e. environmental history
   f. occupational history
   g. personal history

h. past medical history, past surgical history
i. medications

6. a. nervous system
   b. cardiovascular system
   c. gastrointestinal system
   d. genitourinary system
   e. musculoskeletal system

7. patient condition: e.g., exercise tolerance, acceptance into a rehabilitation program
   planning a program to fit that patient's needs

8. realistic goals

9. a. patients, families

10. a. basic information about their disease
    b. respiratory anatomy and physiology (basic)
    c. pulmonary physiology
    d. bronchial hygiene
    e. environmental factors
    f. avoidance of infection
    g. fluid intake
    h. nutrition
    i. medication

11. positioning of the patient to allow gravity to drain secretions; can be done by patient (if family is participating other methods such as chest percussion and vibrations can also be accomplished)

12. 30 to 45 min

13. in the morning before breakfast, or 1 to $1\frac{1}{2}$ hours before bedtime

14. family or primary caregiver

15. a. amount
    b. consistancy
    c. color

16. pursed-lip breathing

17. diaphragmatic breathing

18. a. improve ventilation
    b. prevent atelectasis
    c. decrease work of breathing
    d. increase cough efficiency
    e. increase strength of respiratory muscles
    f. help patient to relax
    g. mobilize secretions and maintain chest mobility

19. use the basic principles of range of motion techniques combined with diaphragmatic pursed-lip breathing with each step

20. a. walk a premeasured distance
    b. take resting pulse

c. start off with left foot; patient walks at stride that he or she is comfortable with, counting out I:E ratios and using diaphragmatic pursed-lip breathing
d. rest when necessary

20. a. prior to stair-climbing, patient should be breathing rhythmically, using I:E ratios that will match climbing effort
    b. patient instructed to exhale while stepping up and to inhale when foot comes to rest on each step
    c. patient can stop and rest at any time while on stairs; pause between each step

21. a. deep inspiration
    b. closed glottis: building up of intrathoracic and intra-abdominal pressures
    c. open glottis
    d. rapid expulsion of air

22. three short easy coughs, followed by three huffs. This should be done a minimum of 3 to 4 times/day.

23. shortness of breath with a full stomach and requiring energy to eat and for the body to metabolize food; poor nutrition

24. look at eating habits, calories consumed, fluid intake, and identify dietary needs

25. maintenance of muscle metabolism for daily living and increases resistance to infection

26. less than or equal to 55 mmHg

27. 1 to 2 l/min

28. a. high-pressure cylinder ("H" or "E")
    b. liquid bulk oxygen system with portable system
    c. oxygen concentrator

29. IPPB, ultrasonic nebulizer, mini-nebulizer, metered dose inhaler, oxygen therapy, continuous aerosol therapy, bronchial hygiene, and mechanical ventilation

30. a. wash with mild detergent
    b. rinse
    c. soak in white distilled vinegar (two parts vinegar, three parts distilled water) for 20 minutes
    d. rinse
    e. drain
    f. let dry on a clean cloth or towel

31. d, f, a, c, e, b

32. a. assess pulmonary status and reduce deficient areas

b. evaluate and monitor equipment, use, care, and provide corrective measures and reinforcement (encouragement)
c. breathing training and exercise
d. summary of visit to be sent to physician

33. a. vital signs
b. overall assessment
c. oxygen usage
d. check all equipment
e. instruction
f. cleaning procedure

PRACTICE QUIZ

1. Which of the following problems associated with chronic obstructive lung disease presents the greatest burden to society?
   a. poor personal hygiene
   b. increase number of hospital admissions
   c. sexual dysfunction
   d. severe dyspnea
   e. decreased activity

2. When assessing sputum, the clinician should consider all of the following, *except*:
   a. color
   b. amount
   c. consistency
   d. salt content
   e. none of the above

3. Personal history should include which of the following?
   a. use of tobacco
   b. drinking habits
   c. sleeping habits
   d. eating habits
   e. all of the above

4. Which of the following may be covered in the education program?
       I. Energy conservation tips
      II. Oxygen therapy
     III. Care and cleaning of equipment
      IV. Good nutrition
   a. I and II
   b. II and III
   c. II only
   d. II, III, IV
   e. I, II, III, IV

5. Which of the following should *not* be considered when evaluating dyspnea?
   a. duration and degree
   b. association with body position
   c. style of clothing
   d. precipitation and relieving factors
   e. none of the above

6. Cough can be inhibited by:
       I. Excessive secretions
      II. Impairment of musculature force
     III. Decreased volumes and flow rates

IV. Dynamic airway collapse
a. II, III, IV
b. I, III, IV
c. III and IV
d. II and IV
e. I, II, III, IV

7. Which of the following is the major goal of a comprehensive pulmonary rehabilitation program?
   a. improve the patient's activities of daily living
   b. decrease the cost of the patient's medication
   c. reverse the patient's disease
   d. promise the patient he or she can return to work at the same job
   e. help the patient save money to pay the hospital bill

8. As a respiratory care practitioner, your role in the rehabilitation program should include:
   I. Assist in delivering therapy
   II. Education
   III. Order medication for therapy
   IV. Chest assessment
   V. Evaluation of home situation
   a. I, III, IV, V
   b. I, II, III, IV, V
   c. II, III, V
   d. I, II, IV, V
   e. III, IV, V

9. A method of determining pulmonary dysfunction include all of the following except:
   a. pulmonary function studies
   b. patient interview
   c. chest radiograph
   d. laboratory data
   e. physical examination

10. The education aspect of pulmonary rehabilitation program should:
    a. be on a 12th grade level
    b. be generalized to all patients
    c. be directed to the patient alone
    d. give the patient some magazines to read
    e. none of the above

11. Studies have shown that physical endurance in COPD patients:
    a. will continue to decrease throughout the course of the disease
    b. can be increased by graded exercises
    c. can be increased by graded exercises only with the use of supplemental oxygen
    d. will increase as sexual activity increases
    e. will remain the same throughout regardless of exercise

12. Exercise programs are designed to:
    a. lower Pa_{CO_2}
    b. raise heart rate
    c. lower $\dot{V}$ max
    d. raise $\dot{V}$ max
    e. raise Pa_{O_2}

13. Exercise consists of which elements?
    I. Duration

    II. Frequency
   III. Distance
   IV. Intensity
  a. I and IV
  b. I, III, IV
  c. II, III, IV
  d. I, II, IV
  e. I, II, III, IV

14. Pursed lip breathing is primarily intended for the patient with:
  a. trauma
  b. neurologic deficits
  c. pneumothoraces
  d. all patients who are tachypneic
  e. bronchiolar collapse

15. A chronic hypercapnic patient is being given oxygen at home at 2 LPM via nasal cannula. The patient is instructed not to set the flow rate any higher, because:
  a. a faster flow is not beneficial
  b. nasal cannulas do not function at flow rates above 2 LPM
  c. hyperoxia may occur leading to lung disease
  d. the oxygen will replace the carbon dioxide
  e. excessive oxygen is dangerous and may depress breathing

16. A COPD patient sits on the edge of the bed, leaning over a bedside table using his accessory muscles at a rate of 32 breaths per minute. This breathing pattern is called:
  a. tachypnea
  b. eupnea
  c. apnea
  d. bradypnea
  e. dyspnea

17. To assess and report the effectiveness of chest physical therapy, the respiratory care practitioner should evaluate which of the following?
    I. Amount of mucous production
   II. Breath sounds
   III. Chest radiograph
   IV. Pulmonary function testing
  a. I only
  b. I, II, III
  c. I and III
  d. I, III, IV
  e. II, III, IV

18. You are instructing a patient in the cleaning of his home care equipment. You tell him to wash, rinse, and dry his equipment, and once a day to soak his equipment in vinegar solution. In doing this, he will be:
    I. Sterilizing his equipment
   II. Retarding bacterial growth
   III. Killing all gram-negative organisms and spores
   IV. Sanitizing his equipment
  a. I and III
  b. II only
  c. I, II, III
  d. II and IV
  e. II, III, IV

19. A respiratory care practitioner is instructing a patient for a home care program. What signs of respiratory infection should the patient be taught to be aware of and learn to recognize?
     I. Changes in color, consistency, and amount of sputum
     II. Pulse increase of 20 percent over normal during exercise
     III. Cough changes
     IV. Persistent dyspnea at rest and with daily activities
    a. I and IV
    b. II and IV
    c. II, III, IV
    d. I, III, IV
    e. I, II, III, IV

20. Your rehabilitation patient informs you that his home has two flights of stairs that he must climb several times a day. You instruct him to:
    a. sell his house and move
    b. to breathe in rhythm with stair-climbing, with expiration covering at least twice as many steps as inspiration
    c. to breathe in rhythm with stair-climbing, with inspiration covering at least twice as many steps as expiration
    d. to take one step at a time, with a resting period at each step
    e. to stay on the bottom floor

ANSWERS TO PRACTICE QUIZ

1.	b	11.	b
2.	d	12.	d
3.	e	13.	d
4.	e	14.	e
5.	c	15.	e
6.	a	16.	a
7.	a	17.	b
8.	d	18.	d
9.	b	19.	d
10.	e	20.	b

UNIT 3

STUDY GUIDE
AND
EXAMINATIONS

$Chapter\ 22$

STUDY SCHEDULES

The following study schedules are based on an 8-week preparation period. The authors see this as a minimum of time needed for adequate preparation for the national examinations. An extension of the 8-week time period is recommended. These schedules allow a select amount of time for each chapter. This 3-day schedule may be adjusted as areas of weakness and strength become apparent. The general procedure for each chapter includes a first-day reference review, a second-day chapter completion, and the use of the practice quiz on the third day to assess the need for further study. Reference sources are varied and multiple for each chapter. No single reference provides all needed material to complete the workbook. The authors suggest the use of at least one comprehensive text, to be supplemented with other texts as needed.

SAMPLE STUDY SCHEDULE CRTT EXAMINATION

SUNDAY	MONDAY	TUESDAY	WEDNESDAY	THURSDAY	FRIDAY	SATURDAY
Chapter 1 Review References	Complete Chapter	Practice Quiz	Chapter 2 Review Reference	Complete Chapter	Practice Quiz	
Chapter 3	Complete Chapter	Practice Quiz	Chapter 4	Complete Chapter	Practice Quiz	
Chapter 5	Complete Chapter	Practice Quiz	Chapter 6	Complete Chapter	Practice Quiz	
Chapter 7	Complete Chapter	Practice Quiz	Chapter 8	Complete Chapter	Practice Quiz	
Chapter 9	Complete Chapter	Practice Quiz	Chapter 10	Complete Chapter	Practice Quiz	
Chapter 12	Complete Chapter	Practice Quiz	Chapter 13	Complete Chapter	Practice Quiz	
Chapter 14	Complete Chapter	Practice Quiz	Chapter 19	Complete Chapter	Practice Quiz	
Chapter 21	Complete Chapter	Practice Quiz	Review Pharmocology and all Calculations	Review	Relax	Exam

SAMPLE STUDY GUIDE FOR RRT EXAMINATION

SUNDAY	MONDAY	TUESDAY	WEDNESDAY	THURSDAY	FRIDAY	SATURDAY
Chapter 9 Review References	Complete Chapter	Take Practice Quiz	Chapter 11 Review References	Complete Chapter	Take Practice Quiz	
Chapter 12	Complete Chapter	Take Practice Quiz	Chapter 13 Review References	Complete Chapter	Take Practice Quiz	
Chapter 14 Review References	Complete Chapter	Take Practice Quiz	Chapter 15 Review References	Complete Chapter 15	Complete Chapter 15	Practice Quiz Chapter 15
Chapter 17 Review References	Complete Chapter 17	Complete Chapter 17	Take Practice Quiz Review Weaknesses Chap. 17	Chapter 18 Review Reference	Complete Chapter 18	Complete Chapter 18
Take Practice Quiz Chapter 18	Chapter 19 Review References	Complete Chapter 19	Complete Chapter 19	Practice Quiz Chapter 19		
Chapter 20 Review References	Complete Chapter 20	Complete Chapter 20	Practice Quiz Chapter 20	Chapter 21 Review Reference	Complete Chapter 21	Practice Quiz Chapter 21
Chapter 17 Review	Complete Chapter 17 Review Calculation	Complete Chapter 17	Practice Quiz Chapter 17	Take Practice Quiz on any area of concern	Review areas of concern	
Chapter 17 Review Calculation	Review Calculation	Review As Needed	Rest	Rest	Rest	Exam

Chapter 23

CRTT PRACTICE EXAMINATION

1. Convert 78°F to Celsius.
   a. 25.5 C
   b. 30°C
   c. 45.6°C
   d. 52°C
   e. 122°C

2. A man weighing 220 pounds has a weight in kilograms of:
   a. 44 kg
   b. 110 kg
   c. 100 kg
   d. 150 kg
   e. 220 kg

3. The absence of molecular motion and heat is termed:
   a. freezing
   b. Kelvin
   c. evaporation
   d. molecularization
   e. absolute zero

4. The term that describes the patient body position as lying horizontal and face down is:
   a. Fowler's
   b. Trendelenburg
   c. prone
   d. supine
   e. axel

5. The process of using the hands and sense of touch to detect physical signs of the patient's condition is known as:

    a. inspection
    b. observation
    c. palpation
    d. auscultation
    e. tactile fremitus

6. Which of the following is True about tactile fremitus?
    I. The patient should repeat the phrase "99."
    II. Areas of increased transmission are the only areas of concern.
    III. The hand should be pressed firmly on the chest.
    IV. The examiner should use fingertips only.
    V. It is often too painful for the patient.
    a. I, III, IV
    b. II, III, V
    c. I, II, III
    d. I and III
    e. I only

7. Which of the following comprises the sternum?
    a. the body
    b. the scapula
    c. the manubrium
    d. the xiphoid process
    e. a, c, and d

8. Which of the following is/are True about the ribs?
    I. there are 12 pairs of ribs
    II. there are 7 false ribs
    III. there are 3 true ribs
    IV. there are 7 true ribs
    V. there are 2 floating ribs
    a. I, II, III, V
    b. I, II, III
    c. I, IV, V
    d. II, IV, V
    e. I only

9. The pleural layer that lines the thoracic wall is termed the _____ pleura.
    a. parietal
    b. thoracic
    c. visceral
    d. pulmonary
    e. costal

10. The bifurcation of the trachea is termed?
    a. angle of Louis
    b. the carina
    c. the bifurcation angle
    d. the hilar region
    e. none of the above

11. Which of the following compose the respiratory unit?
    I. Alveoli
    II. Terminal bronchioles
    III. Respiratory bronchioles
    IV. The alveolar ducts and sacs

V. The subsegmental bronchioles
    a. I, III, IV, V
    b. II, III, V
    c. I, II, III
    d. I, III, IV
    e. I, II, III, IV, V

12. Choose the true statements about oxygen.
      I. Colorless, odorless, and tasteless
      II. Density of 1.43 g/l at zero celsius and 760 mmHg
      III. Boils at $-183°$ Celsius
      IV. Makes up 78.08 percent of Earth's atmosphere
      V. Atomic number is 10
    a. I, II, III
    b. II, III, IV
    c. II, IV, V
    d. III, IV, V
    e. I, II, III, IV, V

13. Which of the following is/are regulated by the ICC (DOT) with respect to cylinders?
    a. shipping
    b. filling
    c. marking
    d. labeling
    e. all of the above

14. The cylinder filled with helium should be color-coded:
    a. green
    b. brown
    c. orange
    d. white
    e. black

15. Which of the following are False about the general safe practices with oxygen?
      I. Petroleum-based products should not be used.
      II. Alcohol vapors might ignite in presence of high concentrations of oxygen.
      III. Oxygen will burn.
      IV. Oxygen administered in a croup tent needs no special precautions.
      V. Electrical toys and equipment are not safe in a croup tent.
    a. I, III, IV
    b. I, II, III
    c. I and II only
    d. III and IV only
    e. I, II, III, IV, V

16. The Pin locations for nitrous oxide are:
    a. 2 and 5
    b. 3 and 5
    c. 3 and 6
    d. 1 and 5
    e. none of the above

17. The oxygen safety system that functions to isolate floors or sections of a floor is termed:
    a. station outlet
    b. zone valve
    c. riser valve

    d. floor valve

    e. shut off main valve

18. Which of the following will affect the F_{IO_2} delivered with the usage of a low-flow oxygen delivery system?
       I. Respiratory rate
       II. Ventilatory pattern
       III. Equipment reservoir
       IV. Patient's anatomic reservoir
       V. Tidal volume
    a. I, II, V
    b. II, IV, V
    c. I, II, III
    d. I, II, IV, V
    e. I, II, III, IV, V

19. Your patient has been on a nasal cannula for 8 hours at an F_{IO_2} of 0.28; the patient exhibits a change rate and depth and pattern of breathing. The physician is adamant about the F_{IO_2}. What device can you suggest to better serve the patient's needs?
    a. Venturi mask
    b. nasal catheter
    c. simple mask
    d. nonrebreathing mask
    e. partial rebreathing mask

20. Given a large volume nebulizer, set at 0.40 F_{IO_2}, and driven by an oxygen flow rate of 15 LPM, what is the total flow to the patient?
    a. 40 LPM
    b. 45 LPM
    c. 50 LPM
    d. 63 LPM
    e. 75 LPM

21. The type of manual resuscitator using the spring disk is:
    a. the Ambu E-2
    b. the Laerdal
    c. the Hope II
    d. the Hope
    e. the PMR

22. Which of the following is/are a type of hyperbaric unit?
    a. fixed multiplate unit
    b. hyperbaric plate unit
    c. monoplate unit
    d. oxyplate unit
    e. a and b

23. The oxygen analyzers designed on the Pauling principle would be considered:
    a. paramagnetic
    b. thermoconductive
    c. electrochemical
    d. mass spectrometers
    e. none of the above

24. The cathode of the Clark electrode is commonly made of which material?
    a. platinum

b. silver
c. bronze
d. gold
e. lead

25. Which of the following incorporates gas analyzing principles?
    a. oximeters
    b. transcutaneous oxygen monitors
    c. high flow nebulizing unit
    d. oxyhood
    e. a and b

26. Which of the following is a hazard of aerosal therapy?
    I. Cross contamination
    II. Salt retention
    III. Swelling of hygroscopic sputum
    IV. Fluid overload
    V. Increased urine output
    a. I, II, III
    b. I, III, IV
    c. I, II, III, IV
    d. I, III, IV, V
    e. I, II, III, IV, V

27. The amount of moisture present in normal alveolar air is:
    a. 32 mg/l
    b. 38 mg/l
    c. 40 mg/l
    d. 42 mg/l
    e. 44 mg/l

28. Which of the following devices functions with the use of the piezoelectric principle?
    a. cascade humidifier
    b. Bennet nebulizer
    c. ultrasonic nebulizer
    d. pass-over humidifier
    e. wick nebulizer

29. The patient is on a nasal cannula at 3 LPM; the E cylinder has 1800 PSIG left. How long will it last?
    a. 2 hours and 8 minutes
    b. 2 hours and 48 minutes
    c. 3 hours and 14 minutes
    d. 2 hours and 20 minutes
    e. 2 hours and 12 minutes

30. The PR-2 cycles to expiration when:
    I. Reducing valve is set
    II. A set pressure is achieved
    III. The oxygen source is delayed
    IV. The rate control is set
    V. The flow of gas to the patient falls below 1–3 LPM
    a. I, II, III
    b. I, IV, V
    c. II, III, V
    d. I, II, III, IV
    e. I, II, III, IV

31. A good chest physiotherapy procedure should include:
    a. a review of the x-ray films
    b. vibration techniques
    c. coughing techniques
    d. percussion and correct positioning
    e. all of the above

32. Which of the following would be considered a contraindication for chest physiotherapy?
    a. chest pain
    b. fresh rib fractures
    c. empyema
    d. frank hemoptysis
    e. all of the above

33. The Bird VII with the air mix pushed in will most affect which of these variables:
    a. expiratory time
    b. inspiratory time
    c. sensitivity
    d. nebulization of medication
    e. pressure delivery cycle

34. When delivering an IPPB treatment with a Bird VIII, the unit will no longer cycle into expiration. What should be checked?
    a. the possibility of a leak
    b. the patient's tongue for occlusion of the mouthpiece
    c. the oxygen delivery system
    d. the occlusion of the tubing
    e. the expiratory cycling mechanism

35. The double-lumen endotracheal tube is called:
    a. Cole
    b. Pitt Speak
    c. Bi-Lumen
    d. Carlens
    e. Doublex

36. Which of the following is False about the nasopharyngeal airway?
    I. Should be rotated every 4 hours
    II. Used to aid in bite blockage
    III. Nasal necrosis is of no concern
    IV. Better tolerated than oral airway in alert patient
    V. Airway of choice for the alert patient
    a. I, II, III
    b. II, IV, V
    c. I, II, III, IV
    d. II, III, V
    e. I, II, III, IV, V

37. Airway cuff pressures of less than 5 mmHg will produce:
    a. venous obstruction
    b. arterial flow obstruction
    c. lymphatic flow obstruction
    d. edema
    e. c and d

38. When using the straight laryngoscope blade for endotracheal intubation, the tip is placed where?

a. in the vallecula
b. the aryepiglottic fluids
c. under the epiglottis
d. anterior to the epiglottis
e. none of the above

39. Whihch of the following methods is used to determine correct endotracheal tube placement?
    a. auscultation
    b. x-ray examination
    c. observation
    d. a and b only
    e. a, b, and c

40. A suction catheter should not occupy more than _____ of the internal diameter of the tube being suctioned.
    a. $\frac{1}{4}$
    b. $\frac{1}{3}$
    c. $\frac{1}{2}$
    d. $\frac{3}{4}$
    e. $\frac{2}{3}$

41. Convert the following: 18F = _____ mm.
    a. 2
    b. 3
    c. 4
    d. 5
    e. 6

42. The correct amount of suction vacuum pressure for the adult is:
    a. −40 to −60 mmHg
    b. −60 to −80 mmHg
    c. −80 to −100 mmHg
    d. −80 to −120 mmHg
    e. −120 mmHg and above

43. Which of the following is considered a complication of tracheostomy?
    a. hemorrhage
    b. infection
    c. pneumothorax
    d. subcutaneous emphysema
    e. all of the above

44. Which of the following is/are sporicidal?
    I. ethyl alcohol
    II. acid glutaraldehyde
    III. alkaline glutaraldehyde
    IV. isopropyl alcohol
    V. iodine
    a. I, II, III
    b. II, III
    c. II, III, IV
    d. III, IV, V
    e. V only

45. Which of the following is/are not recommended for sterilization of rubber, metal, and plastic equipment?

      I. autoclave
     II. acid glutaraldehyde
    III. ethylene oxide
    IV. pasteurization
     V. alkaline glutaraldehyde
  a. I and III only
  b. I, II, III
  c. II, IV, V
  d. II, III, IV
  e. I, II, III, IV, V

46. The normal range for serium sodium is:
  a. 3.5 to 5 mEq/l
  b. 99 to 106 mEq/l
  c. 135 to 145 mEq/l
  d. 150 to 159 mEq/l
  e. none of the above

47. Which of the following is the "standard" position of the chest film?
  a. posterior-anterior
  b. anterior-posterior
  c. lateral decubitus
  d. decubitus
  e. lateral

48. The chest film used to detect pleural effusion is:
  a. posterior-anterior
  b. anterior-posterior
  c. lateral decubitus
  d. decubitus
  e. lateral

49. List the following in the order of increasing radiodensity:
     I. Soft tissue
    II. Bones
   III. Air
   IV. Fat
    V. Fluid
  a. I, II, III, IV, V
  b. III, V, I, IV, V
  c. V, III, IV, I, II
  d. V, III, II, I, IV
  e. V, I, II, IV, III

50. Bradycardia is a heart rate of _____ beats/minute.
  a. 100
  b. 120
  c. 80
  d. 65
  e. less than 60

51. TLC − RV = _____.
  a. VC
  b. ERV
  c. FRC

d. IRV

e. none of the above

52. Which of the following diseases are considered to be obstructive?
    I. Bronchiectasis
    II. Pneumonia
    III. Chronic bronchitis
    IV. Asthma
    V. Guillain-Barré
    a. II and IV
    b. II, IV, V
    c. I, III, IV
    d. I, II, IV
    e. I, II, III, IV, V

53. Early in an acute asthma attack, ABGs would yield the following results, *except*:
    I. Increased pH
    II. Decreased pH
    III. Increased Pa_{CO_2}
    IV. Decreased Pa_{CO_2}
    V. Normal to decreased HCO_3
    a. I, II, V
    b. I, IV, V
    c. II, III, V
    d. II, IV, V
    e. II and III

54. In frank pulmonary edema, the sputum would be generally characterized as:
    a. pink and frothy
    b. clear and mucoid
    c. thick and green
    d. yellow and thin
    e. thick and tenacious

55. Which of the following is/are considered restrictive diseases?
    a. Guillain-Barré syndrome
    b. myasthenia gravis
    c. scoliosis
    d. obesity
    e. all of the above

56. Which of the following is considered a $beta_2$ response to stimulation?
    a. vasoconstriction
    b. vasodilation
    c. bronchoconstriction
    d. bronchodilation
    e. increased cardiac rate

57. The disadvantage(s) of tank-type negative pressure ventilation is/are?
    a. cardiovascular systems are adversely affected
    b. nursing care difficult to administer
    c. the patient is not very accessible
    d. an artificial airway is not needed
    e. b and c

58. When determining how a ventilator is cycled, one must consider:
    a. power sources
    b. alarm systems
    c. what terminates inspiration
    d. what ends exhalation
    e. what begins inspiration

59. Which of the following is/are not indication(s) for mechanical ventilation?
    I. Apnea
    II. Acute respiratory alkalosis
    III. Impending respiratory failure
    IV. Acute respiratory failure
    V. Oxygenation
    a. II only
    b. II and IV
    c. I, III, IV, V
    d. I, II, III, IV
    e. I, II, III, IV, V

60. Continuous mechanical ventilation may result in which of the following:
    a. increased cardiac output
    b. enhanced venous return
    c. decreased pleural pressure
    d. decreased mean intrathoracic pressure
    e. increased mean intrathoracic pressure

61. Complications associated with mechanical ventilation include:
    I. Infection
    II. Stress ulcers
    III. Subcutaneous emphysema
    IV. Barotrauma
    V. Renal dysfunction
    a. III and IV
    b. I, IV, V
    c. II, III, IV
    d. I, III, IV, V
    e. I, II, III, IV, V

62. CPAP:
    I. Increases FRC
    II. Impedes venous return
    III. Is used only in control ventilation
    IV. Decreases cardiac output
    V. Increases renal blood flow
    a. I, II, III
    b. I, II, IV
    c. I, III, IV
    d. I, III, IV, V
    e. I, II, III, IV, V

63. On a volume-cycled ventilatory, an increase in airway resistance will:
    a. increase peak airway pressure
    b. increase rate
    c. increase volume
    d. increase flow
    e. alter the I:E ratio

64. The oxygen alarm light on the MA-1 will change from green to red when:
    a. there is a drop in the F_{IO_2} delivered
    b. the line connected to compressed air disconnects
    c. the analyzer is disconnected
    d. there is a drop in the oxygen source pressure
    e. the high-pressure alarm is on silence for 3 minutes

65. On the Bear II ventilator, if only the compressor is functional, what F_{IO_2} will be delivered?
    a. 1.0
    b. 0.6
    c. 0.4
    d. 0.3
    e. 0.21

66. Choose the minimum conditions to begin weaning from mechanical ventilation.
    a. NIF greater than 20 cm H_2O and VC of 3 ml/kg
    b. NIF greater than 40 cm H_2O and VC of 3 ml/kg
    c. NIF greater than 30 cm H_2O and VC of 7 ml/kg
    d. NIF greater than 20 cm H_2O and VC of 15 ml/kg
    e. NIF greater than 15 cm H_2O and VC of 15 ml/kg

67. Which of the following formulas is used to monitor static compliance?

    a. $$\frac{V_T}{\text{plateau pressure} - \text{end expiratory pressure}}$$

    b. $$\frac{V_T}{\text{peak pressure}}$$

    c. $$\frac{\text{peak pressure} - \text{flow}}{\text{plateau pressure}}$$

    d. $$\frac{\text{peak pressure}}{V_T - \text{PEEP}}$$

    e. $$\frac{V_T - \text{peak pressure}}{\text{flow}}$$

68. The following results would indicate the patient is not prepared to be weaned from mechanical ventilation:
    I. $P(A-a)O_2$ less than 300 torr at F_{IO_2} of 1.0
    II. VC greater than 15 ml/kg
    III. NIF greater than -15
    IV. V_D/V_T greater than 30 percent
    V. shunt less than 45%
    a. II only
    b. III, IV, V
    c. I, III, IV
    d. II, III, IV, V
    e. I, II, III, IV, V

69. Which of the following would be the best determinant of the effects of PEEP on the cardiovascular system?
    a. $C(A-a)DO_2$
    b. cardiac output
    c. PaO_2
    d. blood pressure
    e. b and d

70. Which of the following is not a goal of mechanical ventilation?
    a. oxygenation
    b. increased FRC
    c. increased cardiac function
    d. increased distribution of ventilation
    e. b and c

71. Which of the following is not a goal of chest physiotherapy?
    a. to improve ABG results
    b. to relieve dyspnea
    c. to increase awareness of respiratory muscle usage
    d. to improve effectiveness of cough
    e. to aid in the mobilization of secretions

72. What is the correct position to drain the right middle lobe?
    a. Fowler's position, turned left
    b. head down 15 degrees, supine
    c. head down 15 degrees, rotated one quarter onto the left side
    d. head down 15 degrees, rotated one half onto the right side
    e. head down 30 degrees, lying on the left side

73. IPPB is contraindicated in the patient with:
    a. systemic hypertension
    b. untreated pneumothorax (no chest tube)
    c. pulmonary edema
    d. tuberculosis
    e. decreased intracranial pressure

74. Semi-Fowler's position best drains:
    a. the lingula
    b. the apical segments
    c. posterior basal segments
    d. middle lobes
    e. none of the above

75. During a routine IPPB treatment a patient becomes very dizzy and begins to cough up blood. The most appropriate next step would be:
    a. call the nurse
    b. increase the FIO_2
    c. continue the treatment at a lower pressure
    d. discontinue the treatment and notify the physician
    e. suction the patient quickly

76. Which of the following is True about the EOA?
    I. It has 16 holes in the lumen.
    II. It is an emergency airway only.
    III. It is difficult to insert.
    IV. Aspiration of gastric contents is a hazard.
    V. Inadvertent tracheal intubation is not common.
    a. I, II, III
    b. II, III, IV
    c. I, II, IV
    d. II, III, IV, V
    e. I, II, III, IV, V

77. The tracheostomy tube should be changed:

   a. daily
   b. every 8 hours
   c. when obstructed
   d. to clean it
   e. never

78. Which plastic listed here is the most commonly used in the making of artificial airways?
   a. polyvinylchloride
   b. Teflon
   c. nylon
   d. polyethylene
   e. silicon

79. List the following in the correct order to properly prepare the fenestrated tracheostomy tube for patient use:
   I. Place cork in opening of inner cannula.
   II. Remove solid inner cannula
   III. Insert inflation device.
   IV. Deflate cuff.
   V. Place cork in opening of outer cannula.
   a. III, IV, II, V
   b. II, IV, V
   c. II, IV, III, V
   d. I, II, IV, V
   e. II, IV, I

80. Which of the following is the function(s) of the airway cuff?
   a. stabilize the airway
   b. protect the airway
   c. prevent infection
   d. a and c
   e. a and b

81. The standard laryngoscope is designed to be used in which hand?
   a. the right
   b. the left
   c. either hand
   d. neither hand
   e. a and b only

82. The most common complications of extubation are:
   I. Laryngospasm
   II. Glottic edema
   III. Subglottic edema
   IV. Tracheoesophageal fistula
   V. Laryngeal puncture
   a. I, II, III
   b. I, III, V
   c. I, III, IV
   d. II, III, IV, V
   e. I, II, III, IV, V

83. Which of the following is/are a purpose of suctioning?
   a. clear airway of secretions
   b. produce a cough
   c. obtain a sputum sample

    d. stimulate vagal response

    e. all except d

84. Z-79 on the side of an endotracheal tube stands for:

    a. a committee that sets standards for purity of tubes

    b. a designation that the tube has a low pressure cuff

    c. a committee that sets standards for tube usage

    d. a committee that sets standards for tubes and cuffs

    e. all of the above

85. Immediately following extubation, the therapist notices that the patient has inspiratory stridor. This is the cardinal sign of:

    a. glottic edema

    b. bronchospasm

    c. tracheoesophageal fistual

    d. respiratory distress

    e. cuff pressure damage

86. Which of the following should be present during endotracheal extubation procedures?

       I. Racemic epinephrine

      II. Suction source with sterile catheter

     III. Laryngoscope and endotracheal intubation equipment

     IV. Manual resuscitator

      V. Oxygen source

    a. II, III, V

    b. II, III, IV, V

    c. I, II, III, IV

    d. II, III, IV, V

    e. I, II, III, IV, V

87. Magill forceps are generally used in which procedure?

    a. cricothyrotomy

    b. extubation

    c. nasotracheal intubation

    d. tracheostomy

    e. oral intubation

88. When using a tracheostomy tube, what is the function of the obturator?

    a. to break up dried secretions

    b. to aid the patient in speaking

    c. to aid in decannulation

    d. to prevent aspiration

    e. to facilitate tube insertion

89. Which of the following is True of the Carlins endotracheal tube?

       I. It has 16 holes in the lumen.

      II. It has a double lumen.

     III. It is used for emergency intubation.

     IV. The right lumen extends into the right mainstem.

      V. It has a foam cuff.

    a. I and III

    b. II and V

    c. II and IV

    d. III and IV

    e. I, III, IV

90. Which of the following are not considered a part of a CBC report?
    - I. Hematocrit
    - II. Serum sodium
    - III. Hemoglobin
    - IV. Glucose
    - V. Platelet count
    a. I, III, V
    b. II, IV, V
    c. II and IV
    d. II, III, IV, V
    e. I, II, III

91. What x-ray position is used for a portable chest film?
    a. PA
    b. AP
    c. lordic
    d. lateral
    e. transverse

92. Choose the complication(s) associated with chest tube insertion.
    a. infection
    b. pneumothorax
    c. hemothorax
    d. hemorrhage
    e. a, b, and c

93. Where is the chest tube placed to remove air from the pleural space?
    a. 6th to 8th intercostal space
    b. 2nd to 3rd intercostal space midaxillary
    c. 6th to 8th intercostal space laterally, midaxillary
    d. 2nd to 3rd intercostal space anteriorly, midclavicular
    e. none of the above

94. Of the five basic percussion notes, which is produced normally in the lung?
    a. flatness
    b. dullness
    c. resonance
    d. hyper-resonance
    e. tympany

95. The pattern of respiration associated with diabetic ketoacidosis is:
    a. Kussmaul's breathing
    b. Biot's respirations
    c. Cheyne-Stokes respirations
    d. eupnea
    e. diabetic breathing

96. Which of the following terms describes normal breath sounds?
    a. eupnea
    b. wheeze
    c. apnea
    d. vesicular
    e. adventious

97. During chest auscultation the patient should be instructed to breathe in what manner?

I. Deep breaths
II. Through the mouth
III. Through the nose
IV. Slow
V. With a pause at end inspiration
a. I, II
b. II, IV
c. I, II, IV, V
d. I, III, IV, V
e. I, II, III, IV, V

98. Which of the following is/are acceptable sites to take pulse?
I. Radial
II. Brachial
III. Carotid
IV. Femoral
V. Pedal
a. I only
b. I, II, V
c. I, III, IV
d. I, II, III, IV
e. I, II, III, IV, V

99. Which of the following devices produces the highest relative humidity?
a. cool mist jet nebulizer
b. bubble type humidifier
c. vaporizer
d. heated jet nebulizer
e. atomizer

100. Which of the following are segments of the right upper lobe?
I. apical
II. lateral
III. medial
IV. posterior
V. anterior
a. I and IV
b. I, IV, V
c. I, II, IV
d. II, III, IV
e. I, II, III, IV, V

ANSWERS TO THE CRTT PRACTICE EXAMINATION

1. a	9. a	17. c	25. e
2. c	10. b	18. c	26. c
3. e	11. d	19. a	27. e
4. c	12. a	20. d	28. c
5. e	13. e	21. d	29. b
6. e	14. b	22. e	30. b
7. e	15. c	23. a	31. e
8. c	16. b	24. a	32. e

33. b	50. e	67. a	84. d
34. a	51. a	68. b	85. a
35. d	52. c	69. e	86. e
36. a	53. e	70. e	87. c
37. e	54. a	71. a	88. c
38. c	55. e	72. c	89. c
39. e	56. d	73. b	90. c
40. c	57. e	74. b	91. b
41. c	58. c	75. d	92. e
42. d	59. a	76. c	93. d
43. e	60. e	77. c	94. c
44. b	61. e	78. a	95. a
45. a	62. b	79. b	96. d
46. c	63. a	80. e	97. c
47. a	64. d	81. b	98. d
48. c	65. e	82. e	99. d
49. b	66. d	83. e	100. b

Chapter 24

SAMPLE REGISTRY EXAMINATION

1. Venturi masks are often used to treat patients who demonstrate:
   a. eucapnea
   b. tachypnea
   c. exercise hyperventilation
   d. polycapnea
   e. orthopnea

2. In order for a cough to be effective:
   I. Inspiratory capacity must be at least 75 percent of predicted
   II. Intra-alveolar should be greater than 80 cm H_2O
   III. Intra-alveolar should be less than 80 cm H_2O
   IV. Inspiratory capacity must be at least 50 percent of predicted
   V. Peak expiratory flows will be close to 300 LPM
   a. I and II
   b. I and III
   c. III, IV, V
   d. I, II, V
   e. III, IV, V

3. A 46-year-old male received burns on 15 percent of his body and suffered smoke inhalation afterward. His V_D/V_T ratio is 0.7. As a respiratory care practitioner you would recommend:
   a. cool mist therapy via aerosol mask
   b. intubation and mechanical ventilation
   c. intubation and CPAP
   d. antibiotics via aerosol therapy
   e. 40 percent Venturi mask with cool aerosol

4. The Henderson-Hasselbach equation is based on:
   a. a pH of 7.40

b. the law of continuity
c. the law of diabatic heat of action
d. the law of mass action
e. renal excretion of bicarbonate

5. A 23-year-old male admitted to the hospital presents with general weakness and shortness of breath. He has an infection on the plantar surface of his foot which has been cultured for *Clostridium tetani*. Treatment of choice for this individual would be:
   a. mechanical ventilator support
   b. close observation
   c. tetanus vaccine and antibiotic therapy for a gram-positive organism
   d. antibiotic therapy for a gram-negative organism
   e. steroid therapy

6. The normal range of airway resistance in the adult is:
   a. 20 to 30 cm H_2O/l/sec
   b. 1.0 to 10 cm H_2O/l/sec
   c. 0.1 to 0.5 cm H_2O/l/sec
   d. 50 to 100 cm H_2O/l/sec
   e. 0.6 to 2.4 cm H_2O/l/sec

7. Humidity deficit is:
   a. directly proportionate to heat loss of evaporation
   b. the amount of water required to humidify inspired air to body temperature
   c. the ratio between the amount of water present and the amount the air is capable of holding at that temperature
   c. the difference between ambient humidity and dry air
   e. equal to 44 mg/l at body temperature

8. The most appropriate method of evaluating the pulmonary status for a patient with Guillain-Barré syndrome would be:
   a. frequent monitoring of vital capacity and NIF
   b. daily ABGs
   c. pulmonary function test before and after bronchodilator
   d. frequent vital signs
   e. ventilation/perfusion lung scans

9. The appropriate action for ventricular fibrillation would be:
   I. Intravenous administration of Isuprel
   II. Defibrillation
   III. A beta stimulator
   IV. Administration of bretylium
   V. Administration of dopamine
   a. I and V
   b. II, III, V
   c. II only
   d. IV and V
   e. II and IV

10. A capnograph is used for:
    a. measuring closing volumes
    b. measuring CO_2 levels in expired air
    c. measuring O_2 levels in expired air
    d. measuring arterial line pressures
    e. measuring endotracheal cuff pressures

11. Normal shunts are a result of venous admixture in:
    I. Azygos veins
    II. Coronary arteries
    III. Thebesian veins
    IV. Bronchial veins
    V. Pulmonary arteries
    a. II, III, IV
    b. I, III, IV, V
    c. II, III, IV, V
    d. III and IV
    e. IV only

12. By which methods can functional residual capacity be calculated?
    I. Flow-volume loop
    II. Nitrogen washout
    III. Body plethysmography
    IV. DL_{co}
    V. Helium dilution
    a. I, III, IV
    b. II, IV, V
    c. II, III, V
    d. I, IV, V
    e. III, IV, V

13. Two toxic byproducts of ethylene oxide sterilization of polyvinyl chloride are:
    I. Polyhydrine-ethylechlorate
    II. Carbon monoxide
    III. Ethylene chlorohydrine
    IV. Ethylene chlorate
    V. Ethylene glycol
    a. I and IV
    b. III and IV
    c. II and V
    d. I and III
    e. III and V

14. On the Bennett MA-1 ventilator what alarm will activate if inspiratory time exceeds expiratory time?
    a. sigh alarm
    b. high-pressure alarm
    c. disconnect alarm
    d. ratio alarm
    e. low exhaled volume alarm

DATA
Use the following values to calculate questions 15 to 18:

$P_B = 758$ mmHg $P_{H_2O} = 42$ mmHg
$PaO_2 = 75$ mmHg $PaCO_2 = 35$
                          mmHg

$FIO_2 = 0.5$

---

15. What is the PO_2 of moist tracheal air?
    a. 358 mmHg
    b. 379 mmHg
    c. 398 mmHg
    d. 405 mmHg
    e. 459 mmHg

16. What is the P_{AO_2}?
    a. 304 mmHg
    b. 314 mmHg
    c. 324 mmHg
    d. 354 mmHg
    e. 404 mmHg

17. What is the $(A - a)DO_2$?
    a. 350 mmHg
    b. 314 mmHg
    c. 268 mmHg
    d. 239 mmHg
    e. 190 mmHg

18. Which of the following might be the reason for the abnormality in the $(A - a)DO_2$?
    I. Diffusion defect
    II. Shunt
    III. Hyperventilation
    IV. Hypoxia
    V. Ventilation/perfusion mismatch
    a. II and IV
    b. I, II, V
    c. III and IV
    d. II, III, V
    e. I and IV

19. A patient is in the emergency room for treatment of severe bronchospasm due to status asthmaticus. The patient is tachypneic. You would expect the arterial blood gas values to show:
    a. hypoxemia with respiratory alkalosis
    b. normal values
    c. hypocarbia and a normal Pa_{O_2}
    d. hypercarbia and a normal Pa_{O_2}
    e. respiratory acidosis with hypoxemia

20. Which of the following would show up darkest on a chest film?
    a. the heart
    b. air
    c. consolidation of the right lower lobes
    d. atelectasis of the left lung
    e. bronchial tumor

21. All of the following lung diseases are restrictive *except*:
    a. Guillain-Barré syndrome
    b. kyphoscoliosis
    c. cystic fibrosis
    d. myasthenia gravis
    e. pneumonia

22. A regulator attached to an "H" cylinder registers a pressure of 1800 psig. Approximately how many hours remain in the cylinder when the flow rate is set at 8 LPM?
    a. 6 hours, 30 minutes
    b. 8 hours
    c. 11 hours, 45 minutes
    d. 18 hours, 10 minutes
    e. 15 hours

23. Given the following data, calculate oxygen content:

$$Hemoglobin = 14 \text{ gm\%} \qquad PaO_2 = 87 \text{ mmHg}$$
$$PAO_2 = 80 \text{ mmHg} \qquad PaCO_2 = 42 \text{ mmHg}$$
$$SaO_2 = 94\% \qquad P_B = 754 \text{ mmHg}$$

a. 7.8 vol%
b. 12.4 vol%
c. 15.5 vol%
d. 17.9 vol%
e. 19.7 vol%

24. Stimulation for the newborn's first breath includes:
    I. Hypocarbia
    II. Hypoxic drive
    III. Acidosis
    IV. Alkalosis
    V. Thermal changes
a. I, II, III, IV
b. I, II, IV, V
c. I, III, V
d. II, III, V
e. II, IV, V

25. Which of the following could result in a poor cough effort?
    I. Pain
    II. Patient cooperation
    III. Neuromuscular disease
    IV. Spinal cord injury
    V. Increase in airway resistance
a. I, II, III, IV, V
b. II, III, IV, V
c. I, III, IV, V
d. I, II, IV, V
e. I, II, III, IV

26. In what form and where does CO_2 affect the central chemoreceptors?
a. as CO_2 molecule in arterial blood
b. as CO_2 molecule in cerebral spinal fluid
c. as O_2 molecule in cerebral spinal fluid
d. as H^+ in arterial blood
e. as H^+ in cerebral spinal fluid

27. What is the particle range for most pulmonary aerosol applications?
a. 50 to 100 microns
b. 5 to 50 microns
c. 1 to 10 microns
d. 0.5 to 2 microns
e. 0.1 to 0.3 microns

28. On the Bourns BP-200, to establish a tidal volume, which of the following parameters should be used?
    I. Oxygen control
    II. Pressure limit control
    III. Inspiratory time limit
    IV. Flowmeter control
    V. I:E ratio
a. II only
b. II, III, IV, V

c. III, IV, V

d. III and V

e. I, II, III, IV, V

29. During IPPB therapy, which of the following is a physiologic effect?
    I. Decrease the work of breathing
    II. Increase intrathoracic pressure
    III. Manipulate the I:E ratio
    IV. Deliver medication
    V. Increase tidal volume
    a. II, III, V
    b. I, II, IV
    c. III, IV, V
    d. I, II, III, IV, V
    e. I, II, III, V

30. Which of the following ratios depict vascular breath sounds?
    a. 3:1
    b. 2:3
    c. 5:6
    d. 1:1
    e. 1:3

31. Which ventilator is a linear drive constant flow?
    a. Bennett MA-1
    b. Bear 1
    c. Bear Cub
    d. Bourns LS104-150
    e. Siemens Servo 900B

32. Normal CVP pressures is:
    a. 0 to 5 mmHg
    b. 5 to 12 mmHg
    c. 8 to 10 mmHg
    d. 10 to 20 mmHG
    e. 20 to 30 mmHG

33. During resuscitation efforts, evaluation of the pulse should be:
    a. radial artery
    b. brachial artery
    c. carotid artery
    d. temporal artery
    e. femoral artery

34. When administering a mixture of carbon dioxide and oxygen to a patient, which of the following should be evaluated?
    I. Temperature
    II. Respiratory rate
    III. Pulse
    IV. Blood pressure
    V. Patient's color
    a. II and IV
    b. II and III
    c. III and V
    d. I and III
    e. II and V

35. A patient is admitted for a lung compliance study. The patient inspires 500 ml from a spirometer, the intrapleural pressure was measured at -5 cm H_2O pre-inspiratory and 10 cm H_2O at the end of inspiration. The calculated lung compliance would be:
    a. 0.15 l/cm H_2O
    b. 0.5 l/cm H_2O
    c. 0.10 l/cm H_2O
    d. 0.025 l/cm H_2O
    e. 0.25 l/cm H_2O

36. A 1:200 solution of Alupent is needed for a nebulizer treatment. One half cc is mixed with 2 cc of normal saline. The final mixture will have what new dilution of Alupent?
    a. 1:800
    b. 1:400
    c. 1:1000
    d. 1:900
    e. 1:2000

37. Particle size on the ultrasonic nebulizer is determined by:
    a. amplitude
    b. amount of solution in the couplant chamber
    c. output
    d. piezoelectric principle
    e. frequency

38. In a good rehabilitation program, which of the following should be covered educationally with the patient and the family?
    I. Breathing techniques
    II. Oxygen therapy
    III. Care and cleaning of the equipment
    IV. Good nutrition
    V. Energy conservation
    a. I, II, III, IV, V
    b. II, III, IV, V
    c. I, III, IV, V
    d. I, II, IV, V
    e. III, IV, V

39. Which of the following influence a chemical agent's effectiveness?
    I. pH
    II. Temperature
    III. Exposure time
    IV. Flammability
    a. II and IV
    b. I and III
    c. I, II, III
    d. II, III, IV
    e. I, II, III, IV

40. What is meant by a substance that is bactericidal?
    a. It will destroy bacteria, including spores.
    b. It simply impedes growth of bacteria.
    c. It will destroy all living viable bacteria.
    d. It simply impedes the growth of spores.
    e. It will destroy vegetative organisms.

41. Venous return is increased by:

a. isovolumetric IPPB
b. high-volume IPPB
c. blow bottles
d. incentive spirometry
e. expiratory retard

42. A solution that is isotonic in relation to body fluids is:
   a. distilled water
   b. 4% sodium chloride solution
   c. 0.45% sodium chloride solution
   d. 0.9% sodium chloride solution
   e. 10% sodium chloride solution

43. A tracheostomy tube is placed in a patient with a cuff inflated to allow a minimal leak. As the gas in the cuff warms up to body temperature, it may exert sufficient pressure on the tracheal wall to result in necrosis. Which gas law applies to this situation?
   a. Charles' law
   b. Boyle's law
   c. Gay-Lussac's law
   d. Graham's law
   e. Henry's law

44. Complications of suctioning include:
   I. Death
   II. Hypoxia
   III. Decreased hemoglobin
   IV. Dysrhythmias
   V. Infection
   a. I, II, III, V
   b. II, III, IV, V
   c. I, III, IV, V
   d. I, II, IV, V
   e. I, IV, V

45. Which organisms are gram-negative?
   I. *Pseudomonas aeruginosa*
   II. *Staphylococcus aureus*
   III. *Seratia marcescens*
   IV. *Diplococcus pneumoniae*
   V. *Escherichia coli*
   a. I, II, III, V
   b. I, III, V
   c. II and IV
   d. I, III, IV
   e. II, III, IV

46. The recommended treatment of choice for glottic edema is:
   a. sympathomimetic amine administration only
   b. sympathomimetic amines and corticosteroids
   c. sympathomimetic amines, xanthines, and corticosteroids
   d. sympathomimetic amines, xanthines, corticosteroids, and antibiotics
   e. sympathomimetic amines, xanthines, corticosteroids, antibiotics, and anticholinergics

47. An 89-year-old male patient on a volume ventilator continues to clamp down with his mouth on his oral endotracheal tube. He has had his false teeth removed, but the high-pressure alarm continues to sound. The probable cause of and remedy to this problem is:

a. The exhalation line that has become disconnected, causing a large air leak; the remedy is to reconnect the line.

b. The patient is biting on his endotracheal tube; the remedy is to insert a bite block.

c. The patient has bitten a hole in the endotracheal tube and all the air has leaked out; the remedy is to replace the endotracheal tube.

d. The cuff on the endotracheal tube is not working; the remedy is to replace the endotracheal tube.

e. none of the above

48. Immediately after you've extubated a patient he begins to vomit. The first thing the respiratory care practitioner should do is:

a. suction the mouth

b. reintubate

c. resuscitate with a hand resuscitator

d. turn the patient's head to the side

e. immediately call the attending physician

49. Which of the following can cause adult respiratory distress syndrome?

   I. Sepsis

   II. Chest trauma

   III. Near-drowning

   IV. Neurologic trauma

   V. Abdominal surgery

a. I, II, IV, V

b. II, III, IV, V

c. I, II, III, IV, V

d. I, III, IV, V

e. III, IV, V

50. Epiglottitis is best diagnosed by:

a. lateral x-ray of the neck

b. direct visualization of the epiglottis by laryngoscope

c. throat culture

d. blood cultures

e. a ventilation/perfusion study

51. The most common cell associated with lung cancer is:

a. anaplastic (oat-cell) carcinoma

b. adenocarcinoma

c. giant cell carcinoma

d. squamous cell carcinoma

e. sarcoma

52. Negative displacement ventilation works by:

a. generating a low pressure in the alveoli

b. generating a high pressure in the alveoli

c. generating a higher pressure in the airway

d. generating a lower pressure in the airway

e. generating a higher pressure in the chest

53. Factors that can contribute to an asthma attack are:

   I. Exertion

   II. Aspirin

   III. Cold or flu

   IV. Emotional stress

   V. Antigens

a. I, II, IV, V

    b. II, III, IV, V

    c. I, III, IV, V

    d. I, IV, V

    e. I, II, III, IV, V

54. Approximately how many degrees Kelvin equals 106°F?

    a. 127°K

    b. 140°K

    c. 169°K

    d. 296°K

    e. 314°K

55. If 5 liters of oxygen in a Douglas bag at 740 mmHg are compressed to 2 liters, what is the new pressure inside the bag?

    a. 1850 mmHg

    b. 1520 mmHg

    c. 980 mmHg

    d. 850 mmHg

    e. 720 mmHg

56. The portion of the autonomic nervous system responsible for the "fright or flight" response is the:

    a. muscarinic system

    b. nicotinic system

    c. sympathetic system

    d. cholinergic system

    e. parasympathetic system

57. Oxygen transport is carried to the tissues in which of the following ways?

    I. Combined with H^+

    II. Dissolved in plasma

    III. Carbonic anhydrase

    IV. As oxyhemoglobin

    a. I only

    b. I and II

    c. IV only

    d. II and IV

    e. II, III, IV

58. Polarographic oxygen analyzers utilize which of the following principle?

    a. wheatstone bridge

    b. Clark electrode

    c. chemical combinations

    d. Pauling's principle

    e. Bernoulli's principle

59. The trachea normally lies in the midplane of the body between:

    a. C_4–T_1

    b. C_6–T_2

    c. C_6–T_5

    d. C_7–T_4

    e. T_1–T_6

60. A flip-flop device:

    I. Requires only a brief input signal to change output

    II. Requires a memory circuit to give digital readouts

    III. Requires a continuous input signal and alter outputs

IV. Is bistable
V. Is biphasic when accompanied by a monostable signal input
a. I only
b. I and IV
c. III only
d. III and V
e. II only

61. In order to check the validity of the peripheral arterial pressure monitoring:
a. a CVP is inserted
b. pulses are checked frequently
c. a pulmonary capillary wedge pressure should be taken
d. a blood pressure cuff should be used
e. daily arterial blood gases should be drawn

62. Normal pulmonary artery pressure is:
a. 25/8 mmHg
b. 40/20 mmHg
c. 6/0 mmHg
d. 120/80 mmHg
e. 10/2 mmHg

63. On the Bird Mark 7 respirator, inspiratory to expiratory ratio is affected by what control(s)?
a. flow rate
b. pressure selector
c. expiratory timer cartridge
d. all of the above
e. none of the above

64. Hyper-resonance can be found in which of the following?
I. Empyema
II. Atelectasis
III. Acute asthma attack
IV. Compensatory emphysema
V. Congestive heart failure
a. IV only
b. II, III, IV
c. I, II, V
d. III, IV, V
e. III and IV

65. Vital capacity can be defined as:
a. TLC − ERV
b. TV + IRV + ERV
c. ERV + RV
d. IC + RV
e. TLC − FRC

66. On the Bennett PR-2, gas that just passed through the terminal flow control just left the:
a. middle timing accumulator
b. inspiratory nebulizer
c. expiratory nebulizer
d. Bennett valve
e. adjustable regulator

67. When the patient is lying prone with one pillow under the abdomen, this position will drain:

a. posterior segment of the right upper lobe
b. lateral basal segments of the lower lobes
c. anterior segments of the lower lobes
d. posterior basal segments of the lower lobes
e. apical segments of the upper lobes

This case pertains to questions 68 through 70.

CASE

The patient is placed on a mechanical ventilator following an episode of acute pulmonary edema. The clinical data are as follows:

$F_{IO_2} = 0.7$ rate = 15

tidal volume = 0.7 liters

and ABGs after 20 minutes revealed:

pH = 7.10 $P_ECO_2 = 25$ mmHg

$Pa_{CO_2} = 80$ mmHg $HCO_3 = 30$ mEq/l

$Pa_{O_2} = 50$ mmHg

Chest x-ray examination revealed increased fluid, infiltrates in all lung fields.

---

68. Using the Shapiro's clinical shunt equation, calculate the percent shunt.
    a. 51 percent
    b. 23 percent
    c. 5 percent
    d. 82 percent
    e. 33 percent

69. This patient's acid base status is:
    a. respiratory alkalosis with no compensation
    b. compensated metabolic alkalosis
    c. partially compensated respiratory acidosis
    d. compensated respiratory acidosis
    e. mixed acidosis

70. This patient's V_D/V_T ratio is:
    a. 68 percent
    b. 32 percent
    c. 86 percent
    d. 75 percent
    e. 56 percent

71. Removing one lung from an individual would _____ the D_{LCO} as ordinarily measured.
    a. increase
    b. decrease
    c. not change
    d. equal predicted values of
    e. none of the above; it would not be measurable

72. Which of the following are goals for insertion of an artificial airway?
    I. To provide a sealed system for mechanical ventilatory support
    II. To keep the patient from vomiting
    III. To protect the airway from aspiration
    IV. To provide a route for nasogastric feeding
    V. To facilitate suctioning

    a. I, II, IV
    b. II, III, IV
    c. I, IV, V
    d. I, III, V
    e. I and III

73. The major functionally active immunoglobulin in respiratory tract secretions is:
    a. IgA
    b. IgG
    c. IgM
    d. IgE
    e. IgD

74. IN endotracheal tubes in millimeter size represents
    a. inner diameter
    b. outer diameter
    c. inner diameter size plus 2
    d. three times the inner diameter
    e. none of the above

75. Which of the following refers to the correct temperature and time for pasteurization?
    a. 120°C for 30 minutes
    b. 70°C for 30 minutes
    c. 100°F for 60 minutes
    d. 50°C for 120 minutes
    e. 100°C for 10 minutes

76. When using an air-entrainment device, if resistance to flow occurs downstream from the entrainment port:
    I. The total flow from the device decreases
    II. The F_{IO_2} decreases
    III. The F_{IO_2} increases
    IV. The total flow from the device increases
    a. I only
    b. III only
    c. I and II
    d. II and IV
    e. I and III

77. Give the following data for an infant ventilator, what is the tidal volume?
    inspiratory time = 0.5 sec
    expiratory time = 1 sec
    inspiratory flowrate = 7 l/min
    pressure limit = 18 cm H_2O
    a. 5.8 ml
    b. 58 ml
    c. 1.6 ml
    d. 16 ml
    e. 116 ml

78. Inhalation of concentrations of 0.04 percent or less of CO_2 will lead to:
    a. hyperventilation
    b. prevention of postoperative atelectasis
    c. increase in cerebral blood flow
    d. no changes in ventilation status
    e. hypoventilation

79. Nonrespiratory acidosis can be associated with:
    I. Diabetic ketoacidosis
    II. Administration of diuretics
    III. Hypokalemia
    IV. Diarrhea
    V. Vomiting of stomach contents
    a. I and V
    b. I and IV
    c. I, III, IV
    d. I, II,III, V
    e. I, II, IV

80. Bird respirators function by means of which set of opposing forces?
    a. flow versus pressure
    b. time versus pressure
    c. magnetism versus pressure
    d. magnetism versus flow
    e. magnetism versus time

81. Which of the following clinical symptoms can alert the respiratory care practitioner to the possibility of a pneumothorax and/or pneumomediastinum?
    I. Tachypnea
    II. Bradycardia
    III. Deterioration of arterial blood gases
    IV. Decreased compliance
    V. Shortness of breath
    a. II, III, V
    b. III, IV, V
    c. I, III, IV, V
    d. I, II, III, IV, V
    e. II, IV, V

82. Which of the following are of no clinical value in detecting shock?
    I. Swan-Ganz catheter
    II. Systolic blood pressure
    III. Urine output
    IV. Pulse
    V. Disorientation and confusion
    a. I, II, III
    b. II and IV
    c. II, IV, V
    d. I, III, V
    e. I and III

CASE

A 55-year-old man was brought into the emergency room complaining of chest pain radiating to the left arm. He was extremely diaphoretic and seemed short of breath. He had no prior history of any illness, ABGs results on room air were pH 7.30; $Paco_2$ 38 mmHg; Pao_2 55 mmHg; and HCO_3 18.3 mEq/l. Questions 83 to 85 pertain to this case.

---

83. This patient's acid base status is:
    a. respiratory acidosis with hypoxemia

    b. metabolic alkalosis with hypoxemia
    c. metabolic acidosis with hypoxemia
    d. respiratory alkalosis with hypoxemia
    e. mixed acidosis with hypoxemia

84. Treatment to correct the ABG abnormality would be:
    I. Intubate and mechanically ventilate
    II. 40 percent air-entrainment device
    III. Diuretic therapy
    IV. Propranolol
    V. Administration of $NaHCO_3$
    a. II, III, V
    b. I, III, IV
    c. II, IV, V
    d. III and IV
    e. I and V

85. As a result of a myocardial infarction, which of the following is not a complication?
    a. cardiac taponade
    b. acute pericarditis
    c. mural thrombosis
    d. left ventricular failure
    e. none of the above

86. Which of the following devices most accurately reflects left heart pressures?
    a. central venous catheter
    b. arterial catheter
    c. Swan-Ganz catheter
    d. intravenous catheter
    e. right atrial catheter

87. What factor during mechanical ventilation has the greatest influence on cardiac output?
    a. machine pressures
    b. peak airway pressures
    c. mean inspiratory pressures
    d. mean inspiratory flow rate
    e. peak expiratory pressures

88. In high-frequency jet ventilation, mass flow of gas ceases at what level?
    a. alveoli
    b. carina
    c. subsegmental bronchi
    d. terminal bronchioles
    e. respiratory bronchioles

89. A high-pitched wheezing on expiration with pitting peripheral edema and a history of orthopnea are highly suggestive of:
    a. asthma
    b. pulmonary embolus
    c. congestive heart failure
    d. chronic obstructive lung disease
    e. pneumonia

90. How are rate and I:E ratio established on the Bennett PR-2?
    I. Tidal volume
    II. Inspiratory time

III. Rate contol
IV. Expiratory time
V. Fixed I:E ratio
a. I and III
b. II and IV
c. I and IV
d. III and IV
e. III and V

91. Which of the following is the goal of a comprehensive rehabilitation program?
a. improve the patient's activities of daily living
b. decrease the number of admissions to the hospital
c. increase the patient's exercise
d. increase the patient's nutritional status
e. lower the final cost to the patient

92. Sustained maximal inspiration maneuvers are most effective in:
a. treating already existing atelectasis
b. preventing atelectasis
c. treating pneumonia
d. preventing lung infiltrates
e. preventing postoperative hypoxic arrhythmias

93. Which of the following receptors is responsible for the relaxation of the bronchial smooth musculature?
a. alpha receptors
b. $beta_1$ receptors
c. $beta_2$ receptors
d. gamma efferent receptors
e. adentylcyclase receptors

94. The best indicator of hypoxia and the necessity for supplemental oxygen is:
a. the patient's pulse
b. Pa_{CO_2}
c. the patient's respiratory rate
d. Pa_{O_2}
e. the patient's color

95. You are a respiratory care practitioner working in a unit with 100 percent oxygen source and room air source gas. You have no blender. You will have to titrate the gas source so you achieve 45 percent oxygen. How many l/min will you need of each source gas?
a. 7 liters oxygen and 13 liters air
b. 5 liters oxygen and 11 liters air
c. 11 liters oxygen and 5 liters air
d. 13 liters oxygen and 7 liters air
e. 5 liters oxygen and 5 liters air

96. Complication of ventilator care include:
I. Infection
II. Increase production of antidiuretic hormone
III. Atelectasis
IV. Stress ulcers
V. Tension pneumothorax
a. I only
b. IV and V
c. I, III, IV, V

d. II, III, IV, V
e. I, II, III, IV, V

97. The minimum hemodynamic monitoring requirement for a patient who requires PEEP in excess of 5 cm H₂O is:
a. CVP
b. PA pressures
c. ECG
d. cardiac output
e. all of the above

98. Which of the following statements is/are true about the body's normal response to acute hypoxemia?
I. Cardiac output increases.
II. Pulmonary artery pressures increase.
III. A significant change in ventilatory status occurs.
IV. Bradycardia and hypotension occur.
a. I only
b. I and II
c. I, II, III
d. II, III, IV
e. I, II, III, IV

99. P₅₀ refers to:
I. Hemoglobin saturation of PaO₂ that equals 50 mmHg
II. PaO₂ of a blood sample that is 50 percent saturated
III. The reference point to ascertain extent of dissolved oxygen
IV. The reference point to ascertain the position of the oxyhemoglobin dissociation curve
V. A reference value of 37 mmHG
a. I, IV, V
b. II, III, IV
c. I, III, IV
d. II, III, V
e. II and IV

100. At rest, oxygen consumption is approximately:
a. 2500 ml/min
b. 25 ml/min
c. 2.5 ml/min
d. 250 ml/min
e. 200 ml/min

ANSWERS TO THE SAMPLE REGISTRY EXAMINATION

1. b	11. d	21. c	31. d
2. d	12. c	22. c	32. a
3. b	13. e	23. d	33. c
4. d	14. d	24. d	34. b
5. c	15. a	25. a	35. c
6. e	16. b	26. e	36. c
7. b	17. d	27. c	37. e
8. a	18. b	28. b	38. a
9. e	19. a	29. e	39. b
10. b	20. b	30. a	40. c

41. c	56. c	71. b	86. c
42. d	57. d	72. d	87. c
43. c	58. b	73. a	88. b
44. d	59. c	74. a	89. c
45. b	60. b	75. b	90. e
46. b	61. d	76. e	91. a
47. b	62. a	77. b	92. b
48. d	63. d	78. d	93. c
49. c	64. e	79. e	94. d
50. a	65. b	80. c	95. b
51. d	66. b	81. d	96. a
52. a	67. c	82. b	97. a
53. e	68. b	83. c	98. c
54. e	69. c	84. a	99. e
55. a	70. a	85. e	100. d

APPENDIX: COMMONLY USED EQUATIONS AND FORMULAS

1. GAS THERAPY AND LAWS

a. Boyle's Law: $P_1V_1 = P_2V_2$

b. Charles's law: $\dfrac{V_1}{T_1} = \dfrac{V_2}{T_2}$

c. Gay-Lussac's law: $\dfrac{P_1}{T_1} = \dfrac{P_2}{T_2}$

d. Combined gas law: $\dfrac{P_1V_1}{T_1} = \dfrac{P_2V_2}{T_2}$

e. Ideal gas law: $PV = nRT$

f. Dalton's law: $P_{total} = P_1 + P_2 + P_3 + \ldots\ldots + P_1$ where
P = pressure (mmHg), V = volume (ml or l),
T = temperature (°K), n = moles,
R = gas constant (0.0821 l-atm/mole-°K)

g. Law of LaPlace: $P = 2T/r$
where P = pressure (dynes/cm²), T = surface tension (dynes/cm), r = radius (cm)

h. Relative humidity: relative humidity (%) = $\dfrac{\text{absolute humidity}}{\text{capacity}} \times 100\%$

i. Equations relating to the variables FIO_2 oxygen flow, air flow, and total flow using air-entrainment devices or blenders:
FIO_2 = oxygen flow + (0.21 × airflow)/total flow or 0.21 + (0.79 × oxygen flow)/total flow
oxygen flow = total flow × (FIO_2 − 0.21)/0.79
airflow = total flow − oxygen flow
total flow = oxygen flow × 0.79/FIO_2 − 0.21

j. Duration of cylinder flow:
K (l/psi) = 28.3 × volume of gas in full cylinder (ft³)/pressure of full cylinder (psi)

28.3 is factor to convert cubic feet into liters
duration of flow (min) $= K \times$ gauge pressure (psi)/flow rate (l/min)

k. **Temperature:**
$$^\circ F = {^\circ C} + 40 \times 9/5 - 40$$
$$^\circ C = {^\circ F} + 40 \times 5/9 - 40$$
$$^\circ K = {^\circ C} + 273$$

2. MONITORING

a. **Oxygen uptake:**
$$\dot{V}_{O_2} = V_E (F_{IO_2} - F\bar{E}_{O_2})$$

b. **Carbon dioxide output:**
$$\dot{V}_{CO_2} = \dot{V}_E \times F\bar{E}_{CO_2}$$
$$\dot{V}_{CO_2} = \dot{V}_A \times P_{aCO_2}/P_B - P_{A_{H_2O}}$$

c. **Respiratory exchange ratio:**
$$R_E = \dot{V}_{CO_2}/\dot{V}_{O_2}$$

d. **Partial pressure of inspired oxygen:**
$$P_{IO_2} = (P_B - P_{H_2O})F_{IO_2}$$

e. **Alveolar air equation:**
$$P_{AO_2} = P_{IO_2} - P_{aCO_2} [F_{IO_2} + (1 - F_{IO_2}/R_E)] \quad or$$
$$P_{AO_2} = (P_B - P_{H_2O})F_{IO_2} - \frac{P_{aCO_2}}{0.8}$$

f. **Deadspace:**
$$V_D = \left(\frac{P_{aCO_2} - P_{E}_{CO_2}}{P_{aCO_2}}\right) \times V_T$$

g. **Cardiac output (Fick equation):**
$$\dot{Q} = \frac{\dot{V}_{O_2}}{(C_{aO_2} - C\bar{v}_{O_2})} \times 10$$

h. **Shunt equation (classic):**
$$\dot{Q}s/\dot{Q}t = \frac{C_{cO_2} - C_{aO_2}}{C_{cO_2} - C\bar{v}_{O_2}}$$

l. **Shunt equation (clinical):**
$$\dot{Q}s/\dot{Q}t = \frac{(P_{AO_2} - P_{aO_2})\ 0.0031}{C(A-\bar{v})O_2 + (P_{AO_2} - P_{aO_2})\ 0.0031}$$

j. **Alveolar-arterial oxygen gradient:**
$$P(A-a)D_{O_2}$$

k. **Oxygen content of the blood:**
$$C_{aO_2} = (Hb \times 1.34)O_2 \text{ sat} + (0.0031 \times P_{aO_2})$$
$$C\bar{v}_{O_2} = (Hb \times 1.34)O_2 \text{ sat (venous)} + (0.0031 \times P\bar{v}_{O_2})$$
$$C_{cO_2} = (Hb \times 1.34)O_2 \text{ sat (Alveolar)} + (0.0031 \times P_{cO_2})$$
A substitution can be made for P_{cO_2}, which is P_{AO_2}

l. **Arteriovenous oxygen difference:**
$$C(a-\bar{v})O_2 = C_{aO_2} - C\bar{v}_{O_2}$$

m. **Oxygen consumption:**
$$\dot{V}_{O_2} = (C_{aO_2} - C\bar{v}_{O_2}) \times CI \times 10$$

n. **Cardiac index:**
$$CI = CO/BSA$$
$$CO = \text{cardiac output (l/min)}$$
$$BSA = \text{body surface area (m}^2)$$

3. VENTILATION

a. **Alveolar ventilation:**
$$\dot{V}_A = (V_T \times V_D) \times \text{frequency}$$

b. Compliance:
$\Delta V / \Delta P = C$
tidal volume/peak pressure − peep = dynamic compliance
tidal volume/plateau pressure − peep = static compliance

c. Minute ventilation:
$V_E = V_T \times$ frequency

d. Expiratory time:
expiratory time = total time (sec) − tidal volume (l)/inspiratory flow rate (sec)

e. Inspiratory flow rate:
inspiratory flow rate (l/min) = tidal volume (l)/inspiratory time (min) *or*
inspiratory flow rate (l/min) = tidal volume (l) × frequency × I : E ratio/I time

f. Inspiratory time (sec):
inspiratory time (sec) = tidal volume (l)/inspiratory flow rate (l/sec)

g. Airway resistance:
$R_{AW} = \Delta P/$flow rate (l/sec)

h. I : E ratio (time):
60 sec/rate = total time per breath
total time per breath/total of I + E ratio = inspiratory time
total time − inspiratory time = expiratory time

i. Calculation of minimum peak flow rate:
minute ventilation × (I + E ratio)

j. Correction of Paco₂

minute ventilation = present minute ventilation $\times \dfrac{\text{present Paco}_2}{\text{desired Paco}_2}$, *or*

new rate = present rate $\times \dfrac{\text{present Paco}_2}{\text{desired Paco}_2}$

k. Conversion of French to millimeters and millimeters to French:
mm = Fr − 2/4
Fr = (4) × mm + 2

4. DOSAGE CALCULATIONS:

a. $\dfrac{\text{original drug strength}}{\text{amount supplied}} =$

$$\frac{\text{prescribed dosage}}{\text{unknown amount drug to be supplied}}$$

Convert all measurements to the same unit.